HYPOXIA

EDWARD J. VAN LIERE
J. CLIFFORD STICKNEY

HYPOXIA

THE UNIVERSITY OF CHICAGO PRESS

CHICAGO AND LONDON

Library of Congress Catalog Card Number: 63–16722

THE UNIVERSITY OF CHICAGO PRESS, CHICAGO & LONDON

The University of Toronto Press, Toronto 5, Canada

To WEST VIRGINIA UNIVERSITY SCHOOL OF MEDICINE,
which provides the climate for creative work

PREFACE

Scientists, especially physiologists, have manifested an interest in the effects of oxygen deprivation on the animal organism for many years. Lavoisier (1743–94), the brilliant French chemist, first demonstrated the importance of oxygen want to animal life.

World War I (1914–18) aroused an active interest in researches dealing with hypoxia, doubtless because of the use of aircraft. World War II (1939–45) gave still more impetus to investigations on low oxygen tension. During and shortly after the latter war, a great deal of literature was published on hypoxia, especially that produced by high altitudes, anoxic hypoxia. More recently, the exigencies of space medicine have renewed interest in oxygen want.

It is to be remembered that many people in the world dwell at high altitudes. In the United States there are many thousands of people, especially in the Southwest, living at altitudes from 5,000 to over 8,000 feet. In the Andean Mountains there are several millions of native inhabitants born, raised, and living in regions at altitudes over 10,000 feet. Indeed, not far from Lima, Peru, there are about five thousand people (natives and foreign inhabitants, including former residents of the United States) living at an altitude of 14,900 feet, at an average barometric pressure of 446 mm. Hg.

Tibet, the highest country in the world, has a population of approximately four million people. The average elevation is given as 16,000 feet, but this, of course, includes the high peaks. Nevertheless, the capital city, Lhasa, with a population of about fifty thousand, lies at an altitude of somewhat over 12,000 feet.

Not only high altitudes, but, more important, many diseases are associated with some form of hypoxia. In fact, diseases of the heart, circulation, the blood, and the lungs may all cause a condition of oxygen want.

While, as previously mentioned, there has been a tremendous amount of research done in the field of hypoxia, many problems still remain unsolved. The authors hope that this monograph will stimulate further research in this extremely important area. It is hoped further that these researches will add not only to knowledge but to the alleviation of suffering caused by disease.

The authors are under obligation to a number of their colleagues for valuable suggestions and constructive criticism. We wish to thank especially Hugh A. Lindsay and David W. Northup of the Department of Physiology of the West Virginia University School of Medicine for critically reading the manuscript and Wilbert E. Gladfelter of the same department for advising on the section dealing with the nervous system. We appreciate, also, the help of Reginald F. Krause and Daniel T. Watts for consulting in areas concerning biological chemistry and pharmacology, respectively. These men, however, are in no way to be held responsible for errors of commission or omission. The authors alone are responsible for these.

It is also a pleasure to acknowledge the able assistance of our secretary, Mrs. Virginia W. Pence.

We are indebted to the following for permission to use certain figures and data: *Air Service Medical* (U.S. Government Printing Office), the American Medical Association, the American Physiological Society, *Annals of Internal Medicine,* Archives of Psychology, Oxford University Press, W. B. Saunders Company, Society for Experimental Biology and Medicine, the William & Wilkins Company, the *Yale Journal of Biology and Medicine.*

CONTENTS

TABLES

FIGURES

CHAPTER I

INTRODUCTION

HISTORICAL BACKGROUND

It is not the intention of the authors to trace the historical development of the effect of oxygen want on living organisms, since, for the main part, the pertinent discoveries are given throughout this monograph. It may not be out of place, however, to mention a few of the earliest known observations of the effect of hypoxia on man and animals.

Scientific research in oxygen want may be said to have commenced with the studies of Lavoisier. In 1777 he published his paper, "Experiments on the Respiration of Animals and on the Changes Which the Air Undergoes in Passing through the Lungs." Although oxygen actually was discovered by Priestley, it has been said that he merely isolated it; Lavoisier really discovered it.

Man has subjected himself to hypoxic conditions, not only by climbing mountains, but also by rising to great heights in balloons. Experiments with balloons were made as early as 1783 by the Montgolfier brothers. In 1804 a Frenchman, Robertson, reached an altitude of 26,000 feet (7,925 meters) in a balloon and was greatly affected by the oxygen want. Gay-Lussac, the distinguished chemist, ascended in a balloon to a height of 23,000 feet (7,010 meters) and noted only slight effects.

Two of the most famous balloon flights were made in the latter half of the past century. In both instances the balloonists subjected themselves to severe hypoxia; and since these men presumably were unacclimated, it is a marvel that any of them survived the ascent. Glaisher and Coxwell in 1862 made the highest ascent ever made by balloons up to that time. Glaisher gave accounts of this ascent in *Travels in the Air* (5) and an article in *Lancet* (6). These men are said to have attained an altitude of 29,000 feet (8,840 meters) — about the height of Mount Everest, the world's highest mountain. It seems incredible that they ascended to such a great height, and

Haldane (7) has stated that there is some question whether their aneroid barometer was correct. They experienced strange symptoms, such as disturbances of hearing and vision and paralysis of the legs and arms. Glaisher finally became unconscious. Coxwell never lost consciousness, but when he attempted to move his arms he found them paralyzed. However, he had the presence of mind to seize the valve rope with his teeth, which started the balloon downward and thus saved their lives. Publication of these experiments and others attracted the attention of Paul Bert, the brilliant French physiologist, and started him on his studies of the effect of variations of barometric pressure on living organisms.

Perhaps the most famous early balloon ascent and, indeed, the most widely known, is that of the balloon "Zenith," in which three scientists—Sivel, Croce-Spinelli, and Tissandier—made a flight on April 15, 1875. Paul Bert, who was so enthusiastically interested in studies in variations of barometric pressure, induced these men to attempt the flight. It had a tragic ending: two of the men died. Tissandier survived and gave a graphic description of the flight in *La Nature* (1875, p. 337) and in Bert's *La Pression barometrique* (p. 1061). Although provided with bags of oxygen, the three men became so weak after reaching an altitude of 24,606 feet (7,500 meters) that they could not raise their arms to seize the oxygen tube. At a height of 26,250 feet (8,000 meters), Tissandier found it impossible to speak and became unconscious. The instruments showed that the balloon ascended to 28,200 feet (8,595 meters) and then began to descend of its own accord.

Tissandier related that none of the three men showed signs of violent dyspnea but that the heart beats became very rapid. They experienced great muscular weakness without losing consciousness. Complete unconsciousness developed suddenly without any apparent distress and was preceded by a feeling of sleepiness.

Bert was deeply touched with the disastrous outcome of the flight of the "Zenith," but with characteristic vigor he continued his researches of barometric pressure on the animal organism and in 1878 published his work, *La Pression barometrique*. This work deserves wider reading and greater recognition than it has enjoyed.

Bert performed extensive experiments on animals and men and was the first to show that it was the diminished partial pressure of oxygen which produced the physiologic effects at high altitudes. Twenty years later, the distinguished Italian physiologist, Mosso, attempted to explain these effects as being due to the loss of carbon dioxide from the body. This became known as the "Acapnia Theory." Mosso's explanation, although rather widely accepted for a time, suffered a decline; Bert's explanation was regarded as the true one. More recently some physiologists are inclined to accept, in part, Mosso's "Acapnia Theory."

During the past seventy years or so a number of expeditions have been organized for the purpose of studying the physiology of high altitudes. It is worthwhile to call attention to the most important of these, since observations made by members of these expeditions are mentioned many times in this monograph.

Mosso in 1894 made studies on Monte Rosa (15,000 feet—4,572 meters), and since then numerous other workers have made observations on this mountain; a rather extensive study was made by the Durchgeführten Monte Rosa Expedition in 1906. The findings of this expedition were reported by Durig in 1909, in *Physiologische Ergebnisse der im Jahre 1906*. Zuntz, Loewy, Muller, and Caspari led an expedition in 1901; their observations were published in *Hohenklima und Bergwandererungen in ihrer Wirkung auf den Menschen* (Berlin: Bong, 1906).

In 1910 Zuntz and Barcroft and their associates made studies on the Peak of Tenerife (12,000 feet—3,658 meters). Douglas, Haldane, Henderson, and Schneider in 1911 made studies on Pike's Peak (14,100 feet—4,367 meters). This was known as the Anglo-American Expedition. In the winter of 1921–22 Barcroft led an expedition to the Peruvian Andes; most of the observations were made at Cerro de Pasco (14,200 feet—4,327 meters). This is sometimes spoken of as the Expedition of the Royal Society; there were, however, several Americans on this expedition. In 1931 Hartman led an expedition to the Himalayas which is known as the German Himalayan Expedition. In 1935 a group of ten men (led by Dill and Keys) made an expedition to the Chilean Andes; this was known as the International High Altitude Expedition to Chile.

The Himalayan joint committee of the Alpine Club and the Royal Geographical Society sent out expeditions (to the Himalayas) in 1951, 1952, and 1953. In fact, in 1953 Mount Everest was climbed for the first time by an Englishman, Edmund P. Hillary, and a Sherpa, Tensing Norkay.

The data obtained on all the expeditions mentioned have greatly enriched the literature on hypoxia, and the scientific world is indebted to the individual members of these various expeditions for their painstaking observations, often made under the most adverse circumstances.

Besides the work of members of the large organized expeditions to high altitudes, many individuals, working practically alone at high elevations, have made important contributions to our knowledge concerning anoxic hypoxia. The early expeditions to Mount Everest especially, although not organized primarily to gather physiologic data, have taught us a great deal about the effect of extremely high altitudes on man. The early observations of Major Hingston, Colonel Norton, Dr. Somervell, and other, more recent ones are extremely valuable.

DEFINITION OF TERMS

Hypoxia.—The term *anoxemia* was used for many years to express the condition of oxygen want in the body. The word is derived from the Greek (*an* ["privation"] + *oxy*gen + *emia*) and means a deficiency of oxygen in the blood; strictly speaking, it should be used only in that sense. There are, however, conditions in which the body suffers from oxygen want that are not caused by a deficiency of oxygen in the blood.

Barcroft (1) suggested that a general term, *anoxia*—which may be interpreted as "oxygen want"—be used to designate all conditions of oxygen want in the body, regardless of the cause. He suggested, moreover, that three types of anoxia be recognized: "anoxic," "anemic," and "stagnant." Peters and Van Slyke (9) suggested a fourth, "histotoxic anoxia" (Gr. *histo* ["tissue"] + *toxikon* ["poison"]).

The term *anoxia* actually means "without oxygen" and, for this reason, is not without objection. Although the term *anoxia* literally signifies a total lack of oxygen, it has a similarly ambiguous parallel in medical literature, the word *anemia,* which is not interpreted to mean that the individual is bloodless. Nevertheless the term *anemia* is an unfortunate one and should not serve as a pattern.

The most desirable and preferable term is *hypoxia*. It is also derived from the Greek (*hypo* ["under" or "sub"] + *oxy*gen) and means less than a normal amount of oxygen. *Hypoxia* may be combined with the words "anoxic," "anemic," "stagnant," or "histotoxic." We then would have: "anoxic hypoxia," "anemic hypoxia," "stagnant hypoxia," and "histotoxic hypoxia," respectively. In this way the exact type of oxygen deficiency may be expressed.

Oxygen lack, too, is an acceptable expression, although it suggests that oxygen may be totally lacking. Less objectionable are *oxygen want* and *oxygen deficiency*. They are, of course, general terms and do not specify the cause of the insufficient oxygen supply.

Asphyxia.—It is a pity that no clear-cut distinction was made initially in the literature between *hypoxia* and *asphyxia*. The definitions given of these two terms in widely used medical dictionaries are not helpful and, in fact, add to the confusion.

The word *asphyxia* means "without a pulse" (Gr. *a* ["privation"] + *sphyxis* ["pulse"]) and, strictly speaking, should not be used synonymously with *hypoxia*. Asphyxia is so firmly established in the literature, however, that it is often used when oxygen deficiency is meant; for example, the hypoxia produced by carbon monoxide is frequently spoken of as "carbon monoxide asphyxia." One need not be a purist to regard the use of the term *asphyxia* in this sense as unfortunate.

The authors agree with the statement of Gellhorn and Lambert (4) : "It seems important to distinguish sharply between anoxia and asphyxia, because under the clear-cut conditions of physiological experimentations the effects of asphyxia may be fundamentally different from those of anoxia." We are also quite in accord with these authors when they suggest that hypoxia should be considered a condition which results from a diminished oxygen supply to the tissues, while the term *asphyxia* should be employed when there is not only a hypoxia but also an increased carbon dioxide tension in the blood and tissues. Used in this sense, asphyxia is often a frequent consequence of hypoxia.

In summary, the authors believe it to be widely understood that in asphyxial conditions there is an accumulation of carbon dioxide in the lungs and in the tissues of the body. If this actually is the concept of asphyxia that many biologists have, it should not be difficult to accept the distinction between hypoxia and asphyxia previously mentioned; that is, hypoxia designates a diminished supply of oxygen to the tissues; and asphyxia, a condition of hypoxia combined with an increase of carbon dioxide tension in the blood and in the tissues. If this distinction between asphyxia and hypoxia were generally accepted, it would eliminate much misconception.

CLASSIFICATION OF HYPOXIAS

For a recent and comprehensive classification of hypoxias, attention is called to the table on page 8, taken from the *Handbook of Respiration* (2) . This rather elaborate classification is to be used as a guide and a reference. Along with a list of the various types of hypoxias, the causes, mechanisms, and the clinical states associated with hypoxias are given.

The authors of this monograph feel, however, that it would also be helpful to present a more simplified classification, which can be seen at a glance. It is based on the early suggestions made by Barcroft, and those of Peters and Van Slyke as mentioned previously (p. 4).

1. *Anoxic hypoxia (hypoxemia)*.—In this type there is a lack of oxygen in the arterial blood. The tension in the arterial blood is low, and the hemoglobin is therefore not saturated with oxygen to its normal extent. (This is also sometimes called arterial hypoxia.)

2. *Anemic hypoxia (hemic hypoxia)*.—The arterial blood contains oxygen at a normal tension, but there is a shortage of functioning hemoglobin.

3. *Stagnant hypoxia (circulatory hypoxia)*.—Here, although the arterial blood has a normal amount of oxygen held under normal tension, it is not given off to the tissues in sufficient quantities.

4. *Histotoxic hypoxia*.—As the term suggests, the tissue cells are poisoned and therefore unable to make proper use of the oxygen.

Besides classifying hypoxia into four different types, it is also customary to make a distinction between acute and chronic hypoxia.

Acute hypoxia.—This type may be divided into severe, acute hypoxia and mild or moderate hypoxia. The severe type has been called by Schmidt (10) "fulminating hypoxia." We shall, however, refer to it simply as severe, acute hypoxia. It is an extremely rapidly induced type of hypoxia, such as may be caused by inhalation of undiluted physiologically inert gases, such as nitrogen, methane, or helium. A mammal subjected to these gases will become unconscious in from forty-five to ninety seconds and, unless oxygen is given, will collapse.

This type of hypoxia would be produced if, by error, nitrous oxide anesthesia were induced without supplying sufficient oxygen. The condition may be encountered in mines which contain a high content of methane gas or in other places which have vitiated air, such as old wells, holds of ships, silos, or other closed spaces which have been fumigated with poisonous vapors without subsequent proper ventilation.

In mild, or moderately acute, hypoxia the symptoms are produced less rapidly. Experimentally, this type of hypoxia may be produced in several ways: (*a*) by placing the subject in a low-pressure chamber from which air may be withdrawn; (*b*) by the use of a rebreather apparatus; or (*c*) by allowing the subject to breathe oxygen diluted by some inert gas.

In everyday life, aviators, people who live at high altitudes, mountain climbers, and balloonists may all be affected by moderately acute hypoxia. The condition may be produced also by carbon monoxide gas and by certain diseases of the heart, blood and circulation, or lungs.

The symptoms which acute hypoxia may cause are shortness of breath, palpitation, headache, nausea, vomiting, mental confusion,

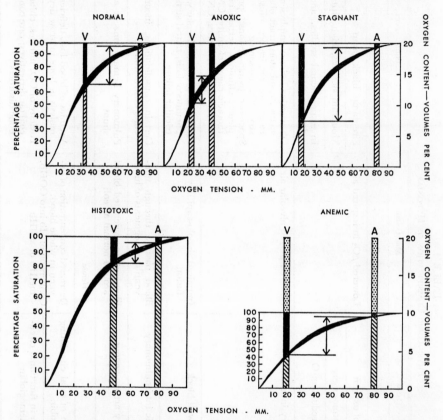

FIG. 1.—Diagram illustrating types of anoxia. Columns representing arterial blood (A) and venous blood (V) are superimposed upon the dissociation curve. The black portion of column represents reduced hemoglobin; shaded portion, oxygenated hemoglobin. Dotted portion of column in the case of anemic anoxia represents the hemoglobin that is lost by hemorrhage or unfit for oxygen transportation, as in carbon monoxide poisoning. The perpendicular arrows denote the volume of oxygen delivered to the tissues from a unit of blood. (From J. H. Means, *Dyspnea* [Baltimore: Williams & Wilkins Co., 1924], p. 67; with additions from Best and Taylor, *Physiological Basis of Medical Practice* [Baltimore: Williams & Wilkins Co., 1939], p. 574.)

muscular weakness and inco-ordination, cyanosis, and sometimes disturbances in vision and hearing. Because of the symptoms which acute hypoxia may produce, it has been suggested by Barcroft (1) that acute hypoxia resembles alcoholic intoxication.

TABLE 1

Physiologic Classification of Hypoxias

Type	Cause	Mechanism	Clinical State
		Anoxic	
Ambient	Dilution of oxygen	Lowered pO_2 in inspired air	Fire damp, black damp
	Rarified atmosphere		Mountain sickness, high altitude blackout
	Selective reduction O_2		In experimental studies, anesthesia accidents
Respiratory	Ventilatory insufficiency	Lowered pO_2 in alveolar air	Obstructive lesions: emphysema, bronchospasm, respiratory tract obstruction, paralysis of respiratory muscles, tetanus, strychnine poisoning Space-occupying lesions: pneumothorax, pleural effusions, certain consolidations, thoracic cage deformity. CNS depression from drugs, anesthetics, CNS lesions
	Alveolar wall block	Impaired alveolo-capillary diffusion	Fibrosis or edema of alveolar wall; infection, pneumoconiosis, mitral stenosis, left ventricular failure
	Physiologic intrapulmonary shunt	Blood passage through non-ventilated segments of lung	Certain consolidations, incomplete bronchial obstruction
	Pulmonary arterio-venous shunt	Shunt of unoxygenated blood around normal alveoli	Pulmonary hemangioma or arterio-venous shunt
		Hemic	
Anemic	Reduction of total circulating hemoglobin	Decreased concentration of oxygen in whole blood.	Anemias of blood loss, deficiency state, hemolysis or bone marrow depression
Toxic	Reduction in functional circulating hemoglobin	Conversion of Hb into COHb, metHb or sulfHb	Toxicity of CO, nitrates, chlorates, various coal tar derivatives; rare congenital metabolic disorders

Category			
Volumetric	Blood volume loss	Low circulating blood flow	Shock association with hemorrhage, burns, trauma or infection
	Volume capacity increase		Peripheral vascular collapse, states with sequestration of blood
Cyanotic congenital cardiac	Anomalous inflow or outflow routes of the heart	Routing of venous blood into left atrium or aorta	Anomalous vena caval drainage, transposition of great vessels, persistent truncus arteriosus
	Absence of one or more cardiac chambers	Mixing of bloods in common cardiac chamber	Cor biloculare, cor triloculare biatriatum
	Abnormal communication between lesser and greater circulations	Ejection of venous blood into left heart or into aorta (right to left shunt)	Fallot type: pulmonary or tricuspid stenosis, or atresia with interatrial or interventricular communication. Eisenmenger type: pulmonary hypertension with "reverse" shunt through atrial septal defect, ventricular septal defect or persistent ductus arteriosus
Minute-flow discrepancy	Myocardial fault	Low cardiac output resulting from diseased myocardium	Heart failure, myocardial infarction, myocarditis
	Constrictive lesion of heart	Low cardiac output resulting from poor diastolic filling	Cardiac tamponade, constrictive pericarditis, arrhythmia, thoracic wall deformity
	Obstructive lesion of heart	Low cardiac output resulting from high resistance to flow	Heart valve lesion, increased pulmonary or systemic vascular resistance
	Relative minute-flow insufficiency	Oxygen demands of tissues in excess of minute-flow	Beriberi, thyrotoxicosis, arterio-venous fistula
Peripheral vascular	Arterial obstruction	Distal ischemia	Coarctation of aorta, atherosclerosis, thrombosis, embolism, arteritis, arteriolitis; laceration, division, extrinsic pressure on artery

TABLE 1 (*Continued*)

PHYSIOLOGIC CLASSIFICATION OF HYPOXIAS

TYPE	CAUSE	MECHANISM	CLINICAL STATE
	Venous stasis	Peripheral congestion	Congestive heart failure, venous obstruction, venous valve incompetence
	Lymph stasis	Low capillary blood flow as a result of high tissue tension	Chronic infection of lymphatics, general edematous states, idiopathic
	Vasospastic states	Distal ischemia resulting from abnormal degree of angiospasm	Raynaud's disease, arterial or venous, spasm, certain cold injuries
Histotoxic			
Enzymatic	Specific enzyme poisoning	Failure of oxygen utilizing enzymes	Cyanide poisoning
Imbalance	Water and electrolyte imbalance	Distorted cellular chemistry	Hyponatremic states

Acute hypoxia, such as is commonly produced by carbon monoxide, may prove rapidly fatal, since unconsciousness develops early without much, if any, warning or respiratory distress. This is the reason people often lose their lives when cars are left running in closed garages; unconsciousness develops so insidiously and painlessly that they are unaware of any danger.

While presumably all the organs of the body are affected by acute hypoxia, the central nervous system and the respiratory and circulatory systems appear to be affected the most. Details of the effects of acute hypoxia on these various organs will be considered later. Mountain sickness, which is produced most frequently by acute hypoxia, will also be considered later.

Chronic hypoxia.—The symptoms associated with chronic hypoxia are produced by long sojourns at high altitudes or by repeated exposures to subnormal supplies of oxygen. Barcroft (1) has suggested that the symptoms produced by chronic hypoxia resemble fatigue, both mental and physical. To avoid reiteration, the mental symptoms will not be discussed here but will be considered in the section which deals with hypoxia and the central nervous system.

The physical symptoms may be mentioned briefly. Even in the acclimatized individual, there may be at high altitudes a dyspnea on exertion, so that the ability to do hard physical work is less than at sea level. Physically, men tire easily at high altitudes, and it is often difficult for them to do a good day's work. Recovery from fatigue, furthermore, is much slower than it normally is at lower altitudes. At extremely high altitudes, such as those encountered in climbing high mountain peaks, physical work is very difficult, so that it may be necessary to rest between virtually each step upward. It has been said that at these extreme altitudes the mountaineer thinks twice before he turns over in bed.

It should be emphasized that what has been said about the physical symptoms of chronic hypoxia probably does not apply to native residents, for example, the Peruvian Indians in the high Andes. It is thought by some that these people may actually have a racial acclimatization.

A chronic mountain sickness may develop after a long sojourn at high altitudes; this will be considered, however, when mountain sickness is discussed. Chronic hypoxia may also produce degenerative changes in certain organs.

EXPRESSION OF THE DEGREE OF HYPOXIA

PERCENTAGE OF OXYGEN

In expressing the degree of hypoxia, the term *oxygen percentage* is often used. This is permissible if it is used to express the actual amount of oxygen present in a known mixture—for instance, a mixture containing oxygen diluted with nitrogen. It is important to recall, however, that altitude does not affect the percentage composition of oxygen of the atmosphere; this has been shown to be true to at least a height of 72,000 feet—21,946 meters (Stevens [12]). It is of interest that calculations based on data in the *Handbook of Respiration* (2) indicate that at 300,000 feet (91,440 meters) the oxygen percentage is 20. It is not, then, the oxygen percentage which changes in rare atmosphere but rather the partial pressure exerted by the oxygen.

It has been pointed out by Horvath, Dill, and Corwin (8) that the conversion of the percentages of oxygen into equivalent altitudes cannot be accomplished by assuming that a given reduction in air pressure corresponds to a proportionate reduction in percentage of oxygen, the total pressure remaining constant. The diluting effects of water vapor and of carbon dioxide must be taken into account. Water vapor exerts a pressure of 47 mm. Hg, and carbon dioxide, 40 mm. Hg under normal conditions.

These authors point out further that it is commonly stated that 10.5 per cent of oxygen at 760 mm. Hg is equivalent to 21 per cent oxygen at 380 mm. Hg. It is usually stated that this corresponds to an altitude of 18,000 feet (5,486 meters). If, however, the pressure exerted by the water vapor and the carbon dioxide be taken into account, the altitude will be approximately 17,000 feet (5,182 meters).

It is of interest that Fenn and his associates (3) have indicated the theoretical impossibility of duplicating exactly the respiratory conditions at altitudes with certain percentages of gaseous mixtures unless the R.Q. (respiratory quotient) is 1.0.

THE PARTIAL PRESSURE OF OXYGEN

According to the mechanical theory of gas pressure, as now understood, each gaseous constituent of the air is capable of exerting its own partial pressure. The partial pressure of all gases decreases with altitude; that is, the higher the altitude, the less partial pressure each gas exerts. The degree of hypoxia, therefore, may be expressed by stating the partial pressure of oxygen in millimeters of mercury. The percentage of oxygen at sea level is 20.96, and the barometric pressure is 760 mm. Hg; so the partial pressure exerted by the oxygen at sea level would be 760 × 0.2096 = 159 mm. Hg. Similarly, the barometric pressure at 18,000 feet (5,486 meters) is approximately 380 mm. Hg; therefore the partial pressure of oxygen would be 380 × 0.2096 = 80 mm. Hg. It is clear, then, that there is a

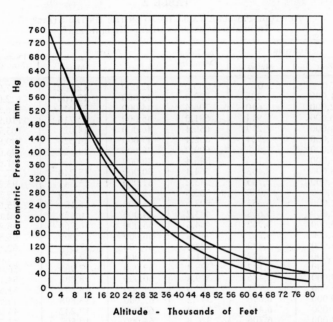

Fig. 2.—Curves showing relation of barometric pressure to height. The upper curve is calculated from the formula given by Zuntz, Loewy, Muller, and Caspari, assuming a mean temperature of 15° C. The lower curve is calculated according to the I.C.A.N. conventional law, assuming standard conditions. (From H. G. Armstrong, *Principles and Practice of Aviation Medicine* [Baltimore: Williams & Wilkins Co., 1939], p. 250.)

direct ratio between barometric pressure and partial pressure of oxygen.

BAROMETRIC PRESSURE

Since air has mass, the higher the altitude, the shorter the column of Hg the air will support. The degree of hypoxia may also then be expressed by giving the height of the mercury column, that is, the barometric pressure. A relationship exists between the altitude and barometric pressure, but this relationship is not a straight line. Figure 2 shows that there is progressively less drop in pressure as the altitude becomes higher; that is, the relationship is exponential.

Approximate Altitudes of Well-known Regions

While it is more accurate and less confusing to express the degree of hypoxia in partial pressures of oxygen in millimeters of mercury or by giving the actual barometric pressure, it is helpful to give the approximate altitude in feet corresponding to these pressures.

TABLE 2

Altitude-Pressure Table Based on the United States
Standard Atmosphere-Feet-Millimeters *

Altitude		Pressure	Altitude		Pressure
Feet	Meters	(Mm. Hg)	Feet	Meters	(Mm. Hg)
0	0	760.0	42,000	12,802	127.9
1,000	305	733.0	43,000	13,106	122.0
2,000	610	706.6	44,000	13,411	116.3
3,000	914	681.0	45,000	13,716	110.9
4,000	1,219	656.4	46,000	14,021	105.7
5,000	1,524	632.4	47,000	14,326	100.8
6,000	1,829	609.0	48,000	14,630	96.0
7,000	2,134	586.4	49,000	14,935	91.6
8,000	2,438	564.4	50,000	15,240	87.3
9,000	2,743	543.2	51,000	15,545	83.2
10,000	3,048	522.6	52,000	15,850	79.3
11,000	3,353	502.6	53,000	16,154	75.6
12,000	3,658	483.2	54,000	16,459	72.1
13,000	3,962	464.6	55,000	16,764	68.8
14,000	4,267	446.4	56,000	17,069	65.5
15,000	4,572	428.8	57,000	17,374	62.5
16,000	4,877	411.8	58,000	17,678	59.6
17,000	5,182	395.4	59,000	17,983	56.8
18,000	5,486	379.4	60,000	18,288	54.1
19,000	5,791	364.0	61,000	18,593	51.6
20,000	6,096	349.2	62,000	18,898	49.2
21,000	6,401	334.8	63,000	19,202	46.9
22,000	6,706	320.8	64,000	19,507	44.7
23,000	7,010	307.4	65,000	19,812	42.6
24,000	7,315	294.4	66,000	20,117	40.7
25,000	7,620	282.0	67,000	20,422	39.8
26,000	7,925	269.8	68,000	20,726	37.0
27,000	8,230	258.2	69,000	21,031	35.2
28,000	8,534	246.8	70,000	21,336	33.6
29,000	8,839	236.0	71,000	21,641	32.0
30,000	9,144	225.6	72,000	21,946	30.5
31,000	9,449	215.4	73,000	22,250	29.1
32,000	9,754	205.8	74,000	22,555	27.7
33,000	10,058	196.4	75,000	22,860	26.5
34,000	10,363	187.4	76,000	23,165	25.2
35,000	10,668	178.7	77,000	23,470	24.0
36,000	10,973	170.4	78,000	23,774	22.9
37,000	11,278	162.4	79,000	24,079	21.9
38,000	11,582	154.9	80,000	24,384	20.8
39,000	11,887	147.6			
40,000	12,192	140.7			
41,000	12,497	134.2			

* From H. G. Armstrong, *Principles and Practice of Aviation Medicine* (Baltimore: Williams & Wilkins Co., 1939), p. 249.

This often orients the reader and allows him, should he be so minded, to make certain comparisons and interpolations which might otherwise be impossible.

It is rather common knowledge, for example, that the city of Denver, Colorado, is situated at an altitude of about a mile (5,280 feet —1,600 meters) ; Colorado Springs, Colorado, at about 6,000 feet (1,829 meters) ; and much of the plateau region of southwestern United States, at an altitude between 5,000 feet (1,524 meters) and 7,000 feet (2,134 meters). It is rather generally known, too, that the altitude of the summit of Pike's Peak is about 14,000 feet (actually 14,100 feet or 4,367 meters). Many readers are familiar with the altitude of Mount Everest, approximately 29,028 feet (8,839 meters) —presumably the highest peak in the world.

VARIABLES OF RESPONSES TO HYPOXIC CONDITIONS

INDIVIDUAL VARIABLES

In discussing the effects of oxygen want on physiologic processes, it is generally recognized that four factors determine the response of an organism to low oxygen tension: (*a*) the suddenness of the production of oxygen want; (*b*) the severity of oxygen want; (*c*) the duration of oxygen want; and (*d*) the physical condition of the body.

ENVIRONMENTAL VARIABLES

There are several variables at high altitudes which, in a measure, may influence physiologic processes. Schneider (11) has listed these as follows: (*a*) lowered atmospheric pressure; (*b*) lowered partial pressure of oxygen; (*c*) temperature; (*d*) humidity; (*e*) increased intensity of sunshine; and (*f*) electrical conditions. It is known that the most important of these factors is the lowered partial pressure of oxygen. It is possible that some of the other factors may influence physiologic processes, but presumably they play subordinate roles.

REFERENCES

1. BARCROFT, J. 1920. *Lancet,* 2: 485.
   ———. 1920–21. *Nature,* 106: 125.
2. DITTMER, D. S., and GREBE, R. M. (eds.). 1958. *Handbook of Respiration,* p. 272. (Proj. 7158; Task 71801) (WADC TR, 58–352).
3. FENN, W. O.; RAHN, H.; and OTIS, H. B. 1946. *Amer. J. Physiol.,* 146: 637.

4. GELLHORN, E., and LAMBERT, E. H. 1939. *The Vasomotor System in Anoxia and Asphyxia.* Urbana, Ill.: University of Illinois Press.
5. GLAISHER, J. 1871. *Travels in the Air.* London: Bentley.
6. ———. 1862. *Lancet,* 2: 559.
7. HALDANE, J. S. 1922. *Respiration,* p. 375. New Haven, Conn.: Yale University Press.
8. HORVATH, S. M.; DILL, D. B.; and CORWIN, W. 1943. *Amer. J. Physiol.,* 138: 659.
9. PETERS, J. P., and VAN SLYKE, D. D. 1932. *Quantitative Clinical Chemistry,* Vol. I. Baltimore: Williams & Wilkins Co.
10. SCHMIDT, C. F. (See *Macleod's Physiology in Modern Medicine,* p. 574. [St. Louis: C. V. Mosby, Co., 1938.])
11. SCHNEIDER, E. C. 1921. *Physiol. Rev.,* 1: 631.
12. STEVENS, A. 1936. *Natl. Geog. Mag.,* 69: 59.

CHAPTER II

EXPERIMENTAL METHODS OF PRODUCING THE HYPOXIAS

Although Paul Bert (4) showed in 1878 that it was the lowered partial pressure of oxygen in the air which produced the physiologic responses at high altitudes, some investigators felt that the low barometric pressure might also be responsible for some of the effects. It has been shown by several workers (2, 4, 16, 23, 27), however, that the reactions characteristic of high altitude can be produced by subjecting the animal organism to a deficiency of oxygen. Lutz and Schneider (23) made quite extensive experiments and produced anoxic hypoxia several different ways; they came to the conclusion that the physiologic responses obtained were quite comparable.

While the latter is doubtless true, several authors have called attention to certain quantitative differences in results obtained when different methods of producing hypoxia are used. It has been suggested, for example, that the acute hypoxia produced with the rebreathing apparatus is not entirely comparable to the changes experienced at high altitudes because of significant differences in the circulation and in the aftereffects. Other differences are also said to occur (18, 28).

ANOXIC HYPOXIA

This type affects the whole body and is one of the most serious forms of hypoxia. It is produced characteristically by high altitudes, although it may be brought about by any process which interferes with the oxygen passing into the blood.

In order to understand clearly the cause of hypoxia produced by low oxygen tensions in the inspired air, it is well to recall what happens under normal conditions. At normal atmospheric pressure of 760 mm. Hg, oxygen exerts a partial pressure of 159 mm. Hg. Under this condition, the partial pressure of oxygen in arterial blood is approximately 100 mm. Hg. At this partial pressure of oxygen, the hemoglobin in the arterial blood is 95 per cent saturated, or, expressed in another way, the quantity combined with hemoglobin amounts to 19 volumes per cent. As the blood passes through the capillary bed, approximately 5 volumes per cent of oxygen are removed, so that the mixed venous blood contains 14 volumes per cent, or a hemoglobin saturation of 70 per cent. The dissociation curve of oxyhemoglobin (Fig. 3) shows that 70 per cent oxygen saturation corresponds, roughly, to a pressure of 40 mm. Hg. The oxygen,

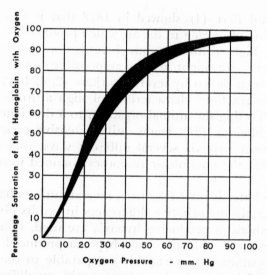

Fig. 3.—The dissociation curve of oxyhemoglobin for human blood. (From J. P. Barcroft, *The Respiratory Function of the Blood* [Cambridge: Cambridge University Press, 1914], p. 226.)

therefore, is carried to the tissues at a relatively high pressure, so that there is a high pressure gradient between the blood capillaries and the tissues.

During anoxic hypoxia, the partial pressure of oxygen and saturation of hemoglobin are both reduced, depending, of course, upon the severity of the hypoxia. As a consequence, the high pressure gradient between the blood in the capillaries and tissues is reduced, so that the capillary blood becomes much less effective in supplying oxygen to the tissues.

Moreover, because of the shape of the oxyhemoglobin dissociation curve, it is recognized that reduction in partial pressure of oxygen in arterial blood is a more prominent feature of incipient hypoxia than is the change in oxygen saturation. Evidence is also available that below a minimal oxygen tension the velocity of oxidative processes in the tissues is proportional to the partial pressure which the oxygen exerts. The lowering, then, of the partial pressure of oxygen in inspired air is, indeed, a serious handicap to the body.

Finally, the increased respirations produced by hypoxia wash the carbon dioxide out of the lungs; consequently the carbon dioxide arterial pressure falls. It is known that one of the important factors in the dissociation of oxygen from oxyhemoglobin is the carbon dioxide tension in the arterial blood (Fig. 4). Since during anoxic

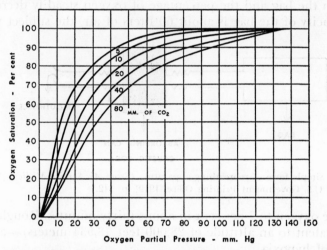

Fig. 4.—Curves of dissociation of the oxyhemoglobin at different pressures of carbon dioxide. Several curves are shown to indicate that the tension of carbon dioxide greatly influences the dissociation of the oxyhemoglobin. (After Bohr.)

hypoxia the carbon dioxide tension is decreased, the hemoglobin does not give up its oxygen readily; and as a consequence the tissues suffer from oxygen want, although there may be adequate oxygen in the blood. As has been pointed out by Wright (35), the tissues in this type of hypoxia are hampered in three ways: (*a*) the rate of oxidation is diminished because of the low tension in the blood; (*b*) there is less oxygen in the blood than normally; and (*c*) the low carbon dioxide tension hampers the dissociation of oxyhemoglobin.

This type of hypoxia may be produced by five different methods: (*a*) use of a rebreather; (*b*) use of a low-pressure chamber; (*c*) dilution of air or oxygen by some inert gas, such as nitrogen or helium; (*d*) artificial pneumothorax; and (*e*) artificial restriction of free influx of atmosphere into the lungs.

A. THE REBREATHER

The principle of the rebreather apparatus is shown diagrammatically in Figure 5. The apparatus consists merely of a bag which may be filled with air and an absorbing can of caustic soda placed between the bag and the mouthpiece

A clip is placed on the subject's nose, and he is allowed to breathe into and out of the bag. The oxygen is used, of course, by the body; and, as the carbon dioxide is removed by the absorbent, the volume of air in the bag and the percentage of oxygen steadily decrease. If the capacity of the bag is about 60 liters of air, the subject will re-

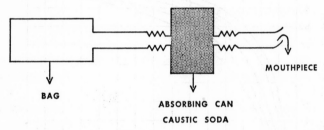

BAG

MOUTHPIECE

ABSORBING CAN

CAUSTIC SODA

FIG. 5.—Simple form of rebreathing apparatus. (From *Air Service Medical* [Washington, D.C.: U.S. Government Printing Office, 1919], p. 342.)

duce the oxygen to 7 per cent in about thirty minutes. Roughly, this is equivalent to an altitude of 28,000 feet (8,534 meters) —a severe degree of hypoxia.

a) *The Flack bag method.*—This apparatus consists of a bag containing about 5 liters of room air. The subject (with a clip on his nose) breathes in and out of the bag. The carbon dioxide is removed by a cylinder, containing a proper absorbent, placed between the bag and the mouthpiece. The arrangement is ostensibly like that shown in Figure 5. The subject breathes out of the bag until the oxygen content is so reduced that he is forced to discontinue breathing; the length of time is noted, and the air in the bag is analyzed for oxygen content.

b) *The Henderson-Pierce rebreather.*—A more elaborate rebreather has been described by Henderson and Pierce (17).

B. THE LOW-PRESSURE CHAMBER

Various types of low-pressure chambers have been described in the literature (1, 3). The simplest means of operating such a chamber is to withdraw the air by means of a suitable pump. At the end of the chamber opposite that at which the air is withdrawn, fresh air should be allowed to enter. To produce a low pressure within the chamber, the air should be withdrawn faster than it enters. Any degree of pressure within the chamber can be produced by manipulation of the intake valve. It is quite necessary to maintain an adequate circulation of the air so that carbon dioxide does not accumulate. This is extremely important. An accurate gauge, preferably a mercury column, should be suitably arranged to determine the barometric pressure within the chamber.

About the time of World War I (1917–19) there were only a few low-pressure chambers in the United States. Today there are many institutions in this country which have excellent low-pressure chambers. West Virginia University, the institution with which the authors are associated, has a modern low-pressure chamber capable of holding eleven men.

In some of these modern chambers the temperature and humidity are carefully controlled. Some have elaborate interiors; that is, they may contain a bed, a chair and table, suitable lights, telephones, and other conveniences, so that one or more individuals may live in them in reasonable comfort for a number of days.

The most important consideration in the construction of an altitude chamber is safety. Every possible precaution should be taken to insure safety. Windows should be provided so that an observer can see clearly the individual in the chamber. It is desirable to be able to communicate by telephone with the subject. The operator should have the control switch near at hand so that the air pump can be stopped immediately if necessary. It is well to have a small oxygen tank available so that, in case of emergency, oxygen can be administered.

These elaborate low-pressure chambers are not necessary for the usual routine experiments on hypoxia where animals are used. For several years the authors (29) employed a relatively inexpensive low-pressure chamber which accommodated two or three individuals or several large dogs. Such a chamber must be constructed of sufficiently heavy material to withstand atmospheric pressure when air is withdrawn. The one in question was made of 5.0 mm. boiler-plate steel with the seams oxyacetylene welded. The windows were made of 12 mm. plate glass, mounted in heavy cast-iron frames. Its construction is not difficult, and it could be made in any reasonably well-equipped welding shop.

Small, inexpensive low-pressure chambers for animal experimentation have been described by Kolls and Loevenhart (21). The authors have such a chamber, which is used for mice, rats, guinea pigs, and small dogs.

c. Dilution of Air or Oxygen by Nitrogen

a) The Dreyer method (8).—This is one of the well-known methods using the principle of air dilution. The apparatus is arranged so that the air which the subject breathes is steadily increasing in percentage of nitrogen. Lutz and Schneider (23) have used this method, the air being delivered to the subject by means of an American model of a Tissot gas mask.

b) The Douglas breathing bag (7).—This bag is widely used to produce anoxic hypoxia. It is made of rubber covered with canvas; the usual capacity is 100 liters of gas, but bags of larger capacity may be obtained. By running compressed air or nitrogen through a gas meter the oxygen concentration can be set at any desired level.

c) Dilution of air or oxygen by use of a flow meter.—The authors have employed a simple method for diluting oxygen with nitrogen, which is especially useful for animal experimentation. An apparatus with which nitrous oxide or ethylene anesthesia is ordinarily administered is used. Oxygen is diluted with nitrogen; and the mixture is allowed to flow into an appropriate bag, which, in turn, is attached to the animal. The bag may be connected either directly with the trachea or with a suitable mask which fits over the muzzle of the animal. A flutter valve is arranged so that the animal exhales to the outside, thus preventing the accumulation of carbon dioxide. The pressure under which the gases are delivered into the bag may be controlled by a suitable lateral valve. The accuracy of this apparatus varies from 0.5 to 1 per cent. It is especially useful when a low-pressure chamber is not available and also for experiments which, for one reason or another, cannot be performed in a low-pressure chamber.

d) Dilution of air in a respiratory chamber with nitrogen.—Obviously, if desired, the air in a respiratory chamber could be diluted with a given quantity of nitrogen or some other inert gas. The carbon dioxide could be removed by a proper absorbent. This method of producing hypoxia is not as widely used as the low-pressure chamber.

d. Production of Artificial Pneumothorax

Hypoxia is occasionally produced experimentally by the establishment of artificial pneumothorax. Pneumothorax cannot be employed successfully with dogs, for in these animals there is imperfect separation of the two halves of the thoracic cavity. The cat and the rabbit, however, are suitable for this type of experiment. It has been observed that after the production of artificial pneumothorax the body adapts itself to this condition much as it does to high altitudes.

This method of producing hypoxia has been criticized since anatomical abnormalities in the body are caused by the collapse of one lung. Grant (9) has clearly shown that the increased values of the formed elements of the blood observed during pneumothorax is a result of hemoconcentration caused by loss of fluid from the vascular bed.

E. RESTRICTION OF INFLUX OF ATMOSPHERIC AIR

There are a few reports in the literature of studies in which restriction of free influx of atmospheric air into the lungs was employed to produce hypoxia. In order to bring this about, the trachea may be compressed to the desired diameter by means of a wire.

EVALUATION OF METHODS

It seems in order here to present briefly a critical appraisal of the different methods of producing experimental anoxic hypoxia. The choice of method depends largely upon the nature of the experiment. Should it be desirable not to hamper the activities of the subject, the use of the Douglas bag to produce hypoxia would be the most satisfactory method. This well-known piece of apparatus is inexpensive, compared with a low-pressure chamber; and, further, it takes up little storage space. It might be pointed out that wearing a mask produces an unphysiologic condition, but most subjects seem not to mind the slight inconvenience it causes.

Any method which makes use of the rebreather for inducing hypoxia may be criticized on the ground that the subject is not exposed to a diminished air pressure. This same criticism applies if the subject is allowed to inhale air or oxygen diluted with some inert gas under normal atmospheric pressure. Some investigators feel that hypoxia produced without changing the atmospheric pressure is not entirely comparable to the changes experienced at high altitudes (p. 17).

In view of this criticism, and for other reasons as well, probably the most satisfactory method of experimentally producing anoxic hypoxia is the use of the low-pressure chamber. If such a chamber is properly constructed, the subject can make himself comfortable and can be observed constantly by the operator.

In working with human beings the psychic factor must be considered. Reliable data cannot be obtained if the subject is apprehensive. He should be made to understand that every precaution has been taken to secure his safety. Valves should be installed which open automatically if the pressure falls too low. A valve which can be controlled within the chamber by the subject in case of an emergency provides a further sense of security. The installation of these safety devices, however, should not make the operator feel that his responsibility is lessened; the subject should be under constant surveillance.

The psychic factor is not so important when working with animals, although it should be borne in mind that, in order to secure trustworthy results, as normal a physiologic state as the experiment permits should be maintained.

Some experimental methods of producing hypoxia, such as the production of artificial pneumothorax or the restriction of the free influx of air into the lungs, as previously mentioned, are unphysiologic. On the other hand, the use of either of these methods for producing hypoxia may give valuable information, for certain disease processes may simulate them. Many human beings suffer from pneumothorax, and, too, several conditions in the thorax may cause pronounced pressure on the trachea.

In the final analysis, while the use of the low-pressure chamber is presumably the most desirable method of producing experimental anoxic hypoxia, there are occasions when the use of other methods to establish this condition are useful.

HEMIC HYPOXIA

This type is, on the whole, less serious than the anoxic type of hypoxia; however, it does affect the entire body. The hemoglobin which is present in the arterial blood is normally saturated with oxygen, and the oxygen tension in the blood is normal; there is then little interference with tissue oxidation. The cause of the hypoxia is a reduction in the volume of oxygen available to the tissues. In less severe conditions, as long as the subject remains at rest the body does not suffer from oxygen want; there are no reserves of oxygen in the blood, however, so the subject's ability to work is greatly decreased.

A. HEMORRHAGE

To produce acute hemic hypoxia, it is necessary to withdraw relatively large quantities of blood from the body. If dogs are used as experimental animals, they may be bled either from the external jugular or by direct puncture of the femoral artery. In order to produce a chronic hemic hypoxia, it is necessary, of course, to withdraw blood from animals at periodic intervals. It has been observed that if there is a reduction of about 20 per cent in the hemoglobin, there will be an increased pulse and respiratory rate.

It should be pointed out that in working with hemic hypoxia the normal blood volume must be maintained. Unless this is done, the experiments may be affected by hypotension produced by the hemorrhage.

B. CARBON MONOXIDE INHALATION

Since carbon monoxide produces a hemic type of hypoxia by combining with hemoglobin, advantage may be taken of this to produce hypoxia by allowing animals to breathe air or oxygen containing a given amount of carbon monoxide. It must be remembered, as has been shown (26), that COHb causes the oxygen curve to shift considerably to the left. As a result, tissue hypoxia is markedly increased for a given reduction of oxygen capacity.

There is some evidence that carbon monoxide produces not only a hemic hypoxia but also a certain degree of histotoxic hypoxia. Be that as it may, carbon monoxide is capable of producing undesirable side effects.

C. OTHER METHODS

Physical or chemical agents used to destroy red blood cells, such as the X ray and phenylhydrazine or other chemicals, are capable of producing side effects which may vitiate studies made primarily on hypoxia. Anemia brought about by dietary control has the same objectionable effects. In order to ascertain the degree of hemic hypoxia, it is, of course, necessary to determine the effective oxygen capacity of the blood.

STAGNANT HYPOXIA

In the stagnant type of hypoxia, which is due to a diminution in circulatory rate, only local areas of the body may be affected, or the whole body may be involved. The blood is normally saturated with oxygen; and the oxygen load, as well as the tension under which it is held, also may be normal. Hypoxia is produced because the amount of oxygen reaching the tissues is not adequate; the slow circulation allows the blood time to give up a larger percentage of its oxygen.

The slow circulation also allows the accumulation of carbon dioxide in the tissues, which facilitates the dissociation of oxygen from the hemoglobin; the oxygen then may be delivered under low pressures. Any measure, of course, which improves the circulation will alleviate the hypoxic state.

Stagnant hypoxia may be produced by impeding the flow of blood to an organ or a system of organs. The diameter of the vessel supplying the tissue under observation may be decreased either by partial

TABLE 3*

TYPES OF HYPOXIAS

TYPE OF ANOXIA	O_2 CAPACITY OF BLOOD (Vol. Per Cent)	ARTERIAL BLOOD			O_2 LOST BY BLOOD IN PERFUSING THE TISSUES (Vol. Per Cent)	VENOUS BLOOD		
		O_2 Content (Vol. Per Cent)	Proportion of Hb Oxygenated at pH_8 7.42 (Per Cent)	O_2 Tension (Mm.)		O_2 Content (Vol. Per Cent)	Proportion of Hb Oxygenated (Per Cent)	O_2 Tension at pH_8 7.39 (Mm.)
None, normal........	20.0	19.0	95	80	4.2	14.8	74	41
Anoxic.............	20.0	14.8	74	**43**	4.2	10.6	53	28
Anemic anemia......	**10.0**	9.5	95	80	4.2	5.3	53	28
Anemic CO poisoning†.............	**15.3**†	14.7	74	80	4.2	10.1	50	28
Stagnant...........	20.0	19.0	95	80	**8.4**	10.6	53	28

* The table illustrates the manner in which the various types of anoxia may produce the same lowered oxygen tension in the venous blood and presumably in the tissues. The figures in boldface indicate the causes of the anoxia. (From D. D. Peters and J. P. Van Slyke, *Quantitative Clinical Chemistry* [Baltimore: Williams & Wilkins Co., 1932], I, 584.)
† The remainder of the hemoglobin is combined with CO.

ligation or by the use of a suitable clamp. Should it be desired to produce a generalized hypoxia, the aorta may be partly ligated or clamped or the aortic valve partly destroyed. It is difficult to produce experimentally the desired degree of hypoxia; better quantitative methods need to be worked out for the production of this type of hypoxia.

It is likely that stagnant hypoxia, theoretically at least, is always associated with some degree of asphyxia; that is, hypercapnia is present.

It should be mentioned that completely ligating a vessel so that the tissues receive no blood at all produces an unphysiologic condition; results obtained from such experiments must be interpreted with care.

HISTOTOXIC HYPOXIA

In this type of hypoxia the cells are not able to utilize the oxygen, although the amount of oxygen in the blood may be quite normal. It is characteristically produced by cyanides. It may theoretically be produced, however, by any agent which depresses cellular respiration.

The mechanism of the action of histotoxic hypoxia is closely associated with the question of cellular oxidation. Space does not permit an exhaustive consideration of this topic here; the reader is referred to the original investigations of Warburg (30, 31, 32), those of Keilin (19), and more recently, those of Quastel (25), Grieg (11), Chance (5), Green (10), and Lehninger (22), whose extensive researches have thrown so much light on problems of cellular oxidation.

It is generally held that a combination of respiratory enzymes (Warburg's *Atmungsferment*) and cytochromes normally constitute the essential oxidizing systems of cells. Schematically this may be represented:

Substrate $\dfrac{\text{Dehydrogenase}}{\text{proteins}}$ Flavin (s) $\rightarrow$ Cytochrome B $\rightarrow$ (Coenzyme Q ?)
$\downarrow$

Cytochrome oxidase $\leftarrow$ Cytochrome A $\leftarrow$ Cytochrome C $\leftarrow$ Cytochrome C_1
(A 3)
$\downarrow$
O_2

(From A. Cantarow and B. Shepartz, *Biochemistry* [3d ed.; Philadelphia, Pa.: W. B. Saunders Co., 1962], p. 382.)

It is thought that Warburg's cytochrome oxidase acts as a catalyzing agent. It has been shown by Warburg that the following compounds all interfere with the ability of cytochromes to take up and release electrons: cyanides, narcotics, alcohol, formaldehyde, acetone, and ethyl urethane. This does not mean, of course, that there may not be other compounds capable of doing the same thing. For example, Watts (34) has shown that many local anesthetic agents (cocaine, procaine, etc.) inhibit the oxidation and reduction of cytochrome C. It is now thought that hypnotics, anesthetics, and narcotic agents block the oxidation-reduction of the cytochromes. (This is often referred to as the principal pathway of biological oxidations.)

A word might be said about the critical oxygen tension of cells. It has been pointed out by Chance (5) that the oxygen affinity of the respiratory system is so high that no changes of rate of respiration occur until the oxygen concentration has fallen to about $4 \mu M/1$ at $25°$ C.

Histotoxic hypoxia is most satisfactorily produced by administering cyanides. In acute experiments, cyanides may be given intravenously. In the authors' experience, only about 1.5–2 mg. per kilo body weight can be given safely to a barbitalized dog. Narcotics, anesthetic agents, and certain other compounds may produce histotoxic hypoxia, but nearly all these produce undesirable side effects; there are few agents, if any, outside of the cyanides, which produce an unequivocal histotoxic hypoxia.

THE HISTOTOXIC ACTION OF CARBON MONOXIDE

It is generally believed that carbon monoxide acts by preventing the normal carriage of oxygen in the blood and not as a direct tissue poison (14, 15). Moreover, according to Killick (20), the percentage saturation of the blood with carbon monoxide represents fairly accurately the degree of hypoxia.

Carbon monoxide, however, is capable of exerting a histotoxic action, since the oxidative enzymes of tissues may be inhibited; but this is thought to be evident only at relatively high partial pressures of the gas. It was reported by Warburg (32) in 1926 that the respiration of yeast was inhibited in a mixture of carbon monoxide with oxygen, but this inhibition was evident only when the partial pressure of the carbon monoxide was nearly five times as high as that of oxygen. That carbon monoxide arrests tissue oxidation by uniting with the iron of a catalyst has been suggested by Warburg (33).

In 1927 J. B. S. Haldane (13), working with rats and using high partial pressures of carbon monoxide, concluded that some substance in the tissue was affected. DeMeio *et al.* (6) in 1934 studied the problem further by comparing the metabolism of isolated tissues in mixtures of oxygen and carbon monoxide with nitrogen and reported that certain tissues showed inhibition with carbon monoxide.

Proof that carbon monoxide does not act as a histotoxic agent is shown by the indifference to carbon monoxide of animals without hemoglobin, such as the cockroach (14). This may be accounted for, however, by the great variance in the degree of affinity of iron-porphyrins for carbon monoxide. It is also claimed that cultures of chick neuroblastic tissues are unaffected by carbon monoxide (12). It should be borne in mind, of course, that adult cells may be affected differently by carbon monoxide than are embryonic cells.

Maurer (24) in 1941 reported the effects of anoxic hypoxia and hypoxia produced by carbon monoxide on the flow of lymph. He obtained comparable results with both methods and suggested, therefore, these results confirmed the belief that carbon monoxide of itself was nontoxic and acted only through its ability to reduce the oxygen-carrying capacity of the blood.

In summary, it may be said that some investigators feel that, although it acts principally by preventing the normal carriage of oxygen, carbon monoxide may also interfere, in a measure, with tissue oxidation.

REFERENCES

1. *Air Service Medical,* pp. 342, 343, 344. Washington, D.C.: U.S. Govt. Printing Office, 1919.
2. BARCROFT, J. 1920. *Lancet,* 2: 485.
   ———. 1920–21. *Nature,* 106: 125.
3. BAUER, L. H. 1928. *Aviation Medicine.* Baltimore: Williams & Wilkins Co.
4. BERT, PAUL. 1878. *La Pression barometrique.* Paris: Masson.
5. CHANCE, B. 1957. *Fed. Proc.,* 16: 671.
6. DeMEIO, R. H.; KISSIN, M.; and BARRON, E. S. G. 1934. *J. Biol. Chem.,* 107: 579.
7. DOUGLAS, C. G. 1911. *J. Physiol.,* 42: 17.
8. DREYER, G. 1920. *Brit. Privy Counc., Med. Res. Counc., Spec. Rept. Ser.,* No. 53, p. 10.
9. GRANT, W. C. 1949. *Amer. J. Physiol.,* 159: 394.
10. GREEN, D. E. 1959. *Advance. Enzymol.,* 21: 73.
11. GRIEG, M. E. 1946. *J. Pharmacol. Exp. Ther.,* 87: 185.
12. HAGGARD, H. W. 1922. *Amer. J. Physiol.,* 60: 244.
13. HALDANE, J. B. S. 1927. *Biochem. J.,* 21: 1068.
14. HALDANE, J. S. 1895. *J. Physiol.,* 18: 201.
15. HALDANE, J. S., and SMITH, J. L. 1896. *J. Physiol.,* 20: 497.
16. HENDERSON, Y. 1919. *Science,* 49: 431.
17. HENDERSON, Y., and PIERCE, H. F. *In: Air Service Medical,* p. 344. Washington, D.C.: U.S. Govt. Printing Office, 1919.
18. KAISER, W. 1928. *Med. Welt.,* 43: 1595.
19. KEILIN, D. 1925; 1936. *Proc. Roy. Soc. London,* B., 98: 312; 100: 129.
20. KILLICK, E. M. 1940. *Physiol. Rev.,* 20: 313.
21. KOLLS, A. C., and LOEVENHART, A. S. 1915. *Amer. J. Physiol.,* 39: 67.
22. LEHNINGER, A. L. 1960. *Fed. Proc.,* 19: 952.

23. Lutz, B. R., and Schneider, E. C. 1919. *Amer. J. Physiol.,* **50**: 228.
24. Maurer, F. W. 1941. *Amer. J. Physiol.,* **131**: 331.
25. Quastel, J. H. 1939. *Physiol. Rev.,* **19**: 135.
26. Roughton, F. J. W. *In: Handbook of Respiratory Physiology,* p. 59. Air University, USAF Sch. Aviat. Med., Sept., 1954.
27. Schneider, E. C. 1924. *Mil. Surg.,* **54**: 328.
28. Schubert, G. 1935. *Physiologie des Menschen im Flugzeug.* Berlin: Julius Springer.
29. Van Liere, E. J. 1936. *J. Lab. Clin. Med.,* **21**: 963.
30. Warburg, O. 1925. *Science,* **61**: 575.
31. ———. 1926. *Naturwissenschaften,* **14**: 759.
32. ———. 1926. *Biochem. Z.,* **177**: 471.
33. ———. 1930. "Herter Lecture." *Bull. Johns Hopkins Hosp.,* **46**: 341.
34. Watts, D. T. 1949. *J. Pharmacol. Exp. Ther.,* **96**: 325.
35. Wright, S. 1961. *Applied Physiology* (10th ed.), p. 212. New York: Oxford University Press.

CHAPTER III

EFFECT OF HYPOXIA ON THE BLOOD

ERYTHROCYTES

Paul Bert in 1878, in his *La Pression barometrique* (13), predicted with rare insight that the blood of animals, as well as of men, living at high altitudes would be found to have greater capacity for carrying oxygen than that of dwellers at lower levels. He believed this to be brought about by the decrease in the partial pressure of oxygen at high altitude and, further, believed this phenomenon to be an important feature in the acclimatization of animals in these regions. In order for this adaptation to take place, however, he thought residence at high altitudes would be required for several generations. He was, of course, in error about the latter point.

In 1882 he was able to prove his hypothesis by the discovery that the blood obtained from animals living at high altitudes in Bolivia actually had greater oxygen-carrying capacity than blood taken from animals at sea level (12). The increased hemoglobin content of the blood of these animals gave it this ability.

A few years later (1890), Viault observed an increase in the number of red blood corpuscles per cubic millimeter in himself and in his companions during a three-week visit in Peru at an altitude of 14,400 feet (4,400 meters) (126). This work gave the final proof of the prediction first made by Bert twelve years before.

Considerable controversy arose over the work of Bert, Viault, and Muntz (93), but their findings have been corroborated repeatedly and are now generally accepted.

Magnitude of Hypoxic Increases in Erythrocytes

An enormous amount of data have been published on the polycythemia produced by high altitudes since the original work of Bert in 1882. In this section, only the acute effects of hypoxia on the increase in the number of red blood cells will be considered. The

31

reader is referred for the chronic effects of hypoxia to chapter x on acclimatization (p. 182).

It was observed by a number of early workers that in many instances hypoxia produced practically an immediate rise in the number of red blood cells in the circulation and also an increase in the amount of hemoglobin. Schneider and Havens (108) as early as 1915, working on Pike's Peak, observed an increase in the number of red blood cells in man after two or three days of residence. Loevenhart and his group (28) reported in the same year that animals subjected to acute hypoxia showed an increase in the number of red blood cells.

In 1945 Hurtado and his associates (62) reported observations made on sixty-seven young individuals who were brought from sea level to various altitudes: 7,920, 10,300, 13,660, and 15,860 feet (2,390, 3,140, 4,165, and 4,835 meters, respectively). A slight polycythemic response was noted, although there was a great deal of individual variation. There is considerable proof now that the increased number of red cells is caused by the hemoconcentration produced by the hypoxia (see p. 37).

POLYCYTHEMIA

The question of decreased oxygen tension or low barometric pressure as the cause of polycythemia naturally arose after it was discovered that a polycythemia was produced by high altitudes. It is obvious that the problem could be solved by subjecting animals to low oxygen tension while maintaining a normal barometric pressure. This can be done readily by diluting the atmospheric air with some inert gas such as nitrogen or by mixing oxygen and some inert gas in the desired proportions.

Sellier (110) in 1894 subjected birds and guinea pigs to a low oxygen tension but maintained a normal barometric pressure. He concluded that the polycythemia produced by high altitudes was caused by low oxygen tension and that the barometric pressure was unimportant. His data, as he himself admitted, however, were inconclusive. In 1913 David (30) did work similar to that of Sellier and came to the same conclusion.

Dallwig, Kolls, and Loevenhart (28) in 1915 felt that these latter data, too, were inconclusive; so they attacked the problem. They used rabbits, young dogs, and white rats. The animals were placed in a chamber so constructed that the oxygen tension could be reduced without changing the normal barometric pressure. It was found that when the animals were subjected to a lowered oxygen tension under normal barometric pressure, polycythemia was produced and, further, that the return to normal was slow (more than a month). They used this as striking evidence in favor of the theory that the blood changes of high altitudes were due essentially to the low partial pressure of oxygen. Their well-controlled and exhaustive experiments, performed on several different species of animals, proved conclusively that polycythemia produced by high altitudes is a function of oxygen want and not of diminished barometric pressure.

CHANGES IN SIZE OF RED BLOOD CELLS

It was stated by Loewy and Wittkower (82) that anisocytosis (inequality in size of the cell) takes place at high altitudes. Smith and his associates (112) in 1924 reported that at an altitude of 11,000 feet (3,330 meters) the individual red blood cells were slightly smaller, although they were capable of holding the same amount of hemoglobin. Bell and Northup (10), working with rabbits which had been given potassium cyanide daily to produce polycythemia, observed no increase in the diameter of the red blood cells.

Several workers, however, have found that at altitude there is a macrocytosis. It has been postulated (33, 44) that this is due to stimulation of the red bone marrow by hypoxia. Hurtado (61) in 1932 found a macrocytosis in the Peruvian natives who lived at high altitudes; he confirmed this finding in later studies (62). Talbott (119) in 1936 reported that there was an increase in the size of the red blood cells in the members of the Chilean High Altitude Expedition after a prolonged residence at altitude. In 1945 Lurie (84) observed a thickness of the red blood cell greater than that found at sea level in dwellers at Witwatersrand, South Africa, at an altitude of 5,740 feet (1,755 meters).

There is considerable evidence, then, that a macrocytosis does appear in subjects who have lived an appreciable length of time at high altitudes. Hurtado *et al.* (62) have pointed out that there is an increase in hemoglobin content of the red blood cells at high altitude and that this increase corresponds to their larger size.

INCREASE IN RETICULOCYTES

That there is a percentage increase in reticulocytes in both man and animals when subjected to hypoxia has been shown by a number of workers (8, 50, 62, 65, 132). Normally there are about 50,000 reticulocytes in a cubic millimeter of blood; that is, they constitute about 1–1.5 per cent of the erythrocytes. They are regarded as young red blood cells. Barcroft (8) reported a reticulocytosis in six Peruvian natives. There was, however, a noticeable individual variation; two natives showed only a moderate increase, but four showed an increase of over 175,000. In the natives there was an increased amount of red bone marrow, so that an excess of red blood corpuscles was discharged into the blood stream.

Experimentally it has been shown that hypoxia may produce a reticulocytosis. Dubin (35) in 1934 subjected rabbits for five days to a barometric pressure of 411 mm. Hg, corresponding to an altitude of 16,000 feet (4,875 meters), and found a 7–10 per cent increase in the reticulocytes. In 1937 Gordon and Kleinburg (50) kept guinea pigs from five to fourteen days at a barometric pressure of about 375 mm. Hg, which corresponds to an altitude of 18,000 feet (5,485 meters), and the reticulocyte count increased by 6–14 per cent. Bell and Northup (10) in 1950 reported that rabbits which had received subcutaneous injections of potassium cyanide 1 mg/kg to 3.3 mg/kg per day showed a statistically significant increase in the number of reticulocytes.

Hurtado et al. have studied reticulocyte response to altitude during what they termed, "temporary," "intermittent," and "chronic" hypoxia. They (62) reported that men dwelling at sea level who were transported to Morococha, altitude of 14,900 feet (4,540 meters), showed a slight rise in the number of reticulocytes in the circulating blood. This was related to the increase in the number of red blood cells. The percentage values did not vary. They found also that flight personnel who had flown sixty to ninety hours monthly at altitudes over 12,000 feet (3,360 meters) showed an increase in reticulocytes. In studying the blood picture in natives residing at Morococha, they found reticulocyte values well above the upper sea-level limit of variation. The highest value observed was 3.3 per cent. In this connection it is of interest that Talbott and Dill (120) at the high altitude of 17,500 feet (5,340 meters) obtained the high count of 3.4 per cent in one of the natives.

Lawrence et al. (80) in 1952 observed no increase in percentage of reticulocytes at 14,900 feet (4,540 meters). On the other hand, at this altitude Merino (86) reported a threefold increase, and Reynafarje et al. (103), a twofold increase. In 1957 Altland and Highman (4) exposed dogs to a simulated altitude of 25,000 feet (7,620 meters) six hours a day five days a week. At the end of two weeks the reticulocyte count was 2.8 per cent.

The increase in the number of reticulocytes has been interpreted as direct evidence of marrow hyperactivity. No one, however, has observed the presence of normoblasts. Hurtado *et al.* (62) have pointed out the fact that no nucleated red cells appear in the peripheral blood, suggesting that the increased erythropoietic activity proceeds in a somewhat orderly manner. In contrast, the condition of polycythemia vera shows a disorder of the entire hemopoietic system.

TIME NEEDED FOR DEVELOPMENT OF INCREASE IN ERYTHROCYTES DURING HYPOXIA

While there has been some divergence of opinion by various workers (1, 32, 38, 97, 103, 108, 112) regarding the exact time necessary for the development of polycythemia at high altitudes, it is generally agreed that it may develop fairly rapidly. It is influenced by the rate and height of ascent, by the physical condition of the subject, and, in a measure, by the amount of physical effort made.

Experimentally, if oxygen want is induced rapidly, there may be a rapid increase in red blood cells and hemoglobin, as was shown with the use of the low-pressure chamber by Gregg, Lutz, and Schneider (55) in 1919. When individuals were subjected to pressures corresponding to altitudes from 15,000 feet (4,570 meters) to 18,000 feet (5,485 meters) at a rate of ascent of 1,000 feet (305 meters) per minute, the erythrocytes and hemoglobin rose within a period of thirty to sixty minutes in 78 per cent of the men examined. It is likely that this was due to hemoconcentration and, perhaps in lesser measure, to the release of red blood cells from certain reservoirs in the body (see chap. v, p. 99).

Experimental work done on animals (28) subjected to hypoxia has, for the main part, corroborated the findings in man; that is, an increase in both red blood cells and hemoglobin was manifested within a relatively short time.

Polycythemia not always present at high altitude.—Reports have been made (92) of individuals whose hemopoietic system did not respond well to increased altitudes. The interpretation was that the tardiness in blood changes was due to the relatively poor physical condition of the subjects. Observations have been made by other workers, however, which indicate that not all apparently normal individuals show a polycythemia at high altitudes. Hurtado (61) has reported several such instances in men living at altitudes between 14,000 feet (4,270 meters) and 16,000 feet (4,875 meters), and Dill has called attention to such a finding in an individual residing at 17,500 feet (5,330 meters) in the Chilean Andes.

There are also reports in the literature which indicate that strenuous exercise at high altitudes may cause a fall in the hemoglobin content of the blood. Cohnheim and Kreglinger (25) in 1909 stated that a hard climb in the Alps to an approximate altitude of 10,000 feet (3,050 meters) produced a distinct fall in the hemoglobin. These apparent paradoxical findings are indeed difficult to interpret. It is known, of course, that extreme physical exertion is capable of destroying red blood cells. It is doubtful, however, that the red blood cells would be destroyed faster than the red bone marrow could produce them under the stimulatory effect of hypoxia.

THEORIES OF THE CAUSE OF HYPOXIC POLYCYTHEMIA

Following the discovery that high altitudes were capable of producing polycythemia, a number of theories were advanced to explain the mechanism of the increased production of red blood cells. Among these were (a) an unequal distribution of erythrocytes throughout the body, (b) a lengthening of life span of the erythrocytes, (c) irradiation by the more powerful sunlight rays at high altitudes, (d) presence of an auxiliary or latent store of red blood cells, (e) an increased concentration of the blood, and (f) an acceleration of hematopoietic activity of the red bone marrow. Each of these theories will be considered briefly; some of them, however, are largely of historic interest.

a) *An unequal distribution of red blood cells throughout the body.*—Experimental evidence has been offered calculated to show that lowered partial oxygen pressure drove the red blood cells to the periphery at the expense of the more deeply situated vessels, so that the total red blood cell count would be unchanged. In 1901 Campbell and Hoagland (20) reported that animals which had been subjected to hypoxia showed more erythrocytes in the vessels of the ear than in those of the mesentery. Foa (43) in 1904, furthermore, reported that the ear veins of rabbits subjected to hypoxia contained more erythrocytes than the blood from an artery. On the other hand, Dallwig, Kolls, and Loevenhart (28) in 1915, working with animals which had been subjected to hypoxia in a low-pressure chamber, found that, within experimental limits, blood withdrawn from the marginal ear vein, carotid artery, or heart had the same count. These latter findings have been accepted, and it is no longer held that hypoxia causes an unequal distribution of red blood cells throughout the body.

b) A lengthening of life span of erythrocytes.—In 1895 Fick (41) suggested that the erythrocytes lived longer at high altitudes and that this probably was the cause of the polycythemia found under these conditions. He offered no experimental evidence for this theory. It has been shown by a number of workers that altitude has no effect whatsoever on the life span of erythrocytes (11, 102, 46).

c) Increased irradiation by the more powerful sunlight at high altitudes.—In 1921 Kestner (70) suggested that it was not the decrease of oxygen pressure in the blood, as was generally supposed, which produced the polycythemia at altitude but rather the increased and more intense irradiation of the rays of the sun. He postulated that the rays formed substances in the air which, when inhaled, stimulated the formation of red blood cells. It was suggested that these unknown substances were nitroxyl compounds. Although environmental factors are mentioned from time to time (68, 105) in connection with changes in the blood picture at altitude, the general consensus is that these factors do not play a significant role.

d) Presence of an auxillary or latent store of red blood cells.—It has been observed by numerous workers that in many instances hypoxia produces practically an immediate rise in the hemoglobin and in the number of red blood cells. This fact puzzled the early investigators; for example, Loevenhart and his co-workers (28) in 1915 definitely stated that their experiments threw no light on this phenomenon. Schneider and Havens (108), working on Pike's Peak in the same year, came to the conclusion that increases in the amount of hemoglobin and in the number of red blood cells seen during the first two or three days were due to the body throwing into the circulation a large mass of reserve blood cells, to blood concentration, and to a stimulation of red bone marrow. They did not know, however, from where the increased blood cells came. Various other investigators made unsuccessful efforts to find blood reservoirs in the body. (For a discussion of blood stores in the body, the reader is referred to chap. v, p. 99.)

It is now known that a significant degree of hemoconcentration takes place during acute hypoxia. It is still believed by some, however, that hypoxia may cause a mobilization of stored blood.

e) A hemoconcentration at high altitudes.—Grawitz (54) in 1895 maintained that the polycythemia produced by hypoxia was more apparent than real and attributed the increase in red blood cells and hemoglobin to a concentration of the blood. He postulated that the body lost more water at high altitudes than at lower levels. His view was challenged by Loevenhart and his collaborators (28).

In the same year that Grawitz published his work, Bunge (17) suggested that vasoconstriction took place at high altitudes and that the blood plasma left the vessels to go into the tissues. There is no evidence, however, that altitude causes a long-continued vasoconstriction. Jacquet (63) in 1901 kept animals at a barometric pressure of 640 mm. Hg, which corresponds to an altitude of about 5,000 feet (1,525 meters), and found that not only the percentage of hemoglobin but also the total mass of hemoglobin increased; the volume of blood, however, remained practically unaltered. Abderhalden, a year later, working with animals at 6,100 feet (1,900 meters), presented evidence to show that there was a hemoconcentration at high altitudes without overproduction.

It was believed by Dreyer and Walker (34) that the change in blood volume was proportional to the area of body surface. They made calculations on Abderhalden's data and concluded that some hemoconcentration had taken place, but an absolute increase in hemoglobin had also occurred. These early workers made their observations at very modest altitudes, about 6,000 feet (1,830 meters) or less, which made their results difficult to interpret.

About 1913 studies on blood volume were made at altitudes well above 6,000 feet (1,830 meters). Schneider and Havens (108), working on Pike's Peak, came to the conclusion that during the first few days there was a significant hemoconcentration. On the other hand, Smith et al. (112), working at an altitude of 11,000 feet (3,400 meters), found no change in blood volume within the first two days at this altitude. Changes did occur a few days later, however.

It is of interest that Lamson (78) in 1920 came to the conclusion that, during acute polycythemia in which sufficient time had not elapsed for increased red blood cell formation to occur, the changes were due to hemoconcentration.

It is now generally held (6, 53, 62) that in the acute phase of anoxic hypoxia, the increase in the number of red blood cells may be a result of hemoconcentration and perhaps, in some animals at least, of a mobilization from blood stores in the body.

f) *An acceleration of hematopoietic activity of red bone marrow.* —The early workers—Bert (13) in 1878, Viault (126) in 1892, and Miescher (89) in 1893—all held that the increase of erythrocytes at high altitudes was due to the low oxygen tension stimulating the red bone marrow.

Miescher felt that the red bone marrow normally existed under a relative oxygen want and that this maintained the bone marrow in a condition of activity, so that the erythrocytes and hemoglobin were being produced constantly. When the body suffered from hypoxia, however, the bone marrow was stimulated to increased activity.

Zuntz *et al.* (133) in 1906 reported histological studies on the bone marrow of dogs at sea level and in animals acclimated to high altitudes. In the latter, a decrease in fat cells and an increase in the blood-forming elements were found.

In 1915 Dallwig, Kolls, and Loevenhart (28), working with animals which had been subjected to low oxygen tensions, found a large increase in hemoglobin per kilo of body weight and a noticeable extension of the red bone marrow. These workers maintained that the low partial pressure of oxygen stimulated the red bone marrow and that their views were closely in accord with those of Miescher (89).

It was shown by Haldane and Priestley (56) in 1905 that before the respiratory center is stimulated by oxygen want the respired air must contain only about 13 per cent of oxygen. Dallwig *et al.* (28) found that the bone marrow was stimulated at 14 per cent oxygen. It was concluded that, while the bone marrow might be slightly less sensitive to oxygen want than the respiratory center, there was little practical difference.

In order to show that bone marrow was not depressed by severe hypoxia, Loevenhart's group kept animals at 6 per cent oxygen for a week; even at this extreme degree of hypoxia the bone marrow was still stimulated. These workers also studied the effect of carbon dioxide on the bone marrow. Animals were allowed to breathe air which contained from 0.5 to 1.0 per cent carbon dioxide. This concentration of carbon dioxide slightly stimulated the bone marrow, but they concluded that it was far less sensitive to carbon dioxide than was the respiratory center.

Since the work of Loevenhart's group (28), a number of investigators have studied red bone marrow histologically during hypoxia. Warren (128) in 1941, and Feigin and Gordon (40) in 1950, making direct marrow examination in animals, found an increased erythroid percentage. Grant (52) in 1951 observed an increased number of colchicine-blocked erythroid mitotic figures.

The sternal marrow of man during hypoxic states, too, has been examined. Merino and Reynafarje (87) in 1949, working with sixteen natives living at an altitude of 14,400 feet (4,400 meters), found 55.6 per cent erythroid cells (normal average value is 20 per cent). Huff *et al.* (60) in 1951 reported that in six human beings the erythroid percentage almost doubled seven days after changing from sea level to 14,900 feet (4,540 meters).

It is of interest here to mention the work of Grant and Root (53) and of Grant (51), who studied the oxygen tension in bone marrow in dogs following hemorrhage. They made the important observation that a vigorous erythropoiesis may occur although the bone marrow pO_2 is not low.

Further proof that the activity of the red bone marrow is stimulated by lowered partial pressure of oxygen is the finding of an increased number of reticulated cells in the circulation at high altitudes. It is known that reticulated cells are young red blood cells. The interpretation is that the red bone marrow is stimulated by the hypoxia and that an increased number of immature red blood cells are entering the circulation.

It should be stated in conclusion, however, that although there is evidence that the stimulation for the polycythemia is the low arterial pO_2, a humoral factor—namely, hemopoietine—is involved in this response (49, 53).

Hemopoietic Factor

It is now recognized that there is a circulating erythropoietic stimulating factor (ESF) detectable in plasma of animals which have been exposed to a low oxygen tension or have been rendered anemic (or have been treated with cobalt). Probably this factor is also found in pregnant, fetal, and newborn animals. There is evidence that the kidney is concerned with the production of ESF. It is thought that ESF acts directly upon the bone marrow, increases rate of red blood cell production and maturity, and, further, leads to the release of erythrocytes from blood forming organs.

There is evidence that its concentration increases shortly after hemorrhage or exposure to hypoxia (or cobalt), and the concentration may remain high until the stimulus is removed.

Blood Volume at Altitude

Many studies on blood volume have been made in acclimatized man and animals, but fewer have been reported during the acute phase of hypoxia. We are concerned here only with acute hypoxia.

The members of the Anglo-American Pike's Peak Expedition

(32) in 1913 made observations on four men during a residence of five weeks (altitude 14,100 feet—4,300 meters). During the first days, three of the subjects showed a diminished blood volume, but this was followed by an increase in the total amount of hemoglobin with a restoration of normal blood volume. In 1941 Asmussen and Consolazio (6) studied two subjects on Mount Evans, which has about the same altitude as Pike's Peak. The blood volume decreased considerably the first three or four days and then rose, but it remained below sea-level value.

Hurtado *et al.* (62) in 1945 determined the blood volume of six subjects two hours after arrival at an altitude of 14,900 feet (4,540 meters). Four showed an increase in blood volume; one indicated but little change; but in one there was a diminution of 8.4 per cent. Determinations made a few days later on five subjects showed that all of them had an increase in blood volume, one as high as 27 per cent. The latter findings would be expected since presumably the red blood cell count had increased.

During chronic hypoxia there is an increase in blood volume both in man and animals. It is generally recognized that residence at high altitudes or exposure to chronic hypoxia produces an increase in the total blood volume largely as a result of the expansion of the red cell mass. (See chap. x, p. 184.)

PLASMA VOLUME AT ALTITUDE

It has been shown by a number of workers that during the acute phase of anoxic hypoxia there may be a significant decrease in the blood plasma volume. In 1945 Asmussen and Nielsen (7) exposed three young men to a simulated altitude of 435–50 mm. Hg, corresponding to about 14,000 feet (4,270 meters), for approximately twenty-four hours. There was a diminution in plasma volume, which was paralleled by an increase in plasma proteins. In the same year Hurtado *et al.* (62) made observations on six subjects two hours after arrival at an altitude of 14,900 feet (4,540 meters). A diminished plasma volume was found in four of the subjects, but two showed a slight rise. After a few days further observations were made on five individuals; two showed a decrease in plasma volume, one as much as 10.9 per cent; three showed an increase, one as high as 13.7 per cent.

In 1950 Huey and Holmes (59), working with a large group of soldiers at an altitude of only 5,280 feet (about 1,610 meters), found a significant decrease in plasma volume. There was no change, however, in the serum protein concentration. Lawrence *et al.* (80) in 1952 also reported a decrease in total blood plasma volume in man at altitude.

Observations on blood plasma volume at altitude have also been made on lower animals. Reismann (100) found a noticeable decrease in the blood plasma volume in dogs; this has also been observed in the rat (45).

Although some of the results, especially in man, were indeterminate, the consensus is that often during the acute phase of anoxic hypoxia there is a decrease in blood plasma volume. This probably does not obtain during conditions of chronic hypoxia in man. (See chap. x, p. 184.)

FACTORS OTHER THAN ANOXIC HYPOXIA PRODUCING POLYCYTHEMIA

Carbon dioxide as an erythropoietic stimulus.—The effect of high carbon dioxide tensions of inspired air on erythrocyte stimulation has been studied both acutely (29, 57, 69, 91) and chronically (28, 36). The acute exposures produced no consistent changes. The longer-term studies made on dogs and rabbits, however, caused a significant increase in the number of red blood cells. Dogs exposed continuously for a week to 0.5–1.0 per cent carbon dioxide showed a 10 per cent rise in the number of erythrocytes (28). Rabbits made to breathe 3–4 per cent carbon dioxide showed an increase of about 20 per cent in the number of red blood cells within four days (36).

In spite of these latter findings, Grant and Root (53) point out that carbon dioxide per se cannot be regarded as a fundamental erythropoietic stimulus, for at high altitudes a lowered partial pressure of carbon dioxide is present; yet there may be an intense erythroid stimulation.

Carbon monoxide.—It was shown by Nasmith and Graham (95) and later by Nasmith and Harrison (96) that carbon monoxide produced a polycythemia in guinea pigs and rabbits. It was necessary to saturate 25–33 per cent of the animals' hemoglobin to produce a marked increase in the red blood cell count. Following an exposure of forty-six days the red blood cells in the guinea pig increased from 5.9 to 8.0 millions per cubic millimeter; in the rabbit the count rose from 7.0 to 10.7 million in twenty-five days. There was a concomitant increase in the hemoglobin. Normoblasts appeared in the circulation a few days after exposure. The effect of carbon monoxide on the number of red blood cells has been reported on other animals, namely, rats (131), mice (19, 73), and dogs (15). It appears that carbon monoxide produces a true polycythemia.

Grant and Root (53) have emphasized that although lower animals develop a striking polycythemia following administration of carbon monoxide, the human subject does not respond to the same degree. (For a discussion of chronic exposure to carbon monoxide see chap. x, p. 199.)

LIMITING FACTOR IN POLYCYTHEMIA PRODUCED BY HYPOXIA

It was pointed out by Lowey and Wittkower (82) in 1937 that the increase in red blood cells at an elevation from 6,000 feet (1,830 meters) upward becomes comparatively unimportant. These authors feel that this diminution in the increase in cells beyond a certain limit is purposive, since if the increase in cells becomes too great, the increased viscosity of the blood caused thereby would make it difficult for the heart to maintain an efficient circulation. This has been denied by Dill (31), who emphasizes that even a noticeable increase in red blood cells has little effect on the resistance to flow of blood because of the axial flow in the arterioles and the ability of the capillary bed to adjust itself to the character of the blood passing through it. (See p. 52.)

It should be pointed out in this connection that there is still an actual increase in the number of red blood cells beyond 6,000 feet. Various observers have reported that the number of red blood cells may rise as high as 7.37 millions per cubic millimeter at great heights, such as 17,500 feet (5,330 meters).

Hurtado *et al.* (62) have pointed out that when arterial saturation reaches a value of about 60–70 per cent, which corresponds to an altitude of approximately 20,000 feet (6,100 meters), a decrease occurs in the percentage of hemoglobin and in the red blood cell count. Talbott (119) in 1936 suggested that this might be associated with a higher rate of destruction of red blood cells. Hurtado and his associates do not believe it is an anatomic variation of the erythropoietic organs, because no plateau is observed in the curve representing the level of polycythemia with increasing degrees of hypoxia. He feels that it may be due to an interference with the production of hemoglobin rather than with the building of the erythrocytic stroma.

Verzar (125) in 1945 and his co-workers suggested a theory to explain the regulation of erythropoiesis at high altitudes. They felt that the initial drop in oxygen saturation of the blood at altitude caused an increased disintegration of erythrocytes and, further, that during the first few days at altitude there was a transient increase in the fragility of the red blood cells. It is known that during hypoxia there is an increase in bilirubin, urobilinogen, and serum iron in the blood. Verzar felt that the increased bilirubin, and perhaps other disintegrative products, provided a stimulus to erythrocytic production. In essence, the theory assumes that the bilirubin content of the blood serves as an erythropoietic hormone and that small amounts are stimulating, while large amounts depress.

In the light of present-day knowledge of the action of erythropoietin, Verzar's theory is probably untenable.

Nature of mechanism of production of hemoconcentration.—As previously mentioned, Grawitz in 1895 held that hemoconcentration at high altitudes could be explained by water loss from the body. This was seriously challenged about twenty years later by Loevenhart and his group (28) and by Schneider and his co-workers (108).

It has been clearly shown, however, that there is a loss of water during anoxic hypoxia. Stickney (114) in 1946 subjected rats for a period of three and one-half hours to simulated altitudes of 4,000, 8,000, 14,000, 18,000, 24,000, and 28,000 feet, corresponding to 1,200, 2,440 4,270, 5,485, 7,315, and 8,535 meters, respectively. He found the body weight loss in rats to be proportional to the altitude up to 28,000 feet. The thresholds for increased total body weight loss, "net loss" (insensible water loss), and fecal excretion lie between 4,000 feet and 8,000 feet; that for urine, below 4,000 feet.

Lawless and Van Liere (79) a year later determined the water content of the cerebrum, kidney, liver, muscles, skin, and adrenal gland in rats which had been subjected to a simulated altitude of 8,000, 18,000, and 28,000 feet, corresponding to 2,440, 5,485, and 8,535 meters, respectively. All of the animals lost a significant amount of weight even at the moderate altitude of 8,000 feet, confirming the work of Stickney. At a simulated altitude of 18,000 feet only the skin and muscle showed a significant water loss. This did not obtain at the two other altitudes tested; the results on the whole, therefore, were indeterminate.

Since the animals all lost a significant amount of weight, and the various organs studied (with the exception noted above at 18,000 feet) did not, it was concluded that hemoconcentration took place. The interpretation was that the body, in order to maintain its homeostatic state, allowed the blood and perhaps the extracellular spaces rather than the tissue cells to lose water.

In 1953 Picon-Reategui *et al.* (98) reported that rats exposed to a simulated altitude of 15,000 feet (4,570 meters) lost up to 20 per cent of body weight within the first week of exposure. The authors stated that the loss of water accounted for 94 per cent of the reduction in the weight of the animals during the first six days at altitude.

There is considerable evidence, then, that certainly in the rat anoxic hypoxia produces a significant water loss in the body. Probably more work should be done on different species of animals.

Valuable studies have been reported on man. Asmussen and Nielsen (7) in 1945 observed that two of three individuals showed a hemoconcentration after being subjected to a simulated altitude of 14,000 feet (4,270 meters) for about twenty-four hours. The hemoconcentration was brought about in part by an increased diuresis. They felt that one-half of the hemoconcentration could be accounted for by loss of extracellular body water, while the remainder was due to the leaking of fluid from the capillaries. They assumed that hypoxia increased the capillary permeability. This assumption could be questioned. (See chap. vii, p. 120.)

POSTEXPERIMENTAL BLOOD CHANGES

In working with animals, Loevenhart's group (28) frequently observed a further increase in the red cell count during the first and second days after removal from the low-pressure chamber. Investigators working with man on the polycythemia produced by high altitudes have also observed this phenomenon. It would appear that the stimulus the red marrow receives from hypoxia persists a little while even though the subject returns to sea level. There is evidence that the plasma level of erythropoietin following exposure to hypoxia is elevated for several hours (118).

Different results have been reported by Tyler and Baldwin (123). In 1925 they reported that rats made polycythemic by exposure to 400 mm. Hg barometric pressure, which corresponds to a simulated altitude of about 16,000 feet (4,900 meters), for a period varying from two to five days lost nearly 50 per cent of the excess red blood cells within a period of six hours after exposure. The authors stressed that there was great individual variation. Their results could be explained on the basis that some of the red blood cells may have returned to the spleen, and also there were probably changes in hemo-concentration.

TIME NEEDED TO RETURN TO NORMAL VALUES

In 1913 Schneider (107) determined the changes in the blood after descent of a man who had lived for a long time on Pike's Peak. He found the percentage of hemoglobin fell slowly from 148 to 132 in thirty days, and to 122 in the following six weeks. The oxygen capacity at the end of ten weeks had diminished 12 per cent. Experimentally, it was shown by Loevenhart's group (28) that after animals were removed from the low-pressure chamber, it often required more than a month for the erythrocytes to reach the level obtained before the exposure to an atmosphere of low oxygen tension. Lowenhaupt (83) in 1942, working with guinea pigs, concluded that recovery from polycythemia induced by anoxic hypoxia appeared to depend on the cessation of increased bone marrow activity rather than on excessive peripheral destruction of red blood cells.

In the past two decades or so it has been shown by a number of investigators (2, 3, 22, 62, 86, 101, 117, 121), working with both men and animals, that the blood picture may not return to normal for weeks or months. Indeed, it has been observed in the laboratories of the authors (116, 124) that in some instances the retention of general adaptation persists longer than six months.

The time it takes for the blood to return to normal following exposure to altitude presumably depends largely upon the amount of polycythemia present. It is of interest that Hurtado *et al.* (62) have pointed out that even when a native of high altitudes comes down to sea level, his blood acquires, after some time, the same morphological characteristics as those found in individuals who have always lived at low altitudes.

HEMOGLOBIN

Since Paul Bert published his *La Pression barometrique* in 1878, it has been known that hypoxia not only produces an increase in the number of red blood cells but also an increase in the amount of hemoglobin. After Bert's original work many investigations were made on this problem. It has been shown conclusively that during hypoxia there is an increase in the total amount of hemoglobin per kilo of body weight.

Dallwig *et al.* (28) in 1915 found that if rats were kept for three weeks at 10 per cent oxygen at atmospheric pressure they had 43 per cent more hemoglobin per kilo of body weight. Their findings corroborated the early reports of Jacquet and Suter (64) made in 1898 and that of Abderhalden (1) in 1902. The members of the Anglo-American Pike's Peak Expedition (32) in 1913 definitely showed

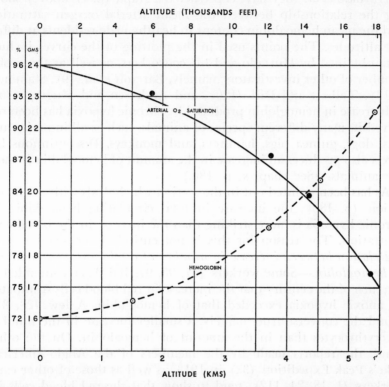

Fig. 6.—Relationship between the mean arterial oxygen saturation (per cent) and the mean hemoglobin content (grams per hundred cubic centimeters) in healthy male residents at different altitudes. (From Hurtado, *et al., Arch. Intern. Med.,* **75** [1945], 284.)

that in man not only the proportion of red blood cells but also the total quantity of hemoglobin in the circulation increased.

Peripheral hemoglobin concentration.—In 1937 Miss Fitzgerald (42) formulated a law that among acclimated inhabitants there is an average rise of about 10 per cent in hemoglobin for every 100 mm. Hg fall in barometric pressure. This rule applies to both sexes.

A classical example of the rise in hemoglobin produced by high altitudes is that of Richards (104), a mining engineer, who, at the request of Haldane, made observations on his own blood at varying altitudes in the Bolivian Andes up to 15,000 feet (4,570 meters). The hemoglobin rose to 130 per cent in four days, and at the end of a month it had risen to 142 per cent; it finally leveled off at 146 per cent in approximately eighty days.

Hurtado et al. (62) have constructed a graph (p. 47, above) showing the relationship between the mean arterial oxygen saturation and the mean hemoglobin content in healthy male residents at different altitudes. The points used in the plotting of the curves include data obtained by Hurtado and his co-workers, as well as those of a number of other investigators, namely, Barcroft et al. (9), Stammers (113), Talbott and Dill (120), and Andresen and Mugrage (5).

Increase in hemoglobin produced by chronic hypoxia has been observed in many different species of animals, such as albino mice and rats, dogs, guinea pigs, hamsters, and monkeys. Discontinuous hypoxia also produces an increase in the amount of hemoglobin in various animals. (See chap. x, p. 180.)

As has been pointed out in the section which deals with acclimatization (p. 180), the increase in total circulating hemoglobin in chronic hypoxia is more striking than the increase in the blood concentration. The reason for this is not entirely understood.

Relation between increase in number of erythrocytes and amount of hemoglobin.—Some workers (47, 96, 97, 106, 127) contended at the turn of the century that the increase in red blood cells stimulated by anoxic hypoxia exceeded that of hemoglobin. A few (28, 37) found the converse true, namely, a smaller increase in the number of erythrocytes than in the amount of hemoglobin. On the other hand, the reports made by the members of the Anglo-American Pike's Peak Expedition (32) in 1913, as well as those of other early workers (1, 18, 24, 112), tend to show that the red blood cells increase in equal proportion with the hemoglobin. Recent work favors this view. Indeed, it would be rather remarkable if this were not true.

EFFECT OF HYPOXIA ON NUMBER OF BLOOD PLATELETS

The effect of hypoxia on blood platelets has engaged the attention of relatively few workers. It has been found that hypoxia causes the number of platelets to increase. A tremendous augmentation at an altitude of 14,000 feet (4,270 meters) was reported by Kemp (66, 67) in 1903. In 1914 Webb, Gilbert, and Havens (129) counted the blood platelets of one hundred college students residing at sea level and obtained an average count of 302,000 per cubic millimeter. The platelet count for one hundred men at the moderate altitude of 6,000 feet (1,830 meters) was found to be 340,000 per cubic millimeter. Koller *et al.* (74) in 1954 found that subjects who ascended by rail to the Jungfraujoch, altitude of 11,342 feet (3,457 meters), showed an increase in the number of thrombocytes in the circulating blood. Also subjects who ascended to Davos, altitude of 5,180 feet (1,508 meters), showed some increase in the number of thrombocytes.

The reason for the increase of blood platelets at altitude is not known, but it has been postulated that hypoxia is capable of stimulating the production of megacaryocytes.

COAGULATION OF THE BLOOD

Since hypoxia increases the number of blood platelets, it is not illogical to assume that the coagulation time would be decreased. Hurtado (61) in 1932 determined the coagulation time of the blood in ninety-five normal Peruvian Indians and found a tendency for a rather short coagulation time at high altitude. He suggested that it was due to an increased blood viscosity, but no correlation between coagulation time and the level of the red cell count has been found.

In 1948 Muralt and Hirsiger (94) found that the prothrombin time (I) of six people living at an altitude of 10,500 feet (3,457 meters) averaged 14.5 per cent longer than that of six individuals at 1,645 feet (540 meters). In a five-man expedition a rise in I of 25 per cent was observed two days after reaching high altitude. In the same year Schonholzer and Von Sinner (109) determined fibrinogen and serum protein levels of six subjects during a ten-day stay at an altitude of 10,500 feet (3,457 meters). The values were higher than those found at 2,440 feet (800 meters).

In 1952 Van Liere and his collaborators (48), working with rats, found that blood coagulation was significantly hastened at a simulated altitude corresponding to an oxygen tension of 10 per cent or less. It was observed, furthermore, that the greater the degree of hypoxia, the shorter the blood coagulation time. Lalli and Sulli (77) in 1956 exposed rabbits for fifteen days to a simulated altitude of 18,-300 feet (6,000 meters). A sharp rise in the number of platelets was noticed (58.8 per cent); there was also an increase in fibrinogen and a decrease in coagulation time.

The effect of asphyxia on blood coagulation time has been reported by Ponka and Lam (99). These authors clamped the trachea of etherized dogs and determined coagulation time. No effect on the clotting properties of the blood was found.

FRAGILITY OF RED BLOOD CELLS

Most of the work reported on the effect of hypoxia on the resistance of red blood cells has been done on partially or well-acclimatized man and animals.

There is experimental evidence that animals subjected to acute severe hypoxia may show a noticeable increase in fragility of the red blood cells. In 1941 Booth (14) allowed dogs to breathe 5 per cent oxygen in nitrogen over a period of several hours. A marked increase in fragility of the erythrocytes was noted. Initial hemolysis occurred in some animals at NaCl solution concentrations as high as 0.70 per cent and in the majority at concentrations well above 0.60 per cent. She concluded that erythrocytes are severely injured by grave degrees of oxygen want. It should be pointed out that following periods of great physical stress, such as are experienced by athletes, hemolysis of the red blood cells is often produced, followed by hematuria.

In 1932 Hurtado (61) determined the fragility of red blood cells in fourteen normal native Peruvian Indians. An increased resistance to hypotonic chloride solution was found. He felt that this was due to the young red blood cells (not nucleated cells). It is of interest in this connection that Minot and Buckman (90) obtained similar results in cases of polycythemia vera.

In 1943 Stickney, Northup, and Van Liere (115) subjected five dogs eight hours daily (except Sunday) to a simulated altitude of 18,-000 feet (5,500 meters) for eighty-eight days. The fragility of the red blood cells was found to be normal. Hemolysis began at 0.46 and was complete at 0.33 per cent. This finding was at variance with the findings of Hurtado and of Minot and Buckman previously mentioned.

Willbrandt and Herrmann (130) in 1944 determined the osmotic resistance of the red blood cells of seven persons who had remained nine days on the Jungfraujoch, altitude around 11,300 feet (3,460 meters). They found that the average osmotic resistance of the red blood cells was increased, which confirmed Hurtado's earlier work.

Hurtado and his associates (62) in 1945 made further studies of the fragility of red blood cells with chronic hypoxia. They studied the red blood cells of natives residing at Oroya, Peru, altitude of 12,-240 feet (3,730 meters). They did not confirm Hurtado's earlier work but, on the contrary, found the fragility of the cells to be essentially normal.

Further work has been reported on animals. In 1947 Tripod (122) kept rats continuously at about 20,000 feet (6,000 meters) for eight days and periodically tested the fragility of the red blood cells. Fragility increased through the sixth day but fell to a low point on the tenth day. Lalli (76) in 1956 exposed rabbits for a period of fifteen days to simulated altitudes of 18,000 feet (5,500 meters), and 21,000 feet (6,400 meters). Some hemolysis was noted.

It appears that red blood cells are relatively resistant to anoxic hypoxia, and it is only when the oxygen tension is greatly reduced that an appreciable degree of hemolysis occurs.

SPECIFIC GRAVITY OF THE BLOOD

As would be expected, the specific gravity of the blood is increased at high altitudes. This is caused by the increase of the number of red blood cells. There is a paucity of data on the specific gravity of the blood during the acute phase of hypoxia. Since it is known that hemoconcentration occurs, some increase in the specific gravity would be expected. There are, however, reports on blood specific gravity during acclimatization in man and animals.

The normal specific gravity of the blood in man may be given as 1.055. It has been observed in man that at Colorado Springs, Colorado, an altitude of approximately 6,000 feet (1,800 meters), the specific gravity of the blood was 1.067; and at Pike's Peak, elevation of 14,100 feet (4,300 meters), it was 1.073.

In the experimentation of Stickney, Northup, and Van Liere reported above, the average value for the specific gravity of the blood increased from 1.0569 to 1.0710 during the period of discontinuous hypoxia; that is, the specific gravity of the blood rose as the number of red blood cells increased.

BLOOD VISCOSITY AT HIGH ALTITUDES

Since there is an increase in the number of red blood cells at high altitudes, it would be expected that the viscosity of the blood would be increased. That this is true has been shown by Hurtado (61), who in 1932 determined the viscosity of the blood in 113 native Peruvian Indians. A Hess viscosimeter was employed, and distilled water used for comparison. The mean value was found to be 8.6; and the variations, from 5.2 to 15.2. This is a distinct increase, since the viscosity at sea level is about 5.1, with variations from 4.7 to 5.9.

The serum viscosity was found to be within normal limits. Hurtado points out that normally the viscosity of plasma exceeds that of serum by 0.2–0.3, but at high altitudes this relationship is reversed. He also found a relationship between the red blood cell count and blood viscosity but none between serum and plasma viscosity and level of red blood cell count.

In 1945 Hurtado and his associates (62) reported a further study. Observations on blood viscosity were made on thirty natives at Oroya, Peru, elevation 12,240 feet (3,730 meters). The mean value found was 8.4, which was about the same as Hurtado reported in 1932. This figure, then, seems well established for the native Peruvian Indians.

It is of interest to pursue the question of blood viscosity at high altitudes somewhat further. It has been shown by Brundage (16) that an increase of one-third in the proportion of red blood cells increased the viscosity of the blood about three times. As pointed out clearly by Dill (31), if the resistance to flow within the body is relatively proportional to the increase of red blood cells, the work of the heart at high altitudes would be out of proportion to any advantage gained by the increased number of erythrocytes.

It has been found, however, that the law of Poiseuille is not applicable to a nonhomogeneous fluid such as blood. When the blood flows through the small arterioles, where the greatest drop in pressure occurs, Fahraeus and Lindquist (39) found that as the diameter of a capillary tube approaches 0.03 mm., the measured viscosity approaches that of plasma. Fahraeus believes that the plasma moves slowly along the periphery in the arterioles but there is an axial flow of red blood cells. Now, when the blood enters the capillary bed, although the resistance to flow in a given capillary must be approximately proportional to the number of red blood cells, some of the capillaries which have been lying dormant may open up so that a large factor of safety is provided. That there are dormant capillaries has been shown by the pioneer work of Krogh (75).

Mendlowitz (85) and Levy and Share (81) have pointed out that a change in hematocrit from 15 to 40 per cent produces only a small increase in in vivo relative viscosity of the blood.

The consensus is, then, that the increase in the number of red blood cells produced by hypoxia does not throw an extraordinary burden on the circulatory system. There is still some divergence of opinion about this, however, and the matter cannot be regarded as entirely settled.

EFFECT OF HYPOXIA ON THE WHITE BLOOD CELLS

In general, it may be said that reduced atmospheric pressure has no important or lasting effect on the number of white blood cells. The differential count, however, may show some variation. There is considerable evidence that there is a relative increase in the number of large lymphocytes at the expense of the polymorphonuclear cells, so that the total count does not materially change. Data have been published on man and on lower animals indicating that there may be a temporary rise in leucocytes when first subjected to altitude.

Effect on animals.—In 1935 Meyer *et al.* (88) studied the effect of reduced atmospheric pressure on the leucocyte count in rats and guinea pigs. Rats were subjected to atmospheric pressures of 422, 352, and 282 mm. Hg, corresponding to approximate altitudes of 15,000, 20,000, and 25,000 feet (4,600, 6,100, and 7,600 meters respectively), and were kept at altitude for a week. The guinea pigs were kept for only twenty-four hours at a level of 422 mg. Hg.

It was concluded that the temporary leucocytosis following reduction in air pressure was due to the emptying of reservoirs of cells, such as those of the spleen, liver, and lungs, and the subsequent leucopenia, to a functional depression of the bone marrow and lymph nodes. These authors stated that the discordant results reported by previous workers could be explained on the basis that it was not recognized that hypoxia first produced a lymphocytosis, followed by a leucopenia. No consistent changes in the differential blood count in their experimental animals could be found.

Cress *et al.* (26) in 1943 subjected rats to a barometric pressure of 400 mm. Hg, corresponding to an approximate altitude of 17,000 feet (5,200 meters), for twelve hours on four successive days. Leucocytosis was observed. The rats were also subjected to carbon monoxide poisoning and hemorrhage (hemic hypoxia); these conditions also produced a leucocytosis. The authors interpreted this to mean that the anoxic hypoxia and the hemic hypoxia caused an excitation of the sympathetico-adrenal system, which produced a discharge of adrenalin. It was assumed that the liberated adrenalin acted directly on the bone marrow. As far as we are aware, however, this latter point has never been proved.

Effect on man.—Hurtado (61) in 1932 determined the leucocyte count in 120 normal Peruvian natives who lived at an altitude of 14,-

890 feet (4,540 meters). The white count varied within limits, but there was a slight tendency for it to be low. He did not find an increase in the lymphocytes. In fifteen cases 28 per cent of the polymorphonuclear neutrophils were found to be immature, although no nucleated red blood cells were observed. The histiocytes in the peripheral blood were increased. Hurtado suggested that, since these cells probably were derived from the reticuloendothelial system, their increase indicated a sign of overactivity of this system.

In 1945 Hurtado and his collaborators (62) made further studies on the white blood count in Peruvian natives who lived at high altitudes. Their findings confirmed Hurtado's earlier work; that is, during chronic hypoxia there was no significant increase in the total number of leucocytes. It was found, however, that the differential count showed a mean percentage increase of lymphocytes. They also reported that when groups of young men were taken to high altitudes in the Andes, a significant rise occurred in the number of white blood cells in over one-third of the men who arrived at a height of 10,300 feet (3,140 meters) or higher. Two men, however, showed a significant decrease.

In 1951 Cullumbine and Kottegoda (27) made observations on six subjects who traveled by train from sea level to a height of 6,000 feet (1,900 meters). Within seven to eight days of commencement of residence at 6,200 feet the concentrations of neutrophils and lymphocyte cells in the blood were increased. These authors emphasize that the increase was not due merely to concentration of the blood by loss of plasma, since the relative fluid loss was much less than the relative increase in the cellular content.

Several explanations may be offered for the temporary leucocytosis which has been observed in both man and animals at altitude. The increased white count may have been due to: (a) the body's reaction to stress (111) produced by the hypoxia, (b) some possible hemoconcentration, and (c) the emptying of certain blood reservoirs in the body into the blood stream. The last is, of course, controversial, since some workers feel that there are no effective blood reservoirs in the body of man. (See chap. v, p. 99.)

OXYGEN CONTENT AND OXYGEN CAPACITY OF BLOOD AT HIGH ALTITUDES

It is necessary to distinguish clearly between *oxygen content* and *oxygen capacity*. The former means the actual amount of oxygen present in the blood under the specified condition, whereas *oxygen capacity* means the amount of oxygen the blood can actually contain if it is exposed to air. The percentage saturation is computed as follows: (oxygen content / oxygen capacity) × 100. Normally, the following relationship exists: (19/20) × 100 = 95 per cent saturation; that is, under normal conditions the arterial blood is 95 per cent saturated with oxygen. It is believed that the increase in hemoglobin and erythrocytes at high altitudes enables the blood to have an increased concentration of oxygen with a subsequent increased oxygen supply to the tissues. The oxygen content of the blood at high altitudes has been investigated by numerous workers.

Hurtado (61) in 1932 reported in the Peruvian natives an oxygen content from 16.5 to 17.5 volumes per cent with an oxygen capacity of 19.2 to 20.0 volumes per cent, which corresponds to an average saturation of 86 per cent in arterial blood. Barcroft, also working with Peruvian natives, obtained virtually the same results. Hurtado's figures show that the oxygen capacity and the degree of saturation (91 per cent) of the arterial blood in lowlanders who ascend to high altitudes are higher than in natives living in such districts. Stammers (113) at Johannesburg, Africa (altitude of 5,700 feet, 1,735 meters), found the saturation in arterial blood within limits of normal lowland values.

It would seem that higher values should be found in the natives than were reported by Hurtado and by Barcroft. Their findings indicate that there are factors of adaptation to high altitudes other than the oxygen content of the blood. In Keys's (71, 72) group the oxygen content of the blood increased an average of 25 per cent. As Keys suggests, this increased oxygen capacity of the blood overcomes, in part, the handicap of low arterial oxygen saturation. Other factors, however, are also at work. He suggests, for instance, that tissues during acclimatization may become habituated to live on oxygen at a lower pressure.

In general, it may be said that the oxygen capacity of the blood increases with the number of red blood cells. For example, the oxygen capacity at sea level is 17.0–18.7; at Colorado Springs (6,000 feet, 1,830 meters), 20.0–21.7; and at Pike's Peak (14,100 feet, 4,300 meters), 27.4 (1a). Dill (31), too, has strongly emphasized that the increase in red cell count is an excellent measure of increase in oxygen-combining capacity. More recent work by several investigators (21, 23, 58) has corroborated the findings of earlier workers. (See chap. x.)

It must be emphasized, however, that while it is believed that the amount of oxygen present in the blood is important, it is still more important that the oxygen be supplied at a definite pressure. It is for this reason that we must look for other factors. The one first suggested by Paul Bert—that in the process of acclimatization the tissues may become habituated to live on oxygen supplied at a relatively lower pressure—may be very cogent.

REFERENCES

1. ABDERHALDEN, E. 1902. *Z. Biol.*, 43: 443.
1a. *Air Service Medical*, p. 143. Washington, D.C.: U.S. Govt. Printing Office, 1919.
2. ALTLAND, P. D. 1949. *J. Aviat. Med.*, 20: 186.
3. ALTLAND, P. D., and HIGHMAN, B. 1952. *Amer. J. Physiol.*, 168: 345.
4. ———. 1957. *J. Aviat. Med.*, 28: 253.
5. ANDRESEN, M. I., and MUGRAGE, E. R. 1936. *Arch. Intern. Med.*, 58: 136.
6. ASMUSSEN, E., and CONSOLAZIO, F. 1941. *Amer. J. Physiol.*, 132: 555.
7. ASMUSSEN, E., and NIELSEN, M. 1945. *Acta Physiol. Scand.*, 9: 75.
8. BARCROFT, J. 1925. *The Respiratory Function of the Blood*, Part I, "Lessons from High Altitudes," pp. 101, 142, 152. Cambridge: Cambridge University Press.
9. BARCROFT, J., *et al.* 1923. *Phil. Trans. Roy. Soc., London*, B, 211: 351.
10. BELL, R., JR., and NORTHUP, D. W. 1950. *Amer. J. Physiol.*, 163: 125.
11. BERLIN, N. I.; REYNAFARJE, C.; and LAWRENCE, J. H. 1954. *J. Appl. Physiol.*, 7: 271.
12. BERT, P. 1882. *C. R. Soc. Biol. (Par.)*, 94: 805.
13. ———. 1878. *La Pression barometrique*. Paris: Masson.
14. BOOTH, M. 1941. *Proc. Soc. Exp. Biol. Med.*, 46: 640.
15. BRIEGER, H. 1944. *J. Indust. Hyg. and Toxicol.*, 26: 321.
16. BRUNDAGE, J. T. 1934–35. *Amer. J. Physiol.*, 110: 659.
17. BUNGE, G. 1895. *Verh. des XIII Kongress Inn. Med.*, p. 192.
18. BURKER, K.; EDERLE, R.; and KIRCHER, F. 1913. *Zbl. Physiol.*, 27: 623.
19. CAMPBELL, J. A. 1934. *Quart. J. Exp. Physiol.*, 24: 271.
20. CAMPBELL, W. A., and HOAGLAND, H. W. 1901. *Amer. J. Med. Sci.*, 122: 654.
21. CHIODI, H. 1957. *J. Appl. Physiol.*, 10: 81.
22. CLARK, R. T., JR., and OTIS, A. B. 1952. *Amer. J. Physiol.*, 169: 285.
23. CLARK, R. T., JR.; OTIS, A. B.; and LEUNG, S. W. 1949. *Amer. J. Physiol. (Proc.)*, 159: 564.
24. COHNHEIM, O. 1913. *Med. Klin.*, 20: 783.
25. COHNHEIM, O., and KREGLINGER, G. 1909. *Z. Physiol. Chem.*, 63: 413.

26. CRESS, C. H.; CLARE, F. B.; and GELLHORN, E. 1943. *Amer. J. Physiol.,* **140:** 299.
27. CULLUMBINE, H., and KOTTEGODA, S. R. 1951. *Ceylon J. Med. Sci.,* **8:** 63.
28. DALLWIG, H.; KOLLS, A.; and LOEVENHART, A. S. 1915. *Amer. J. Physiol.,* **39:** 77.
29. DAUTREBANDE, L. 1938. *Ann. Physiol.,* **14:** 516.
30. DAVID, O. 1912. *Z. Klin. Med.,* **74:** 404.
31. ——. 1913. *Deutsch. Arch. Klin. Med.,* **109:** 129.
31. DILL, D. B. *Life, Heat and Altitude,* pp. 133, 135, 150. Cambridge, Mass.: Harvard University Press.
32. DOUGLAS, C. G., *et al.* 1913. *Phil. Trans. Roy. Soc., London,* B, **103:** 185.
33. DRASTICH and LEJHANEC, cited by A. LOEWY and E. WITTKOWER. 1937. *The Pathology of High Altitude Climate.* London: Oxford University Press.
34. DREYER, G., and WALKER, E. W. A. 1913. *Lancet,* **175:** 1175.
35. DUBIN, M. 1934. *Quant. J. Exp. Physiol.,* **24:** 31.
36. DUFTON, D. 1917. *J. Physiol.,* **51:** V.
37. EGGERS, F. 1897. *Arch. Exp. Path. Pharm.,* **39:** 426.
38. ERLICH and LAZEREUS. 1905. "Anaemia," *Nothnagel's Encyclopedia,* p. 22. Philadelphia and London.
39. FAHRAEUS, R., and LINDQUIST, T. 1931. *Amer. J. Physiol.,* **96:** 562.
40. FEIGIN W. M., and GORDON, A. S. 1950. *Endocrinology,* **47:** 364.
41. FICK, A. 1895. *Arch. Ges. Physiol.,* **60:** 589.
42. FITZGERALD, M. P. 1913. *Phil. Trans. Roy. Soc., London,* B, **103:** 351.
43. FOA, C. 1904. *Laboratorie scientifique international du Monte Rosa* (Turin), **1:** 15.
44. FRANK and HARTMAN, cited by A. LOEWY and E. WITTKOWER (see N. 33 above).
45. FRYERS, G. R. 1952. *Amer. J. Physiol.,* **171:** 459.
46. FRYERS, G. R., and BERLIN, N. I. 1952. *Amer. J. Physiol.,* **171:** 465.
47. FUCHS, R. F. 1908. *Sitzungsb. d. phys.-med. Soz. zu Erlangen,* **40:** 204.
48. GILMORE, B. J.; MACLACHLAN, P. L.; and VAN LIERE, E. J. 1952. *Anesth. Analg.* (Cleve.), **31:** 136.
49. GORDON, A. S. 1959. *Physiol. Rev.,* **39:** 1.
50. GORDON, A. S., and KLEINBERG, W. 1937. *Proc. Soc. Exp. Biol. Med.,* **37:** 507.
51. GRANT, W. C. 1948. *Fed. Proc.,* **7:** 43.
52. ——. 1951. *Proc. Soc. Exp. Biol. Med.,* **77:** 537.
53. GRANT, W. C., and ROOT, W. S. 1952. *Physiol. Rev.,* **32:** 449.
54. GRAWITZ, E. 1895. *Klin. Wschr.,* **32:** 713, 740.
55. GREGG, H. W.; LUTZ, B. R.; and SCHNEIDER, E. C. 1919. *Amer. J. Physiol.,* **50:** 216 and 302.
56. HALDANE, J. S., and PRIESTLEY, J. G. 1905. *J. Physiol.,* **32:** 225.

57. HIMWICH, H. E., *et al.* 1936. *J. Biol. Chem.,* 113: 383.
58. HOUSTON, C. S., and RILEY, R. L. 1947. *Amer. J. Physiol.,* 149: 565.
59. HUEY, D. M., and HOLMES, J. H. 1950. *Fed. Proc.,* 9: 64.
60. HUFF, R. L., *et al.* 1951. *Medicine (Balt.)* , 30: 197.
61. HURTADO, A. 1932. *Amer. J. Physiol.,* 100: 487.
62. HURTADO, A.; MERINO, C.; and DELGADO, E. 1945. *Arch. Intern Med.,* 75: 284.
63. JACQUET, A. 1901. *Arch. Exp. Path. Pharm.,* 45: 1.
64. JACQUET, A., and SUTER, F. 1898. *Korrespondenzblt. Schweiz. Aertze,* 28: 104.
65. KAULBERSZ, J. 1933. *Z. Ges. Exp. Med.,* 86: 785.
66. KEMP, G. T. 1903. *Amer. J. Physiol.,* 10: xxii.
67. ———. 1904. *Bull. Johns Hopkins Hosp.,* 15: 177.
68. KENNEDY, W. P., and MACKAY, I. 1936. *J. Physiol.,* 87: 337.
69. KERTI, F., and STENGEL, F. 1929. *Wien. Arch. Inn. Med.,* 16: 381.
70. KESTNER, O. 1921. *Z. Biol.,* 73: 1.
71. KEYS, A. 1936. *Sci. Monthly,* 43: 289.
72. KEYS, A.; HALL, F. G.; and BARRON, E. S. G. 1936. *Amer. J. Physiol.,* 115: 292.
73. KILLICK, E. M. 1937. *J. Physiol.,* 91: 279.
74. KOLLER, F.; SCHWARZ, E.; and MARTI, M. 1954. *Acta Endocr.,* 16: 118.
75. KROGH, A. 1929. *The Anatomy and Physiology of the Capillaries.* New Haven, Conn.: Yale University Press.
76. LALLI, G. 1956. *Riv. Med. Aero.,* 19: 638.
77. LALLI, G., and SULLI, E. 1956. *Riv. Med. Aero.,* 19: 606.
78. LAMSON, P. D. 1920. *J. Pharmacol. Exp. Ther.,* 16: 125.
79. LAWLESS, J. J., and VAN LIERE, E. J. 1947. *Amer. J. Physiol.,* 149: 103.
80. LAWRENCE, J. H., *et al.* 1952. *Acta Med. Scand.,* 142: 117.
81. LEVY, M. N., and SHARE, L. 1953. *Circulat. Res.,* 1: 247.
82. LOEWY, A., and WITTKOWER, E. 1937. *The Pathology of High Altitude Climate,* p. 40. London: Oxford University Press.
83. LOWENHAUPT, E. 1942. *J. Lab. Clin. Med.,* 27: 874.
84. LURIE, H. I. 1945. *Quart. J. Exp. Physiol.,* 33: 91.
85. MENDLOWITZ, M. 1948. *J. Clin. Invest.,* 27: 565.
86. MERINO, C. F. 1950. *Blood,* 5: 1.
87. MERINO, C. F., and REYNAFARJE, C. 1949. *J. Lab. and Clin. Med.,* 34: 637.
88. MEYER, O. O.; SEEVERS, M. H.; and BEATTY, S. R. 1935. *Amer. J. Physiol.,* 113: 167.
89. MIESCHER, F. 1893. *Korrespondenzblt. Schweiz. Aertze,* 23: 809.
90. MINOT, G. R., and BUCKMAN, T. E. 1923. *Amer. J. Med. Sci.,* 166: 469.
91. MIURA, H. 1936. *Tohoku J. Exp. Med.,* 30: 72.
92. MOLEEN, G. A. 1910. *J. A. M. A.,* 67: 477.
93. MUNTZ, A. 1891. *C. R. Soc. Biol. (Par.)* , 112: 298.

94. MURALT, V. G., and HIRSIGER, W. 1948. *Helv. Physiol. Pharmacol. Acta,* 6: 626.
95. NASMITH, G. G., and GRAHAM, D. A. L. 1906. *J. Physiol.,* 35: 23.
96. NASMITH, G. G., and HARRISON, F. C. 1910. *J. Exp. Med.,* 12: 282.
97. OLIVER, G. 1901. *A Contribution to the Study of Blood and Blood Pressure.* London: H. K. Lewis.
98. PICON-REATEGUI, E., *et al.* 1953. *Amer. J. Physiol.,* 172: 33.
99. PONKA, J. L., and LAM, C. R. 1948. *Proc. Soc. Exp. Biol. Med.,* 68: 334.
100. REISMANN, K. R. 1951. *Amer. J. Physiol.,* 167: 52.
101. ———. July 1951. *USAF Sch. Aviat. Med.,* Proj. Report No. 1.
102. REYNAFARJE, C.; BERLIN, N. I.; and LAWRENCE, J. H. 1954. *Proc. Soc. Exp. Biol. Med.,* 87: 101.
103. REYNAFARJE, C.; LOZANO, R.; and VALDIVIESE, J. 1959. *Blood,* 14: 433.
104. RICHARDS, J. 1913. *Phil. Trans. Roy. Soc., London,* B, 103: 316.
105. ROBERTS, J. I. 1948. *J. Trop. Med.,* 51: 254.
106. SCHAUMAN, D., and ROSENQUIST, E. 1898. *Z. Klin. Med.,* 35: 162.
107. SCHNEIDER, E. C. 1913. *Amer. J. Physiol.,* 32: 295.
108. SCHNEIDER, E. C., and HAVENS, L. C. 1915. *Amer. J. Physiol.,* 36: 380.
109. SCHONHOLZER, G., and VON SINNER, F. 1948. *Helv. Physiol. Pharmacol. Acta,* 6: 639.
110. SELLIER. 1894–95. *Thèse Doc. Med. Bordeaux.*
111. SELYE, H. 1946. *J. Clin. Endocr.,* 6: 117.
112. SMITH, H. P., *et al.* 1924. *Amer. J. Physiol.,* 71: 395.
113. STAMMERS, A. D. 1933. *J. Physiol.,* 78: 21P.
114. STICKNEY, J. C. 1946. *Proc. Soc. Exp. Biol. Med.,* 63: 210.
115. STICKNEY, J. C.; NORTHUP, D. W.; and VAN LIERE, E. J. 1943. *Proc. Soc. Exp. Biol. Med.,* 54: 151.
116. STICKNEY, J. C., and VAN LIERE, E. J. 1942. *Amer. J. Physiol.,* 137: 160.
117. ———. 1942. *J. Aviat. Med.,* 13: 170.
118. STOHLMAN, F., Jr., and BRECHER, G. 1959. *Proc. Soc. Exp. Biol. Med.* 100: 40.
119. TALBOTT, J. H. 1936. *Folia Haemat. (Lpz.)* , 55: 23.
120. TALBOTT, J. H., and DILL, D. B. 1936. *Amer. J. Med. Sci.,* 192: 626.
121. THORN, G. W., *et al.* 1942. *Amer. J. Physiol.,* 137: 606.
122. TRIPOD, J. 1947. *Arch. Int. Physiol.,* 55: 59.
123. TYLER, D. B., and BALDWIN, F. M. 1935. *Proc. Soc. Exp. Biol. Med.,* 33: 165.
124. VAN LIERE, E. J.; STICKNEY, J. C.; and NORTHUP, D. W. 1948. *Amer. J. Physiol.,* 155: 10.
125. VERZAR, F. 1945. *Hohenklima-Forschungen des Basler Physiologischen Institutes.* Basel: Schwabe.

126. VIAULT, F. 1890. *C. R. Soc. Biol.* (*Par.*) , 111: 917.
127. VOORNHELD, H. T. von. 1902. *Arch. Ges. Physiol.,* 92: 1.
128. WARREN, C. O. 1941. *Amer. J. Physiol.,* 135: 249.
129. WEBB, G. B.; GILBERT, G. B.; and HAVENS, L. C. 1914. *Colorado Med.,* 11: 4.
130. WILLBRANDT, W., and HERRMANN, E. 1944. *Helv. Physiol. et Pharmacol.,* 12 (Suppl. III) : 47.
131. WILLIAMS, I. R., and SMITH, E. 1935. *Amer. J. Physiol.,* 110: 611.
132. WOLFER, R. 1934. *Schweiz. Med. Wschr.,* 15: 120.
133. ZUNTZ, N., and LOEWY, A. 1906. *Hohenklima und Berwanderungen.* Berlin: Bong & Co.

CHAPTER IV

CHEMICAL CHANGES IN THE BLOOD
DURING HYPOXIA

A considerable amount of work has been reported on the acid-base balance of the blood during anoxic hypoxia, but less has been reported on other chemical changes which take place during this condition.

Acid-base balance of the blood.—It is important to discuss in some detail the effect of hypoxia on the acid-base balance of the blood. This problem is intimately related to the chemical changes in the blood brought about by the hyperpnea produced by anoxic hypoxia; so some reiteration will be necessary when the effect of hypoxia on the chemistry of respiration is discussed (p. 132).

The early view was that anoxic hypoxia was associated with acidosis, which gave rise to the so-called acidosis theory. In 1910 Ryffel (70), however, could find no excess of lactic acid or of any other abnormal acids in the urine or blood of subjects who had been exposed either to a low-pressure oxygen tension in a respiration chamber or to high altitudes. It appeared, then, that the "acidosis theory" could not be explained on the basis of accumulation of abnormal acids in the blood.

On the other hand, in 1915 Hasselbalch and Lindhard (37), using a low-pressure chamber, found that low oxygen pressures produced a diminution in the excretion of ammonia. They felt that the acidosis of high altitudes was due to diminished formation of ammonia by the body.

In 1919 Haldane, Kellas, and Kennaway (35) found that if oxygen tension were lowered even slightly, a pronounced diminution in the excretion of acid and ammonia occurred and that the urine became alkaline in reaction. This made the "acidosis theory" no longer tenable, and it gave way to the "alkalosis theory." These illuminating experiments threw a great deal of light on the chemical changes which take place in the body during hypoxia and helped explain certain alterations in breathing during anoxic hypoxia, as well as the changes which take place during acclimatization.

Henderson (39, 40) and later Haggard and Henderson (34) independently reached the same conclusion as did Haldane and his co-workers, namely, that there is an alkalosis at high altitudes (in spite of a reduced alkaline reserve in the blood). These and other studies led to the modern conception of the chemical changes which take place in the blood during anoxic hypoxia.

The changes which interest us here, however, are only those which influence the acid-base balance of the body. It is known that the hyperventilation produced by hypoxia produces a lowering of the alveolar carbon dioxide tension and, consequently, a lowering of the carbon dioxide arterial tension. This means an alkalosis is produced. The kidneys, in an effort to maintain an acid-base balance, secrete more base. Sundstroem (79), in 1919, was one of the first workers to make a relatively complete study of the excretion of acids and alkaline elements at high altitudes. He reported some increases in the excretion of sodium and potassium.

It is thought that the excretion of bicarbonate by the kidney continues until the plasma bicarbonate is reduced by nearly the same proportion as the carbon dioxide tension; hence, it is also thought that there is only a slight increase in the pH of the blood. Whether or not there actually is an appreciable change of hydrogen-ion concentration in the resting body during anoxic hypoxia has been of great interest to a number of physiologists.

Barcroft and the members of his expedition to the Peruvian Andes in 1921–22 were greatly interested in this problem. In his monograph Barcroft (6) states that his expedition group desired a well-equipped laboratory for the express purpose of studying changes in hydrogen-ion concentration. The results they obtained, however, were not clear-cut, but their data did indicate slight increases of pH (0.00–0.15). Barcroft felt that they had offered no evidence that the blood was more acid at high than at low altitudes when the body was at rest. During exercise, however, they found marked differences; at higher altitudes less work produced changes in the hydrogen-ion concentration.

Koehler, Brunquist, and Loevenhart (54) allowed young pigs to breathe air containing 5–8 per cent oxygen (38–40 mm. oxygen tension) and obtained a pH increase of 0.11–0.13. In 1932 Henderson and Radloff (42) reported work on the acid-base balance of the blood during progressive decrease of oxygen. They found that while the oxygen was above 8 per cent there was an alkalosis but if the oxygen fell below 8 per cent an acidosis was produced.

Observations by Keys et al. (53) have shown that the blood becomes more alkaline up to an altitude of 12,000 feet (3,360 meters), which corresponds to a barometric pressure of 483 mm. Hg; above this altitude there is either no further change or a return to normal. From the available evidence it may be said, then, that until severe degrees of hypoxia are produced there is an alkalosis of the blood, which is only partly compensated for by a fall in plasma bicarbonate.

It is known that in extreme hypoxia the alkalosis is replaced by an acidosis which becomes more marked as death approaches. The low oxygen tension probably interferes with the proper combustion of the carbohydrates in the tissues, and the lactic acid formed produces an intense acidosis. As death approaches, the respiratory center fails, so that carbon dioxide is no longer given off by the lungs; and this, added to the increased carbon dioxide accumulation in the tissues, causes an extreme reduction in the pH of the blood. Loevenhart and his co-workers (54) found that anoxic hypoxia can produce more marked acidosis in the body than any other condition. In their experiments with pigs they obtained a pH as low as 6.7, and the carbon dioxide combining power was depressed to 9.8 volumes per cent.

It should be mentioned, however, that Loevenhart and his associates (54) always felt, in spite of the soundness of the "alkalosis theory," that anoxic hypoxia was fundamentally an acidotic process and that as soon as oxygen want appeared, acid production in the cell began. The effect was masked, however, by the loss of carbon dioxide in the initial hyperventilation period.

In the experiments reported by Loevenhart's group, no determination was made as to whether the acidosis was due to alkali loss or to the increased production of acid metabolites. They could not, however, find sufficient lactic acid in the blood to account for the severe acidosis. On the other hand, Macleod (60), working on hypoxia and shock, reported distinct increases in lactic acid production in the blood. The validity of his results has been challenged.

It is obvious that more work is needed to determine the actual cause of the intense acidosis seen in the terminal stages of acute anoxic hypoxia. There is considerable evidence from a number of reliable investigators that the acidosis cannot be accounted for by accumulation of lactic acid. It seems that other acids must be sought. It would be well to investigate the amounts of acetoacetic acid and beta-hydroxybutyric acid present. In the light of recent work on the chemistry of muscle contraction, the presence of phosphoric, adenylic, glycerophosphoric, pyruvic, and perhaps other acids should be investigated.

Alkaline reserve.—It was shown as early as 1904 by Galleoti (30) that the titration alkalinity of the blood was diminished by exposure to low pressures either in a steel chamber or at high altitudes.

According to Peters and Van Slyke (67), there is little change in the alkaline reserve during the first hour or so of anoxic hypoxia—merely a decrease in carbon dioxide tension, owing to the accelerated respiration, and a consequent increase in pH. After a few hours the alkaline reserve begins to fall—the extent, of course, depending upon the severity of the hypoxia. It already has been mentioned that Loevenhart's group (54) found the carbon dioxide combining power depressed to 9.8 volumes in the terminal stage of anoxic hypoxia.

Formation of lactic acid.—Although the effect of hypoxia on lactic acid production in the body has been considered briefly in the discussion of the acid-base balance of the blood, it is of interest to consider this in somewhat more detail. Since it is known that lactic acid develops in the blood during exercise, it is not illogical to suppose that its production might increase during oxygen want. As a matter of fact, as early as 1891 Araki (2) reported that in acute oxygen want large quantities of lactic acid were produced in the body. In 1908 Boycott and Haldane (13) believed that the hyperpnea seen during anoxic hypoxia was produced by the increased production of lactic acid sensitizing the respiratory center to carbon dioxide.

That at moderately high altitudes, 10,000 feet (3,050 meters), lactic acid does not accumulate in the blood was shown by Barcroft et al. (7) in their expedition to Monte Rosa. At 15,000 feet (4,570 meters), Barcroft observed a suggestion of an increase in lactic acid production, although there was no certain indication. In fact, it was rather generally accepted that oxygen want produced an increase in lactic acid during hypoxia; and this, in part, gave rise to the "acidosis theory" previously discussed. Macleod (60) in 1921 believed that there was an excess of lactic acid during hypoxia and that this aided in neutralizing increased base. Sundstroem (79), on the other hand, claimed that there was no increase of lactic acid production at high altitudes.

Experimentally (51) it has been shown in the turtle that complete hypoxia for several hours may cause an increase of the lactic acid in the blood to almost 1,000 mg. per cent. The turtle, unlike a mammal, can withstand complete hypoxia for about thirty hours. The results obtained from the turtle are not of practical interest. They do show, however, that during severe hypoxia there may be a great rise in blood lactates.

In 1943 Henderson and Greenberg (41) reported that only when the oxygen in the inspired air became less than 7 per cent did an increase in lactic acid in the blood develop.

The important observations of Bock, Dill, Edwards, Keys, and their co-workers (11, 22, 23, 53) have added to our knowledge concerning the production of lactic acid at high altitudes. They found that after severe exercise at an altitude of 12,000 feet (3,660 meters) the blood lactate was lower than after comparable exercise at sea level; that following exercise at 15,000 feet (4,570 meters) it was still lower; and that even at the great altitude of 20,000 feet (6,095 meters) the lactic acid was barely above the normal level. Dill (21) states that while these findings at present cannot be explained, the fact that the blood lactate is not elevated at high altitudes presumably serves as a safeguard against overexertion of the body. He points out that if the body at high altitudes could produce such severe disturbance in the acid-base equilibrium as it can at sea level, grave injury might be caused.

Lactate-pyruvate ratio.—This is not the place to discuss in detail the formation of lactic and pyruvic acid and the significance of the lactic-pyruvate ratio. It is in order, however, to discuss the effect of hypoxia on this ratio.

Huckabee (46, 47) has pointed out that under normal conditions changes in blood lactate correspond closely to changes in blood pyruvate. During anoxic hypoxia, however, an excess amount of lactate relative to pyruvate is produced. This excess lactate formation commences when the arterial oxygen saturation falls below 65 per cent. Ivy and his colleagues (28) in 1949 reported that exposure to hypoxia at a simulated altitude of over 15,000 feet (4,570 meters) produced an increase of lactic and pyruvic acids and a rise of the lactic-pyruvic ratio.

The cause of liberation of lactates in severe hypoxia is not entirely understood. Korner (55) has suggested that it may be the result of increased activity of the sympathetico-adrenal system. Greene and Phillips (33), however, have demonstrated that dogs which have been subjected to total preganglionic sympathectomy upon exposure to hypoxia still liberate a smaller, but significant increase in blood lactate.

Blood sugar.—In 1857 Claude Bernard (10) noticed that the urine of animals which had been poisoned by carbon monoxide contained sugar. Since his original observations this has been verified by many workers. The glycosuria apparently results from mobilization of liver glycogen, since it does not occur if the animals have been starved previous to the exposure of carbon monoxide (41).

Kellaway (52) in 1919 came to the conclusion that mobilization of sugar during hypoxia was caused by the effect of oxygen want on the central nervous system. Although evidence was available that the output of epinephrine was accelerated, he felt that this was not the cause of the increased blood sugar.

In 1926 Mikami (62), working with rabbits, concluded that the increase in blood sugar (and urine sugar as well) was roughly proportional to the degree of hypoxia. As a matter of fact, Munzer and Palmer (65) many years before, working with men, had reached the same conclusion. Mikami also showed that intravenous injection of alkali inhibited the hyperglycemia and, further, that it prevented the fall in arterial carbon dioxide associated with carbon monoxide poisoning. His work suggests that the acid-base balance of the blood may play a part in the production of hyperglycemia.

In 1933 Buresch (15) reported that rabbits which were exposed daily to carbon monoxide showed an increase in their blood sugar level. In the same year Boedicker (12), however, reported opposite findings.

Schulze (72) in 1936, working with mice and using carbon monoxide to produce hypoxia, concluded that the adrenals were stimulated by hypoxia and that they were responsible for the immediate rise in blood sugar. His view, then, was opposed to that of Kellaway.

The effect of complete hypoxia on the blood sugar of the turtle has been reported by Johlin and Moreland (51). Turtles, which are extremely resistant to hypoxia, were kept in an atmosphere of pure nitrogen up to twenty-eight hours. The glucose rose from 50 mg. to 1,200 mg. In a subsequent paper (63), Moreland reported that alkali lowers the high blood sugar produced by complete hypoxia in the turtle but causes a further increase in the lactate, so that there is a reduction of the sugar-to-lactate ratio. This finding confirmed, in part, the previous work of Mikami (62).

Gellhorn and Packer (31) have reported studies on the glycogenolytic action of epinephrine. They observed that short periods of hypoxia (7 per cent oxygen) acted antagonistically to insulin hypoglycemia, whereas prolonged periods (two hours) aggravated hypoglycemia. The glycogenolytic action of epinephrine increased during a short period of hypoxia but was lost after a prolonged period. This presumably was not due to depletion of the glycogen reserves of the liver.

Forbes (27) in 1936 reported observations on blood sugar and glucose tolerance at altitudes up to 20,144 feet (6,140 meters) in acclimatized subjects in rest and at work. At 17,520 feet (5,340 meters) glucose-tolerance tests were given. Although blood sugar rose slightly with altitude, there was no conclusive proof that high altitudes caused its rise; and during work the behavior of blood sugar was approximately the same at all altitudes. In two of three subjects the glucose tolerance was greatly decreased at 17,500 feet (5,340 meters).

McQuarrie and Ziegler (56) in 1939, working with dogs, found that hypoxia prevented insulin convulsions in spite of the fact that the blood-sugar level in insulinized dogs subjected to hypoxia was lower than in those animals treated with insulin alone. Gellhorn *et al.* (32) confirmed these findings and came to the conclusion that in all species studied hypoxia prevented insulin convulsions. They explained that the convulsions produced in insulinized rats which were subjected to hypoxia were of a hypoxic rather than of a hypoglycemic nature. They regarded this specific sensitivity to hypoxia as characteristic of small animals, which are known to have a high metabolic rate. McQuarrie *et al.* (58) in 1939 found that hypoxia produces hyperglycemia in normal dogs but causes a fall in blood sugar in adrenalectomized animals.

A considerable amount of work has been done on the acute effects of hypoxia on the blood sugar of dogs, goats, and sheep in the laboratory of the authors. The animals were exposed to hypoxia for a period of fifteen minutes. In 1948 Stickney, Northup, and Van Liere (76), working with dogs, found that exposure to a simulated altitude of 24,000 feet (7,300 meters) produced a significant rise in blood sugar, 6 mg/100 ml. Animals subjected to a simulated altitude of 28,000 feet (8,500 meters) showed a rise of 41 mg/100 ml. When the animals were exposed to 32,000 feet (9,700 meters), their blood sugar rose to 56 mg/100 ml. In essence, the more severe the hypoxia, the greater the rise in blood sugar.

Data on the effect of hypoxia on goats (78) and on sheep (77) were also reported. Sheep exposed to a simulated altitude of 24,000 feet (7,300 meters) showed a rise of 10.8 mg/100 ml. At 28,000 feet (8,500 meters) the value found was 15.4 mg/100 ml. Goats were found to be somewhat more sensitive to hypoxia as far as the effect on blood sugar was concerned. When these animals were subjected to a simulated altitude of 24,000 feet (7,300 meters), the blood sugar rose 40.1 mg/100 ml; at 28,000 feet (8,500 meters), the value found was 59 mg/100 ml.

It is of interest to point out that the resting blood sugar of sheep and goats is considerably less than it is in dogs.

To summarize the effect of hypoxia on blood sugar: effective degrees of hypoxia produce a significant rise in the blood sugar level in many animals. More work is needed, however, on the effect of hypoxia on the blood sugar in man.

Serum proteins.—Hurtado and his colleagues (50) in 1945 determined the concentrations of serum proteins on fifty subjects at sea level and after arrival at high altitudes. They found a definite rise directly related to the level of altitude. Increases of 2.9, 4.0, 5.3, and

7.9 per cent were found at altitudes of approximately 8,000 feet (2,440 meters), 10,000 feet (3,050 meters), and 16,000 feet (4,875 meters). This temporary increase in serum protein can probably be accounted for by the hemoconcentration known to occur at altitude.

Asmussen and Nielsen (4) in the same year subjected three human beings to a simulated altitude of 435–50 mm. Hg, which corresponds to about 14,000 feet (4,270 meters). They observed an increase in plasma protein concentration. In 1948 Muralt and Notter (66) determined several protein concentrations in the blood of six subjects living at an altitude of about 11,350 feet (about 3,457 meters). A rise was observed in all protein values, but the nonprotein nitrogen remained unchanged.

Stickney et al. (75) in 1943 determined the plasma protein concentration in the five dogs used in the experiment reported in chapter iii (see p. 50, above). It was found that the plasma protein concentration in these partially acclimatized dogs decreased 9.69 per cent, which was statistically significant.

Huey and Holmes (48) in 1950 made determinations of serum proteins on a large number of individuals (fifty soldiers, thirty-two male students, and twenty-two females) at 5,280 feet (about 1,600 meters). At this modest altitude no values significantly different from those obtained at sea level were observed.

Nonprotein nitrogen.—Armstrong (3) exposed animals to a simulated altitude of 18,000 feet (5,500 meters) daily for four hours; no change was noted in the amount of nonprotein nitrogen in the blood. The work was repeated on man at lower levels, 12,000 feet (3,600 meters), and again no change was noted.

Sodium chloride.—Armstrong (3), using the same procedure as he did when nonprotein nitrogen was studied, found that anoxic hypoxia apparently had no effect on the amount of sodium chloride in the blood. Ferguson and Smith (26) exposed unanesthetized dogs to a simulated altitude of 30,000 feet (9,100 meters) and found no change in plasma sodium concentration. It was observed by Sundstroem (79) in 1919 that at the beginning of residence at high altitudes there was a definite initial retention of chlorides. This means, of course, that some undetermined cation had to be retained. The entire question of electrolytes in hypoxia needs further probing, with concurrent study of cations and anions.

Guanidine.—Andes et al. (1) found no change in the level of guanidine in dogs after exposure to a simulated altitude of 24,000 feet (7,315 meters) for periods up to seven and one-half hours. Short exposures (one-half hour) at 28,000 feet (8,535 meters) likewise had no effect.

Potassium.—a) Effect of asphyxia. It has been shown by several workers (17, 20, 44, 64, 84) that generalized asphyxia of an animal causes a stimulation of the adrenals and a liberation of potassium from the tissues. Mullin *et al.* (64) reported an increase in the blood potassium in tetany and in asphyxia in dogs. They could not account for the increase on a basis of loss of body fluid or a potassium shift from the red blood cells to the plasma. The interpretation was that it came from the active muscle tissue or from the liver. It was suggested that the elevated potassium level might serve to increase the irritability of the central nervous system and speed synaptic conduction during asphyxia.

Cattel and Civin (17) in 1938 found in the cat that from four to five minutes of complete asphyxia caused a rise in blood potassium to 38 mg/100 cc. (Normal range is from 10–30 mg/100 cc.) This returned to normal within two to three minutes after normal respiration was resumed.

In 1936 Houssay and his co-workers (44, 45) reported that the potassium rise produced by asphyxia could be eliminated by sectioning the splanchnics or by performing either adrenalectomy or hepatectomy. They reported further that ischemia, produced by stimulating the peripheral end of the vagus until the heart stopped, produced a rise in blood potassium and that hemorrhage did likewise. The rise in blood potassium produced by hemorrhage could be prevented only by hepatectomy. They concluded that the asphyxia stimulated the adrenals to secrete more epinephrine and that this caused the liver to mobilize the potassium.

Fenn (24) has pointed out that it is not certain that all the potassium comes from the liver, since a loss due to asphyxia has been reported in the heart (18, 19) and in the skeletal muscle of the cat (5, 25). He feels that while probably all the tissues tend to give up some potassium during asphyxia, most comes from the liver as a result of a specific adrenalin mechanism.

b) Anoxic hypoxia: Sundstroem (79) in 1919 found that at high altitudes there was an increase in the excretion of potassium. Hall *et al.* (36) in 1936 reported that the blood potassium of rabbits which were transported to high altitudes was greatly reduced; that of the llama, however, was only slightly lowered. The authors pointed out that the animals were excited when the control samples were taken at sea level. This was unfortunate, since true normal values might not have been obtained. It was reported by McQuarrie and his collaborators (57) and by Ziegler (83) in 1940 that dogs made to breathe 5–9 per cent oxygen in nitrogen for several hours showed a decrease in the blood potassium.

More recent work by Ferguson and Smith (26) corroborates the findings of earlier workers. Unanesthetized dogs were subjected to a simulated altitude of 30,000 feet (9,145 meters) for ninety minutes. A noticeable decrease (about 19 per cent) in plasma-potassium concentration during the periods of acute decompression was observed. The major decrease occurred during the first thirty minutes. During the post-decompression period, plasma-potassium concentration rose and in about half of the experiments exceeded the pre-decompression level.

In summary, it appears that, while asphyxia causes an immediate increase in blood-potassium level, anoxic hypoxia causes a decrease.

Bilirubin.—In general, it may be said that polycythemia associated with constant or intermittent hypoxia tends to produce proportional elevation in the serum bilirubin. The majority of workers agree that there is an absolute increase in destruction of the red blood cells during hypoxia. It has been shown (61) that the hemolytic index (mg. daily urobilinogen excretion per 100 gm. total hemoglobin) remains unchanged, which indicates that the relative rate of hemoglobin destruction is probably not increased at altitude. It is of interest that the life span of the red blood cells during hypoxia is unchanged at altitude (9, 68, 29).

Hurtado (49) in 1932, using Van den Bergh's indirect method, found a rise in bilirubin in the blood of twelve native Peruvian Indians living at high altitudes. In a subsequent paper (50), he reported that intermittent hypoxia also may produce slightly higher values in serum bilirubin. This was found to be true in certain flight personnel and also in railroad workers who labored at high altitudes but spent considerable of their time at sea level. He observed that some individuals who dwell at high altitudes showed an increase of serum bilirubin as high as 100 per cent. He also found a small amount of urobilin in the urine. (For further discussion concerning effect of chronic hypoxia on bilirubin see chap. x.)

Tanaka and Homma (81) in 1936, working with rabbits, reported that severe degrees of hypoxia, corresponding to altitudes of 16,500 feet (about 5,000 meters) or more, caused a decrease in the excretion of bilirubin. It is of interest that Hurtado (50) found degrees of retention of injected bilirubin higher than that of men at sea level in four natives of Morococha, Peru, who had all previously shown an increase in serum bilirubin.

Rich (69) observed that rats subjected to low oxygen tension also showed a diminished ability to secrete intravenously injected bilirubin. Campbell (16) has suggested that prolonged hypoxia may be an important factor in causing hepatic insufficiency from the point of view of excretion of pigment. It has been suggested, too, that the bilirubinemia in residents at high altitudes may be produced by defective liver function (50, 61) and that at altitude there is a higher threshold for bilirubin excretion (82).

The entire matter of hyperbilirubinemia during hypoxia is not fully understood. Hurtado (50) feels that it is caused by several factors, but the two most important probably are: (*a*) increased rate of pigment formation, and (*b*) decreased power of hepatic cells to excrete pigment due to the hypoxia.

In summary: presumably there is an absolute, and not a relative, increase in the amount of red blood cell destruction during hypoxia. Actually the liver does a reasonably good job in excreting the pigment, considering that there is so much more to get rid of because of the polycythemia. It is not fully understood why the liver does not secrete more pigment than it does. Perhaps it is simply working at full capacity, but it is also possible that the hypoxia affects the hepatic cells.

Blood lipids.—As far as the authors are aware, the effect of oxygen want on blood lipids has not been reported in man; for the main part, work of this nature has been performed on rabbits.

A number of workers (14, 38, 43, 73, 74) have shown that anemic hypoxia, that is, hemorrhage, produces a lipemia. It is generally agreed that the increase in blood lipids is confined to the plasma. In 1920 Horiuchi (43), working with rabbits, showed that a single acute hemorrhage (45 cc.) or repeated bleeding results in a marked lipemia; return to normal values required from fourteen to eighteen days.

Sundstroem and Bloor (80) in the same year reported that short exposures to atmospheric pressures from 350 to 400 mm. Hg, corresponding to altitudes of 20,000 to 17,000 feet (6,100 to 5,200 meters), caused an average decrease in plasma phospholipids of 13.2 per cent. It was thought that the decrease was due to an enrichment of the erythropoietic organs, that is, a redistribution of phospholipids from the blood-forming organs.

Schmensky (71) found that blood cholesterol increased at high altitudes. Whereas normally it is found in the blood at a concentration of 180 mg. per cent; at Davos, altitude of 5,100 feet (about 1,525 meters), he found it to be elevated to 200 mg. per cent and from 350 to 480 mg. per cent in some natives. The cause of this rise is not clear. Guzman-Barron (8), however, claims that hypercholesterolemia does not occur in acclimated inhabitants in the Andes. Hurtado (49) reached the same conclusion.

The work reported by Starup (74) in 1934 is of especial interest. Working with rabbits, he found that a hemorrhage of one-fifth to one-sixth of the blood volume produced a lipemia which involved all the blood lipids; neutral fat was affected the most; cholesterol next; and lecithin last. A marked lipemia was found to result from the administration of phenylhydrazine, from the intravenous injection of distilled water, or from exposure to a reduced barometric pressure of from 300 to 360 mm. Hg. corresponding to altitudes of 24,000–19,000 feet (7,300–5,800 meters). He concluded that the immediate cause of the lipemia was oxygen tension being reduced both when the atmospheric pressure was lowered and when anemia was produced by the various methods previously outlined.

MacLachlan (59) in 1939 showed that there is a wide species variation in response to oxygen want as far as blood lipids are concerned. The blood-plasma lipids of cats and dogs exposed to oxygen want for short periods were not affected either during the fasting state or during the active absorption from the intestine. In the rabbit, however, there was a fall in plasma lipids after three hours of hypoxia (254 mm. Hg); this fall was due mainly to a decrease in neutral fat content. Normal levels were established in six hours. It was suggested that the difference in response between the rabbit and the dog or cat might be due to different abilities to utilize fats.

Since rabbits do not respond in the same way as other mammals studied, it is not permissible to draw conclusions concerning the possible effect of oxygen want on the blood lipids in man. This phase of the work deserves further study.

REFERENCES

1. ANDES, J. E., et al. 1940. J. Lab. Clin. Med., 26: 530.
2. ARAKI, T. 1891; 1892; 1893; 1894. Hoppe Seyler Z. Physiol. Chem., 15: 335; 16: 201; 17: 311; 18: 1.
3. ARMSTRONG, H. G. 1939. Principles and Practices of Aviation Medicine, p. 289. Baltimore: Williams & Wilkins Co.
4. ASMUSSEN, E., and NIELSON, M. 1945. Acta Physiol. Scand., 9: 75.

5. BAETJER, A. M. 1935. *Amer. J. Physiol.,* 112: 139.
6. BARCROFT, J. 1925. *The Respiratory Function of the Blood,* Part I, "Lessons from High Altitudes," p. 93. Cambridge: Cambridge University Press.
7. BARCROFT, J., *et al.* 1914. *Phil. Trans. Roy. Soc., London,* B, 206: 49.
8. BARRON, G., cited by C. MONGE, *et al.* 1935. *An. Fac. Ciencias Med. Lima* (3 reports), 18.
9. BERLIN, N. I.; REYNAFARJE, C.; and LAWRENCE, J. H. 1954. *J. Appl. Physiol.,* 7: 271.
10. BERNARD, CLAUDE. 1857. *Lecons sue les des substances toxiques et medicamenteuses.* Paris: J. B. Bailliere et fils.
11. BOCK, A. V.; EDWARDS, H. T.; and DILL, D. B. 1932. *J. Clin. Invest.,* 11: 775.
12. BOEDICKER, W. 1933. *Arch. Hyg.,* 109: 124.
13. BOYCOTT, O. E., and HALDANE, J. S. 1908. *J. Physiol.,* 37: 355.
14. BOYD, E. M., and STEVENS, J. W. 1937. *J. Biol. Chem.,* 122: 147.
15. BURESCH, H. 1933. *Arch. Hyg.,* 109: 211.
16. CAMPBELL, J. A. 1928. *Lancet,* 2: 84.
17. CATTELL, M., and CIVIN, H. 1938. *J. Biol. Chem.,* 126: 633.
18. CLARK, A. J.; GADDIE, R.; and STEWART, C. P. 1934. *J. Physiol.,* 82: 265.
19. DENNIS, J., and MOORE, R. M. 1938. *Amer. J. Physiol.,* 123: 443.
20. DENNIS, J., and MULLIN, F. J. 1938. *Proc. Soc. Exp. Biol. Med.,* 38: 560.
21. DILL, D. B. 1938. *Life Heat and Altitude,* p. 172. Cambridge, Mass.: Harvard University Press.
22. DILL, D. B.; TALBOTT, J. H.; and CONSOLAZIO, W. V. 1937. *J. Biol. Chem.,* 118: 649.
23. EDWARDS, H. T. 1936. *Amer. J. Physiol.,* 116: 367.
24. FENN, W. O. 1940. *Physiol. Rev.,* 20: 377.
25. FENN, W. O., *et al.* 1939. *Amer. J Physiol.,* 128: 139.
26. FERGUSON, F. P., and SMITH, D. C. 1953. *Amer. J. Physiol.,* 173: 503.
27. FORBES, W. H. 1936. *Amer. J. Physiol.,* 116: 309.
28. FRIEDEMANN, T. E., *et al.* 1949. *Quart. Bull. Northw. Univ. Med. Sch.,* 23: 438.
29. FRYERS, G. R. 1952. *Amer. J. Physiol.,* 171: 459.
30. GALLEOTI, G. 1904. *Arch. Ital. Biol.,* 41: 80.
31. GELLHORN, E., and PACKER, A. C. 1939. *Proc. Soc. Exp. Biol. Med.,* 41: 345.
32. GELLHORN, E.; PACKER, A. C.; and FELDMAN, J. 1940. *Amer. J. Physiol.,* 130: 261.
33. GREENE, N. M., and PHILLIPS, A. D. 1957. *Amer. J. Physiol.,* 189: 475.
34. HAGGARD, H. W., and HENDERSON, Y. 1920; 1921. *J. Biol. Chem.,* 43: 3 and 20; 47: 421.
35. HALDANE, J. S.; KELLAS, A. S.; and KENNAWAY, E. L. 1919–20. *J. Physiol.,* 53: 181.

36. HALL, L. G.; DILL, D. B.; and BARRON, E. S. G. 1936. *J. Cell. Comp. Physiol.*, **8:** 301.
37. HASSELBALCH, K. A., and LINDHARD, J. 1915. *Biochem. Z.*, **68:** 295.
38. HEKI, M. 1930. *J. Biochem. (Tokyo)*, **11:** 369.
39. HENDERSON, Y. 1919. *Science*, **49:** 431.
40. ———. 1920. *J. Biol. Chem.*, **43:** 29.
41. HENDERSON, Y., and GREENBERG, L. A. 1934. *Amer. J. Physiol.*, **107:** 37.
42. HENDERSON, Y., and RADLOFF, E. M. 1932. *Amer. J. Physiol.*, **101:** 647.
43. HORIUCHI, Y. 1930. *J. Biol. Chem.*, **44:** 363.
44. HOUSSAY, A. B.; MARENZI, A. D.; and GERSCHMAN, R. 1936. *Rev. Soc. Argent. Biol.*, **12:** 434.
45. ———. 1937. *C. R. Soc. Biol. (Par.)* , **124:** 382, 383, 384.
46. HUCKABEE, W. 1958. *J. Clin. Invest.*, **37:** 244.
47. ———. *Ibid.*, p. 264.
48. HUEY, D. M., and HOLMES, J. H. 1950. *Fed. Proc.*, **9:** 64 (Part I) .
49. HURTADO, A. 1932. *Amer. J. Physiol.*, **100:** 487.
50. HURTADO, A.; MERINO, C.; and DELGADO, E. 1945. *Arch. Intern. Med.*, **75:** 284.
51. JOHLIN, J. M., and MORELAND, F. B. 1933. *J. Biol. Chem.*, **103:** 107.
52. KELLAWAY, C. H. 1910. *J. Physiol.*, **53:** 211.
53. KEYS, A. 1936. *Sci. Monthly*, **43:** 289.
54. KOEHLER, A. E.; BRUNQUIST, E. H.; and LOEVENHART, A. S. 1925. *J. Biol. Chem.*, **64:** 313.
55. KORNER, P. I. 1959. *Physiol. Rev.*, **39:** 687 (Part I) .
56. McQUARRIE, I., and ZIEGLER, M. 1939. *Proc. Soc. Exp. Biol. Med.*, **39:** 525.
57. McQUARRIE, I., *et al.* 1940. *Chin. Med. J.*, **58:** 26.
58. McQUARRIE, I., *et al.* 1939. *Proc. Soc. Exp. Biol. Med.*, **42:** 513.
59. MACLACHLAN, P. L. 1939. *J. Biol. Chem.*, **129:** 465.
60. MACLEOD, J. J. R. 1921. *Amer. J. Physiol.*, **55:** 175.
61. MERINO, C. F. 1950. *Blood*, **5:** 1.
62. MIKAMI, S. 1926–27. *Tohoku J. Exp. Med.*, **8:** 237.
63. MORELAND, L. B. 1937. *J. Biol. Chem.*, **117:** 471.
64. MULLINS, F. J.; DENNIS, J.; and CALVIN, D. B. 1938. *Amer. J. Physiol.*, **124:** 192.
65. MUNZER, E., and PALMER, P. 1894. *Z. Heilk.*, **15:** 185.
66. MURALT, G., VON, and NOTTER, B. 1948. *Helv. Physiol. Pharmacol. Acta*, **6:** 649.
67. PETERS, J. P., and VAN SLYKE, D. D. 1923. *Quantitative Clinical Chemistry*, I, 967. Baltimore: Williams & Wilkins Co.
68. REYNAFARJE, C.; LOZANO, R.; and VALDIVIESEO, J. 1959. *Blood*, **14:** 433.
69. RICH, A. R. 1930. *Bull. Johns Hopkins Hosp.*, **47:** 338.
70. RYFFEL, J. H. 1909–10. *J. Physiol.*, **39:** 20.
71. SCHMENSKY, cited by A. LOEWY and E. WITTKOWER. 1937. *The Pathol-*

ogy of High Altitude Climate, p. 49. London: Oxford University Press.

72. SCHULZE, E. 1936. *Arch. Exp. Path. Pharm.*, **180:** 649.
73. SCHWARTZ, H., and LICHTENBERG, H. H. 1937. *J. Biol. Chem.*, **121:** 315.
74. STARUP, U. 1934. *Biochem. Z.*, **270:** 74
75. STICKNEY, J. C.; NORTHUP, D. W.; and VAN LIERE, E. J. 1943. *Proc. Soc. Exp. Biol. Med.*, **54:** 151.
76. ———. 1948. *Amer. J. Physiol.*, **154:** 423.
77. ———. 1950. *Fed. Proc.*, **9:** 122.
78. ———. 1951. *Amer. J. Physiol.*, **167:** 559.
79. SUNDSTROEM, E. S. 1919. *Univ. Calif. Publ. Physiol.*, **5:** 121.
80. SUNDSTROEM, E. S., and BLOOR, W. R. 1920. *J. Biol. Chem.*, **45:** 153.
81. TANAKA, H., and HOMMA, M. 1936. *Bull. Naval Med. Ass.* (Japan), Abst. Sec., **25:** 14.
82. URTEAGA, O. 1942. *An. Fac. Med. Lima*, **25:** 89.
83. ZIEGLER, M. R. 1940. *Proc. Soc. Exp. Biol. Med.*, **43:** 165.
84. ZWEMER, R. L., and PIKE, F. H. 1938. *Ann. N.Y. Acad. Sci.*, **37:** 257.

CHAPTER V

EFFECT OF HYPOXIA ON THE HEART AND CIRCULATION

THE HEART RATE

1. *Acute effects.*—It is well known that acute hypoxia produces an acceleration of the heart beat (4, 63, 66, 67, 122, 142). It was shown by Lutz and Schneider (101) in 1919 that if subjects were allowed to breathe pure nitrogen, an acceleration of the heart within five to fifty-five seconds (in 66 per cent of all cases within fifteen seconds or less) would be observed. Experiments by the same authors performed in a low-pressure chamber, in which the barometric pressure was lowered at a rate corresponding to an ascent of 1,000 feet (305 meters) a minute, showed a quickening of the pulse in 26 per cent of all subjects at tensions of oxygen equivalent to an altitude of 4,000 feet (1,200 meters) or less.

Barcroft (9) has stated that altitudes above 10,000 feet (3,050 meters) quicken the pulse in unacclimatized individuals at rest. Schneider and Truesdell (144) have shown that the heart rate slowly and gradually increases until the oxygen tension is equivalent to that of about 446 mm. Hg barometric pressure, which corresponds to an altitude of about 14,000 feet (4,270 meters). After this altitude has been reached there are greater increments in heart rate for each 1,000 feet (305 meters) of ascent. At a barometric pressure of 428.6 mm. Hg, corresponding to an altitude of about 15,000 feet (4,570 meters), the increase averaged fifteen beats. At a pressure of 379.4 mm. Hg, corresponding to an altitude of 18,000 feet (5,485 meters), it averaged twenty beats.

Schneider (142) emphasizes that there is a good deal of individual variation at 14,000 feet (4,270 meters); some subjects show a slight increase in cardiac rate, while others show rises of ten beats or more. If the individual suffers from mountain sickness, there is pronounced acceleration of the pulse; but after the attack wears off, this subsides. It is generally agreed that the greatest augmentation of the heart rate occurs in those who are not in good physical condition. In healthy individuals Schneider and his co-workers (143) did not find the pulse extraordinarily labile at high altitudes. They also observed that the heart works at high altitudes at an increased rate in all positions with about the same differences as at low altitude.

McFarland (107) in 1937 reported that, in an ascent by train from sea level to an altitude of 14,890 feet (about 4,500 meters), six subjects showed an increase in the basal pulse rate from an average of 65 beats to 75.7 beats. In the standing position there was an increase from 78.3 to 89.5 beats. In a fifty-minute airplane flight, starting at sea level and reaching an altitude of 15,000 feet (4,570 meters), observations on four subjects showed a distinct increase in pulse rate in all. In one subject the pulse rose from 60 to 89 beats per minute; in a second subject, from 100 to 116; in a third, from 68 to 86; and in a fourth, from 72 to 115. It may well be, however, that anxiety contributed somewhat to the increased pulse rate.

Dripps and Comroe (39) in 1947, working with human subjects, reported that a significant increase in pulse rate occurred when the concentration of oxygen in the inspired air was reduced from 20.9 to 18 per cent. Their findings are pretty much in accord with those reported by Schneider and his co-workers in 1919 (101).

It was shown by several early workers (71, 101, 141) that if the constant level of low oxygen be maintained for an hour or more, the pulse rate in many instances, although not in all, becomes retarded. These early observations were confirmed by Rahn and Otis (129) in 1947. They showed that the maximum elevation of pulse rate following acute exposure is not sustained, and some fall toward the resting value occurs during the first hour of exposure. (See Table 4.)

A number of workers (6, 39, 66) have shown that the heart rate may be doubled in animals breathing from 7 to 8 per cent oxygen (corresponding to an altitude well over 22,000 feet—6,705 meters).

Cause of increased heart rate: The cause of the increased heart rate during hypoxia is not fully understood. Barcroft (9) pointed out in 1925 that in the resting animal hypoxia produces cardiac quickening until the central nervous system commences to lose its grip. It was not known how much of the effect was due to loss of vagal tone or to increase in sympathetic control. Sands and DeGraff (138) in the same year reported that the pulse rate was increased by reduced tonic activity of the vagal cardio-inhibitory center and, to a lesser degree, by increased activity of the sympathetic cardioaccelerator center.

Wright (170) has written that cardiac acceleration produced by hypoxia is due to direct effects of oxygen lack on the sinoauricular node, and, furthermore, this is coupled with effects due to the reflex secretion of adrenaline from the adrenal glands. A number of workers (5, 6, 39, 43, 162) have suggested that the change in heart rate during hypoxia is initiated at the chemoreceptors of the aortic and carotid bodies. This was challenged by Bernthal and his associates (16) in 1951 and by Daly and Scott (31) in 1958.

The first-named investigators, working with dogs, recorded changes in heart rate during hypoxic stimuli to the carotid chemoreceptors and found that the direct reflex change in heart rate initiated by hypoxia produced a moderate slowing. They concluded that cardiac acceleration of generalized hypoxia does not arise chemoreflexively

TABLE 4

PULSE RATE CHANGE, IN PERCENTAGE OF GROUND-LEVEL VALUE,
DURING PROGRESSIVE EXPOSURE: MAN*
(Pulse Rate Index at Ground Level: 100)

EXPOSURE TIME (Minutes)	ALTITUDE (Feet and Meters)				
	12,000 3,658	16,000 4,877	18,000 5,486	20,000 6,069	22,000 6,705
10	113	111	107	124	131
20	115	110	109	112	126
30	113	103	108	117	124
40	106	103	111	107	. . .
50	104	101	108	. . .	. . .
60	99	105	104	. . .	. . .

* H. Rahn and A. B. Otis, *Amer. J. Physiol.*, 150 (1947): 202. From *Handbook of Circulation*, WADC Technical Report 59–593 (October, 1959), p. 162.

from the carotid bodies and that this applied to the aortic chemoreceptors as well.

Daly and Scott also reported that hypoxic stimulation of the carotid bodies produced bradycardia in dogs. They pointed out that in spontaneously breathing dogs there may be an increase, a decrease, or no change in pulse rate. They felt that the increase is due to the reflex stimulation from the lungs over the vagi nerves and that this tachycardia masks the bradycardia.

In 1954 Nahas *et al.* (118) studied the heart rate in five sympathectomized, non-narcotized dogs which had been made to breathe 8 per cent oxygen in nitrogen. They observed that the changes in heart rate were of smaller magnitude than those observed in intact animals. Adrenalectomized dogs subjected to the same conditions did not show these changes.

In summary, it may be said that the mechanism causing an increase in heart rate during hypoxia still is not known. A number of workers feel that the change is initiated at the chemoreceptors of the carotid and aortic bodies; this has been denied by other workers. More work is obviously needed on this problem.

2. *Aftereffects on the heart rate.*—The aftereffects of hypoxia on heart rate are different from those of respiration (p. 135). They depend upon the length of time the individual has been exposed to hypoxia. If he has been exposed for only an hour or so, the heart returns to its normal rate at once; if, however, the sojourn at high altitudes has been long enough for acclimatization to take place, the cardiac rate may be subnormal for many days after the subject's return to a low altitude, as has been shown by a number of early workers (40, 77, 140, 156).

3. *Effect of exercise on the pulse rate at high altitudes.*—The effect of exercise upon the pulse rate at high altitudes depends on whether or not acclimatization has taken place. In the non-acclimatized individual relatively mild exercise will produce the same symptoms at high altitudes as will severe exercise at low altitudes, namely, a forcible and rapidly beating heart with concomitant breathlessness. (For a discussion of the effects of exercise on pulse rate in acclimatized individuals see chap. x.)

EFFECT OF PROGRESSIVE HYPOXIA ON HEART AND CIRCULATION

A number of workers (55, 56, 63, 138, 142, 145, 163) have studied the effect of progressive hypoxia on the heart and circulation. These studies have shown, for the main part, that under those conditions the heart accelerates, the systolic pressure is either maintained or gradually falls, and the pulse pressure remains unchanged or increases.

Sands and DeGraff (138), in their studies of the effect of progressive hypoxia on the heart and circulation in the dog, concluded that the circulation was improved until the oxygen in the inspired air reached 9 per cent; when the oxygen percentage was diminished below this point, a circulatory crisis occurred.

They pointed out that hypoxia has two opposing effects on the heart. On the one hand, it produces a reduction in the effective venous pressure, which reduces cardiac filling, and it also causes an abbreviation of the systolic phase of ejection. On the other hand, hypoxia raises the initial tension in the left ventricle and also increases the velocity of ventricular ejection. These two opposing factors during the course of the early stages of progressive hypoxia remain evenly balanced and tend to maintain or increase slightly the normal systolic discharge.

Sands and DeGraff cite three factors to account for an increase in the minute-flow of the blood through the body during hypoxia: (*a*) an increased systolic discharge, (*b*) an increased rate of the heart beat, and (*c*) a reduced peripheral resistance. This beneficial influence of hypoxia, however, persists only until the concentration of oxygen reaches 9 per cent.

As mentioned previously, when the hypoxia becomes more severe, a circulatory crisis occurs. There is first a decline of systolic and diastolic pressures and a reduction in pulse pressure. Beginning signs of failure of the circulation become manifest because of reduction in the minute-output of the heart. The heart becomes slower, the ejection phase becomes still more abbreviated, and circulatory collapse becomes imminent. Since the combination of these factors causes the cardiac output steadily to diminish, the blood pressure soon drops to a point incompatible with the life of the animal.

Sands and DeGraff state that there is some evidence that the stimulating effects of hypoxia up to the point of the circulatory crisis (which occurs at 9 per cent oxygen) may be accounted for by the fact that hypoxia either depresses the vagi or stimulates the accelerator mechanism. When the vagi are cut, the cardiac acceleration produced by hypoxia is often, but not always, absent, indicating that the accelerating mechanism may be stimulated.

Wiggers (164) in 1941, reviewing the effect of progressive hypoxia on the heart and circulation, points out that some laboratory investigators (35, 65, 82) have concluded that oxygen lack has no stimulating action on the ventricles and that dilatation and depression result when blood is about one-half saturated with oxygen. His views are not in accord with this concept, and he calls attention to the work of Sands and DeGraff and that of Strughold (153).

Wiggers also emphasizes that during hypoxia the ventricles eject the blood with a greater economy of effort, as judged by a criterion reported in his publication of 1928 (167) and later corroborated on the human subject (49). He summarizes the effects of progressive hypoxia on the heart and circulation as follows: A progressive decrease in respired oxygen volumes to about 12 per cent (a period he calls hypoxia, corresponding to blood oxygen saturation to about 75 per cent and to altitudes to 15,000 feet—4,570 meters) increases the flow of blood by redistribution of blood flow and by cardiac acceleration. He attributes the increased cardiac rate to decreased vagal tone, to increased accelerator nerve activity, and perhaps to some direct effect on the S-A node. During this period the vigor of ventricular contractions increases, the period of systolic expulsion shortens, and the effective venous pressure falls slightly.

When the oxygen in the inspired air falls below 12 per cent (which he calls the "true period of hypoxia"), a greater stroke volume occurs, the velocity of ejection increases further, and the economy of effort is enhanced. When the oxygen declines to 7 or 6 per cent (corresponding to an arterial-blood oxygen saturation between 50 and 35 per cent and to altitudes up to 30,000 feet—9,100 meters), a

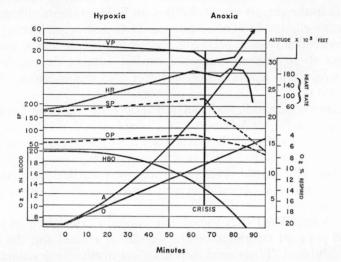

FIG. 7.—The effect of progressive anoxia on the heart and circulation. Graph showing the relation of percentage of oxygen respired (O) to altitude (A) and oxygen saturation of blood (Hb) and division into stages of venous pressure (VP), heart rate (HR), systolic (SP) and diastolic (DP) pressures in dogs during progressive hypoxia and anoxia. (From C. J. Wiggers, *Ann. Intern. Med.*, 14 [1941], 1239.)

coronary crisis occurs. The arterial pressure declines abruptly, the pulse pressure is reduced, the systolic pressure decreases, the venous pressure rises greatly, and various types of conduction and rhythm disturbances occur. Wiggers feels that the circulatory crisis is essentially an acute congestive heart failure due to the depressant effect of hypoxia on the myocardium.

CARDIAC OUTPUT

1. *Anoxic hypoxia.*—The effect of hypoxia on cardiac output has been extensively investigated. Some of the early workers reported that hypoxia had little or no effect on cardiac output, and some

found a decrease. Some of the early literature in this field will be reviewed briefly. Observations on cardiac output by the Anglo-American Pike's Peak Expedition in 1911, by means of a recoil board and measurement of pulse pressure, showed that the volume of the heart strokes continued practically the same on Pike's Peak (elevation of 14,100 feet—4,300 meters) as at low altitudes. Kuhn (94) in 1913, working at an altitude of 11,000 feet (3,355 meters) ; Hasselbalch and Lindhardt (77) in 1916, working at a simulated altitude of 12,000 feet (3,360 meters) ; and Doi (35) in 1921, producing acute hypoxia in the cat, all reported either an indeterminate change or no significant change in cardiac output. Lutz and Schneider (101) in 1919 concluded from experiments performed in a low-pressure chamber that there was an increased cardiac output during hypoxia. Later work with a rebreather, however, did not confirm this finding (145) .

The work of Sands and DeGraff (138) in 1925 has been commented upon. In 1926 Dreyer (38) , working with a cardiometer on decerebrate cats, found that hypoxia which lowered arterial oxygen saturation from 50 to 80 per cent caused an augmented cardiac output. Kisch (89) , in the same year, using overventilation in curarized dogs to produce an arterial oxygen saturation of 70 per cent, also found an increase in cardiac output.

Jarisch and Wastl (82) found that when the arterial blood was less than 60 per cent saturated, cardiac dilatation ensued and the output was diminished. Their work was done on urethanized animals, and vagotomy and thoracotomy had been performed. Gremels and Starling (65) , in the same year, working with a heart-lung preparation, found that hypoxia first produced no change and then a diminution in the systemic output of the heart.

Harrison and his co-workers (76) criticized the results of the investigators who reported that hypoxia decreased cardiac output on the grounds that their observations were made mostly on anesthetized animals and that nearly all work involved thoracic operations which entailed shock. Furthermore, the studies reported on man were concerned with blood flow in only one part of the body, and indirect and unreliable methods were used.

In 1927 Harrison and Blalock (74) showed that severe hypoxia of short duration caused an increase in the minute-cardiac output. It was also shown that a rapidly produced anemia led to increased cardiac output. The work suggested that the minute-cardiac output might be inversely proportional to the tissue oxygen tension. If the arterial blood were less than 70 per cent saturated with oxygen, the minute-cardiac output was always increased. In the same year Harrison *et al.* (76), using the Fick method, found that cardiac output in normal unanesthetized dogs first showed an increase when the arterial blood was saturated about 75 per cent. They designated this the "anoxemia threshold." In a subsequent paper (75), the conclusion was reached that the circulatory response to hypoxemia was independent of the nervous system and endocrine glands but was due to a vascular action. They also produced some evidence which indicated that the tension of oxygen in the heart muscle was possibly the most important factor in the control of the circulatory volume.

Harrison and his co-workers (76) definitely felt that if the oxygen saturation fell below 75 per cent, cardiac output increased. In support of their views they point out, first, that their findings have been uniform throughout their work, which is in contrast to that of other workers; second, that the Fick method which they employed to determine cardiac output is conceded to be very accurate; and, lastly, that they used normal unanesthetized manipulations.

Other investigators have fully corroborated the findings of Harrison and his co-workers. Grollman (66) in 1930 made observations on two subjects on Pike's Peak. He reported that the heart output per minute increased steadily for about four or five days, reaching a maximum of about 48 per cent above its sea-level value, and then gradually declined to its normal level as the hemoglobin concentration was increased. Christensen (24) in 1937 reported findings made on the cardiac output of members of the Chilean Expedition. His work agreed qualitatively with Grollman's, but quantitatively he did not find the same relations between circulatory rate and hemoglobin concentration as did Grollman.

In 1954 Nahas *et al.* (119) reported that cardiac output in the dog was significantly elevated after a five-minute exposure to 8 per cent oxygen. During the past decade a number of workers (12, 37, 52) have shown that there is a relationship between cardiac output and arterial saturation.

It is of interest to mention briefly the effect of chronic hypoxia on cardiac output. Rotta (135) in 1947, working with native residents in Peru at 14,900 feet (4,540 meters), reported a slightly greater cardiac output (about 8.5 per cent). However, in more recent studies (136, 137) using the method of right heart catherization, no difference could be found in the resting cardiac output of acclimatized individuals.

2. *Anemic hypoxia.*—The work of Harrison and Blalock in 1927 has been mentioned. Chiodi *et al.* (23) in 1941 studied the effect of

acute carbon monoxide poisoning on the cardiac output of dogs. They reported a slight increase with HbCO saturations ranging up to about 30 per cent. However, from that level up to 50 per cent saturation, cardiac output increased as much as one-half. In 1954 Sunahara and Beck (154) produced anemia in anesthetized dogs and found that when a critical level was established, a further decrease in hematocrit caused a proportional increase in cardiac output. When the hematocrit was returned to normal, cardiac output decreased. The authors concluded that arterial oxygen content is the primary factor in the regulation of cardiac output in the intact animal.

It is now generally accepted that both hemic hypoxia and anoxic hypoxia may produce an increase in cardiac output. Some investigators feel that this increase plays an important role in the ability of an individual to withstand hypoxia and to become acclimatized to high altitudes (24, 34, 66, 80, 103, 104).

Mechanism of increased cardiac output: The exact cause of increased cardiac output during hypoxia is, as yet, not fully understood. Wiggers (164, 166) feels that the work of Strughold (153), who used "controlled circulation" (i.e., heart rate, arterial diastolic pressure, venous pressure, and alveolar carbon dioxide kept constant) in dogs, gave convincing proof that hypoxia initially increases systolic discharge. Strughold demonstrated that a significant increase in diastolic size occurred without change in venous pressure. He concluded that the dilation was due to a decrease in myocardial tonus and that the lengthening of the cardiac fibers had a beneficial action on the stroke volume in accordance with Starling's Law of the Heart.

Wiggers (166) feels that the hypoxic stimulation of the chemoreceptors reflexively increases the cardiac rate and that the increased epinephrine discharge causes a vasoconstriction. He states, also, that certain degrees of hypoxia (below 12 per cent) stimulate the cardiac muscles directly, an effect similar to that of minute doses of epinephrine. Forber and Evans (48) have questioned the latter view. They maintained that in no single set of experiments have all the extracardiac factors been rigorously excluded. They point out further that experiments in the heart-lung and isolated heart preparations (19, 65) during hypoxia have not supported this view. These authors, working with completely isolated hearts of cats, reported that increases in cardiac output (of purely cardiac origin) by the isolated heart under hypoxia are seen only when CO_2 is absent from the ventilating gas. They concluded that the augmented cardiac output is due to elevation in pH and that there is no evidence of a direct stimulating effect of hypoxia on the myocardium.

Nahas *et al.* (119), working with dogs, felt that the increased heart rate contributed largely to the increased cardiac output produced by hypoxia and that there was also a significant elevation of stroke volume.

Recently Gomori *et al.* (59) concluded from their work on anesthetized dogs that the adrenal glands play no part in the increase of cardiac output during hypoxia. They were unable to demonstrate the existence of a neural or endocrine mechanism which would account for the increase in cardiac output. They believe that hypoxia gives rise to local vasodilatation; this would produce an increased cardiac filling and would probably account for the augmented output. They quote the work of Patterson and Starling (124) to support their view. Some physiologists, however, would not agree with their interpretation.

In summary, it may be said that the exact mechanism of increased cardiac output during hypoxia is not known. However, it is not unlikely that sympathetic activity is increased during hypoxia and that both epinephrine and norepinephrine are liberated. If this be true, the pulse rate would increase, and probably the heart would beat more forcibly; there would also be an increased vasoconstrictor tone, and the arterial pressure would rise. All of these factors could account for an increased cardiac output.

BALLISTOCARDIOGRAPHY DURING HYPOXIA

A number of investigators have measured cardiac output during hypoxia by means of the ballistocardiograph. Starr and McMichael (151) in 1948 studied the cardiac output and cardiac rate using this instrument in twenty-one subjects at sea level and at simulated altitudes from 16,000 (4,875 meters) to 18,000 feet (5,485 meters) in a pressure chamber. It was observed that cardiac output increased 14 per cent per beat. Galdston and Steele (53) measured cardiac output ballistocardiographically in young, healthy men in a reclining position. Cardiac output was increased when they breathed 10 per cent oxygen (simulated altitude of approximately 17,500 feet —5,330 meters). Similar results were obtained by Franzblau *et al.* (50) in ten young, normal males, working at approximately the same altitude.

In 1951 Scarborough *et al.* (139), using sixteen normal subjects, found that the increased cardiac output produced by hypoxia (oxygen saturation from 85 to 70 per cent) was largely due to cardiac acceleration. The authors reported that the ballistocardiograms were normal in form and remained so throughout the period of hypoxia. Masini *et al.* (102) in 1953 subjected sixteen healthy subjects to various degrees of hypoxia: 10, 7, and 5 per cent oxygen. They reported an increase in the cardiac index (minute-volume of blood per square meter of body surface) . The stroke volume showed little change. It was observed that the pattern of the ballistocardiogram in healthy subjects always remained within the normal limits.

In 1960 Moss (116) studied the pattern of the ballistocardiogram in six normal subjects. It is recognized that the slope of the initial systolic deflection (H-I wave) on the acceleratory ballistocardiogram reflects the rate at which the cardiac ejection force is generated. When the subjects breathed 10 per cent oxygen for twenty minutes this rate was significantly increased.

In summary, it may be stated that in most instances, but not in all, the ballistocardiograph demonstrates that hypoxia is capable of producing an increase in cardiac output. Furthermore, hypoxia has little, if any, effect on the pattern of the ballistocardiogram.

BLOOD-VOLUME FLOW

A number of workers have reported experiments on both man and animals which concern blood-volume flow in various parts of the body during anoxic hypoxia and hemic hypoxia.

Experiments performed on man.—As early as 1914 Schneider and his colleagues (143) made some observations on Pike's Peak on the blood flow through the hand and reported an increase in the circulation. Several years later, however, using the rebreather method (145) , a decreased flow was observed. Freeman *et al.* (51) in 1936, working on shock, studied the effects of oxygen deficiency on peripheral flow in the hand and obtained variable results. Making somewhat similar studies on man two years later, Gellhorn and Steck (57) used from 7.6 to 9.8 per cent oxygen mixtures and also reported variable results.

Abramson and his co-workers (2,3) in 1941, employing the venous occlusion plethysmograph, reported peripheral vascular responses to general hypoxia in normal adult males. The majority of the subjects showed an increase in the rate of blood flow through the forearm and leg, although a decrease in hand circulation generally occurred. The latter was not considered especially important, since the hand is apt to respond to all types of vasoconstricting stimulation. Abramson and his collaborators (1) in 1943 reported that anemia in man produced a vasoconstriction of the hand. They observed, however, that anemia caused the blood flow through the muscles to increase.

In 1958 Sunahara and Girling (155) measured the blood flow through the forearm and hand during and after exposure of normal human subjects to 225 mm. Hg (corresponding to a simulated altitude of about 30,000 feet—9,100 meters) with maintenance of arterial oxygen saturation. Hand-blood flow was reduced significantly in all subjects, but forearm-blood flow was unaffected. These authors felt their studies indicated that reduced barometric pressure increases sympathetic activity of the blood vessels of the skin in man.

Black and Roddie (18) in 1958, using the venous occlusion plethysmograph, studied the effect on blood flow through the forearm of breathing 5–10 per cent oxygen in nitrogen mixture. They found it increased, but the addition of CO_2 to the inspired air abolished the effect. They concluded that the fall in vascular resistance in the forearm during hypoxia is more due to hyperpnea than lack of oxygen.

Recently work has been reported on the effect of hypoxia on peripheral venous tone. Eckstein and Horsley (42) measured venous tone by the plethysmographic method in nine unanesthetized young men breathing mixtures containing 11.5 and 7.5 per cent oxygen. When the latter percentage was used, a significant decrease in venous distensibility occurred.

Simonson (144) in 1960 reported the effects of breathing 10 per cent oxygen (in 90 per cent nitrogen mixture) on impedance plethysmographic pulse tracings from the forehand. Forty-two young, healthy men (18–30 years) and fifty-eight older men (55–65 years) were studied. In the older men there were greater changes of extracranial circulation, especially in amplitude. The authors interpreted this as a loss of stability in peripheral circulation during stress. Perhaps this finding explains, in part at least, why several workers reported variable results in studying peripheral blood flow during hypoxia.

Litwin and Aviado (98), working with an isolated lobe of the lung, found that blood volume increased when ventilated with 5 per cent and 10 per cent oxygen mixtures. The effect was more pronounced with the more severe grade of hypoxia. Fishman (47) recently has critically reviewed the problem of pulmonary blood flow during acute hypoxia in both man and animals and emphasizes the great difficulty in working on this problem. He points out that there is no unanimity concerning the effects of acute hypoxia on the pulmonary blood volume of the isolated lung preparation. He points out, also, the difficulty of measuring pulmonary blood volume in man. Using the indirect method there is evidence, however, that pulmonary blood volume remains unchanged during moderate grades of acute hypoxia.

Experiments with animals.—Working with morphinized and chloralized dogs, Bernthal (15) reported that low alveolar oxygen produced an initial decrease in flow of blood in the regions supplied by the brachial and femoral arteries. This was followed by an increased flow above the preadministration level. The injection of sodium cyanide (histotoxic hypoxia) also caused a decrease in blood flow. If the regions described above were denervated, mixtures low in oxygen content did not decrease the blood flow. The author concluded that there are both central and peripheral mechanisms constantly at work.

It has been reported that in hemic hypoxia there is increased blood flow in the muscles of the dog (78) and in the muscles of the rabbit (32).

Litwin and Aviado (98) in 1960 subjected forty-seven anesthetized dogs to 5 per cent oxygen and observed a vasoconstriction of the perfused hind leg. Vasodilatation occurred during reoxygenation.

Splanchnic blood flow.—Bernthal (15) in 1930, studying blood flow volume in dogs anesthetized with morphine and urethane, observed that low oxygen mixtures decrease the volume of blood flow in the superior mesenteric artery. Sodium cyanide (histotoxic hypoxia) caused an increase in flow. If the region supplied by the superior mesenteric artery were denervated, low oxygen mixtures caused an increased blood flow, provided constant artificial respiration was used. The blood-volume flow decreased if spontaneous changes in ventilation were allowed. The author concluded that there are two mechanisms involved, as there are in the regions supplied by the brachial and femoral artery. Bernthal cautioned, however, that the superior mesenteric arterial flow cannot safely be used as an indication of the flow in abdominal viscera in general.

In 1951 Myers (117), studying splanchnic blood flow estimated by the bromosulfalein method, found an increase in anemia approximately proportional to the increase in cardiac output. Rabinowitz *et al.* (128) also studied the effect of hemic hypoxia on splanchnic blood flow. Acute anemia was produced in anesthetized dogs by withdrawal of blood and its simultaneous replacement with an equal volume of 6 per cent dextran. It was found that the splanchnic blood flow (and cardiac output) increased immediately after production of the anemia.

Recently Fischer *et al.* (46), working with dogs, have shown that the hepatic artery flow changes with the degree of hypoxia. Mild hypoxia in most cases enhances blood flow and depresses resistance in the hepatic artery. Severe hypoxia (blood saturation less than 40 per cent) produces a marked constriction of the hepatic artery. They feel that this constriction is probably induced by some stimulation adrenergic in character.

In summary, Sands and DeGraff (138), in their studies on the effect of progressive hypoxia on the heart and circulation as mentioned previously (p. 79), came to the conclusion that there was an increase in the minute-flow through the body during anoxic hypoxia. They pointed out that this was brought about by three factors: (*a*) increased cardiac rate, (*b*) increased systolic discharge, and (*c*) decreased peripheral resistance. When the literature is reviewed, it may be seen that not all investigators have always found an increased blood flow during hypoxia in certain parts of the body. The results show considerable variation, and at times a decrease may be found; this probably is to be expected, since hypoxia may act as a general stimulus.

In studying the influence of hypoxia on blood flow, interpretations must be made with care, especially if only one part of the body is studied. Bainbridge (8) has shown, for example, that an increase in blood flow through the hands may be counterbalanced by vasoconstriction elsewhere, presumably in the splanchnic area. Attention has been called to the difficulties in determining the blood volume of the lungs during acute hypoxia. Obviously more work is needed on the effect of hypoxia on the blood flow in the body.

CORONARY CIRCULATION

In 1925 Hilton and Eicholtz (81) showed that there was an improved flow of blood through the coronary vessels during anoxic hypoxia, so that blood flow through the heart increased even though there were no changes in arterial pressure. The results reported by these workers have been confirmed by a number of investigators using various techniques.

It is now known that the volume of coronary flow increases greatly when the oxygen is reduced to 8 or 9 per cent. Indeed, it has been shown (83) that hypoxia is a more powerful coronary vasodilator than preparations such as sodium nitrite, amyl nitrite, and histamine and xanthine derivatives. It was shown by Green and Wegria (64) in 1940 that preliminary ventilation with a gas mixture containing from 5 to 7 per cent oxygen increased coronary flow a hundred fold. More recently Hackel *et al.* (70) subjected anesthetized dogs for five minutes to severe degrees of hypoxia (as low as 5 per cent); the mean coronary blood flow increased from 125 to as high as 500 cc/100 gm of left ventricle per minute, a tremendous increase.

Working with open-chest anesthetized dogs, Feinberg *et al.* (45) in 1957 reported that coronary flow increased with increasing severity of hypoxia at the same level of cardiac work.

Both anoxic hypoxia and hemic hypoxia increase coronary flow. Case *et al.* (22) in 1954 studied the effect of a graded acute anemia on coronary arterial resistance and on ventricular function in dogs by replacing blood with dextran. Coronary resistance decreased progressively and markedly as the hematocrit was lowered. Ventricular curves were not depressed because the coronary dilatation compensated for the decrease in oxygen content down to a hematocrit of 32 per cent. At 23 per cent the ventricular function curve was depressed, and at 17 per cent a frank failure with a descending limb was obtained. In a subsequent paper these authors (22) reported further work on the degree of coronary vasodilatation and adequacy of ventricular function.

It has been firmly established, then, that both anoxic hypoxia and hemic hypoxia increase coronary blood flow.

Mechanism of increased coronary flow.—Green and Wegria (64) in 1942, working in Wiggers' laboratory, found that both asphyxia (produced by interrupting artificial respiration) and local ischemia in an area of the myocardium increased coronary flow. They concluded that hypoxia causes relaxation of the walls of the coronary vessels. In 1954 Wiggers (165) concluded from his own work that augmented coronary flow was due to vasodilatation and, further, that the intensified cardiac contractions aided venous flow.

Hackel and Clowes (68) in 1956 studied coronary blood flow and myocardial metabolism during hypoxia in adrenalectomized-sympathectomized dogs. They concluded that the increase in coronary blood flow is not necessarily mediated by either the cardiac sympathetic nerves or the adrenal glands. They expressed the opinion that local metabolic factors are the primary determinants of coronary blood flow.

Berne *et al.* (14) in 1957, working on open-chest dogs and in fibrillating heart preparations, found that reduction of oxygen of arterial blood produced increased coronary blood flow only when coronary sinus oxygen levels fell below approximately 5.5 volume per cent. It was found that a moderate lowering of arterial oxygen content does not decrease coronary resistance by a direct action on the vessel walls but rather that the vasodilatation appears to be related to myocardial hypoxia.

There appears to be no general agreement as to the mechanism for the enhancement of coronary flow during hypoxia. Regardless of the exact mechanism, increased coronary blood flow during hypoxia obviously is of great benefit to the organism.

CONDUCTION OF THE NORMAL CARDIAC IMPULSE

Early electrocardiographic studies (43, 44, 63, 105, 106) were reported which indicated that hypoxia delayed conduction of the normal cardiac impulse. In a series of papers in 1925 Resnik (131) reported that studies made on dogs suggested that the S-A node was highly sensitive to hypoxia and that there was a brief period in which impulse formation was accelerated. This period was rapidly followed, however, by a progressive slowing of the intrinsic rate of the heart. Hypoxia, furthermore, first produced a shortening and later, a lengthening of the A-V conduction. Resnik believed that the changes in conduction were brought about by hypoxia directly affecting the myocardium.

It was observed by Harris and Randall (73) in 1944 that impairment of conduction was not apparent until the percentage of oxygen in inspired air was reduced to approximately 8 per cent. Indeed, during moderate degrees of hypoxia the conduction rate is often increased. In a later paper Harris and his co-worker (72) observed that during moderate degrees of hypoxia the P-R interval was shortened, as was the QRS, but severe degrees caused a lengthening.

Coffman, Lewis, and Gregg (25) in 1960, using the electrocardiograph, studied the effect of prolonged periods of hypoxia on A-V conduction in dogs with extracorporeal circulation. They reported that myocardial hypoxia for 100 minutes was the limit for the return of A-V conduction. Rodriquez (132) in 1961, working with dogs which had been subjected to repeated hemorrhages (10 per cent of the blood volume), found a marked decrease in the ventricular conduction velocity.

Recently Bagdonas *et al.* (7) studied the effects of ischemia (stagnant hypoxia) and anoxic hypoxia on the conducting system of the dog's heart. Electrodes were placed at various locations within and on the heart. The Purkinje system was found to be the most resistant. There was no recordable electrical activity after 40 minutes of ischemia. After 120 minutes of severe hypoxia electrical activity in the atrium was depressed; the specialized conducting system distal to the A-V node was not markedly affected. The authors felt that because of the striking differences between the effect of hemic hypoxia on the conduction system distal to the A-V node, a lack of oxygen was probably not as important as factors such as the retention of metabolites, changes in blood pH, and electrolyte concentrations occurring during ischemia. It is of more than passing interest that ventricular fibrillation always occurred with ischemia but not with anoxic hypoxia.

It is known that moderate degrees of hypoxia may produce a vagal hyperactivity (160); and doubtless this could account, at least in part, for the delayed conduction. Severe degrees of hypoxia probably produce a delayed conduction by directly affecting the conduction tissue.

EXCITABILITY AND REFRACTORY PERIOD OF THE VENTRICLES

Harris and Matlock (72) in 1947 observed that moderate degrees of hypoxia (5–7 volume per cent oxygen) lowered the threshold of excitability of the ventricles but severe degrees caused the threshold to rise rapidly. They observed, also, that the refractory period was somewhat shortened at moderately hypoxic levels but pronounced hypoxia lengthened the refractory period by 15 per cent.

Recently Rodriques (132) subjected dogs to repeated hemorrhages (10 per cent of the calculated blood volume); she reported that in 60 per cent of the experiments there was a lowering of the threshold of excitability. She observed, further, that the refractory period was either shortened or remained unchanged.

CHEMISTRY OF HEART MUSCLE

It is in order to consider briefly the effect of hypoxia on the chemical changes in the heart muscle.

Glycogen.—The problem of glycogen in cardiac muscle has interested many workers. One difficulty is that investigators have described more than one type of glycogen. For example, Merrick and Meyer (110, 111) in 1954, after determining the glycogen content in hearts of dogs, rats, mice, and goldfish which had been subjected to hypoxia, came to the conclusion that there were two forms of extractable glycogen, representing two physiological entities. One type described was soluble in trichloroacetic acid, and the other was insoluble in this reagent. Recently Meyer and Purdy (113) have also recognized two forms of glycogen. These two forms of glycogen are spoken of as free and bound glycogen. It remains to be demonstrated, however, whether there are actual structural differences in the two types.

Be that as it may, it is generally accepted now that hypoxia increases the rate of breakdown of glycogen in the heart (21, 30, 69, 95, 114) and also increases glycolysis. It is of interest that experiments suggest that the high resistance to hypoxia of some animals, especially the goldfish, may be associated with the high glycogen content of the heart. Merrick (109) has shown that the goldfish heart has the highest normal value of glycogen of any known vertebrate heart (23.25 mg/g of heart tissue). He believes that cardiac glycogen is an emergency stand-by used by the heart during periods of anoxic stress.

Cordier and Dessaux (28) in 1951 allowed rats to breathe pure nitrogen which caused death in two to three minutes; 90 per cent of normal glycogen content disappeared from the heart muscle. When placed in an atmosphere of nitrogen and carbon dioxide, death was caused in three to five minutes, and the glycogen content fell to 40 per cent. When the rats breathed a mixture of 50 per cent carbon dioxide, 20 per cent oxygen, and 30 per cent nitrogen, the glycogen was only slightly reduced. They concluded that mobilization of glycogen induced in the heart muscle by lack of oxygen is inhibited by carbon dioxide and that this inhibition is probably due to general depression by CO_2 of cellular metabolism.

Hackel *et al.* (69) in 1954 found that 10 per cent oxygen had but little effect on the carbohydrate uptake, whereas 5 per cent oxygen resulted in decreased coefficients of extraction for glucose, lactate, and pyruvate. However, total utilization was maintained, since the arterial concentrations of these substances were increased. Complete hypoxia resulted in marked depression of the coefficients of extraction.

Recently Meyer and Purdy (113) placed rats in an atmosphere of nitrogen until convulsions appeared; the animals were allowed to recover from twenty minutes to fifteen hours. Both free and bound cardiac glycogen were decreased by the hypoxia, but resynthesis was rapidly restored, within forty to sixty minutes.

A number of workers have studied the effect of hypoxia on glycogen in the perfused heart or have worked with certain isolated portions of the heart.

Winburg (168) in 1955 studied the effect of hypoxia on the contractility of isolated cardiac muscle as influenced by glucose. His results suggested that during prolonged hypoxia glucose may be used as a substrate for the energy production necessary to maintain the functional integrity of the contractile mechanism. In a later paper (169) he investigated the influence of glucose on contractile activity of the isolated papillary muscle of the ventricle of the cat during and after hypoxia. He observed that under aerobic conditions glucose was not required in the medium for the maintenance of contractile strength. However, under anaerobic conditions strength decreased rapidly and after thirty minutes of hypoxia contractions ceased. Reintroduction of oxygen after fifteen minutes of hypoxia resulted in full recovery of contractile strength.

Recently Cornblath et al. (29) studied glycogenolysis and phosphorylase activity by subjecting perfused rat heart to glucagon and hypoxia. Both glucagon and hypoxia greatly stimulated glycogenolysis and lactate production. Hypoxia reduced cardiac glycogen by more than 80 per cent with a proportionate production of lactate within about fifteen minutes.

Other metabolic changes.—A number of workers (54, 60, 95, 112, 157) have studied metabolic changes other than those concerning glycogen in the heart muscle during hypoxia. Recently Berne (13) pointed out that adenosine is an effective vasodilator. From experiments performed on the isolated cat's heart and on the intact heart of the dog, he postulated that during hypoxia myocardial nucleotides give rise to adenosine; this substance readily diffuses out of cardiac cells and induces vasodilation. Assuming that his interpretation is correct, it is obvious that this mechanism would be helpful to cardiac muscle laboring under the stress of hypoxia.

Gangloff et al. (54) subjected rats to a simulated altitude of 24,000 feet (7,315 meters) 8 hours a day for a total of 250 hours. No significant differences in creatine and creatinine were found, but creatine phosphate was increased from 40 to 70 per cent.

Recently Gott (60), studying anoxic arrest in the dog, observed that the heart goes into rigor in about forty-five minutes with completion at sixty-five minutes. Phosphocreatine was depleted in about five minutes.

Electrolyte changes.—Studies have been reported on tissue electrolyte changes in the heart during hypoxia (17, 26, 90, 99, 121, 130). Reeves (130) in 1961 subjected rats four hours a day (five days a week) for from twenty-six to twenty-eight weeks. No change was found in the potassium content of the heart in the experimental animals. Biddulph et al. (17) in 1960, also working with rats, exposed them to 8 per cent oxygen for one hour. No significant changes were found in sodium, potassium, or chloride ions in the ventricular muscles. In the auricular muscles, however, there were significant increases in sodium and chloride in these animals.

Water distribution.—In 1952 Lemley and Meneely (95) studied the effect of hypoxia on the distribution of tissue fluid in the heart of the rat. The animals were exposed for one hour to 7 per cent oxygen; the oxygen percentage was then lowered to 3 per cent, which proved fatal in 0–15 minutes. Significant increases in the total water and extracellular water of the ventricles were observed. There was, however, a significant decrease in the intracellular water.

ELECTROCARDIOGRAPHIC TRACINGS

The most common finding with the electrocardiogram under hypoxic conditions is that the T-wave is either decreased or inverted. During severe degrees of hypoxia there may be a slowing of the conduction rate, as evidenced by the lengthening of the P-R interval, that is, the time it takes the impulse to travel from the S-A node to the A-V node. At times there may be other changes in the electrocardiographic tracing, such as a deformity of the QRS complex. A number of early investigators (62, 85, 96, 134) have shown that normal individuals who had been subjected to a generalized hypoxia showed an S-T deviation in their electrocardiogram.

It was pointed out by Harris and Randall (73) in 1944 that, as hypoxia develops, the girth of the chest is increased during expiration. The change in the R-wave can be produced artificially by inflating the chest and is not necessarily associated with hypoxia. It is likely due to rotation of the heart. On the other hand, the elevation of the T-wave during hypoxia appears to be of cardiac origin, since it cannot be produced by inflation of the lungs. The authors mentioned above feel that it is probably due to a dilatation of the heart.

Luft (100) recently has pointed out the changes in the electrocardiogram in Lead II which occur in an individual who has been at an altitude of 16,400 feet (5,000 meters) for five minutes. There was an increase in heart rate and a reduction in the height of the T-wave from 0.46 to 0.33 mv.; after one minute at an altitude of 24,600 feet (7,500 meters) there was a decrease to 0.23 mv. At the latter altitude there was a slight depression of the ST segment, and the P-wave was higher. All these changes disappeared within thirty seconds following the administration of oxygen.

Hemingway (79) in 1944, making studies on useful consciousness, subjected thirty-one subjects to a stimulated altitude of 35,000 feet (19,670 meters) while breathing oxygen. The oxygen supply was disconnected, and the average arterial oxygen saturation of the men fell to 56.6 per cent. The electrocardiogram showed suppressed T-waves and extra systoles; the subjects showed evidence of a circulatory crisis.

In 1948 Minut-Sorokytina *et al.* (115), working with human beings in an altitude chamber, noted a change in the electrocardiogram at a simulated altitude of about 13,950 feet (4,250 meters). There was an increase in the height of the P and R-waves, notching of the P-wave, sinus tachycardia, and occasionally ST depressions.

During recent years Penaloza and his co-workers have made exhaustive observations on the effect of altitude on the electrocardiogram. In 1958 he and his associates (125) studied the changes in the electrocardiogram produced by altitude by comparing records taken on ten normal subjects at sea level (Lima, Peru) and at Morococha (14,900 feet—4,540 meters) from one to 30 days after their arrival. Although the changes were variable, they were usually of three types: (*a*) shifts to the right of the frontal plane QRS axis, (*b*) T-wave voltage increases in the limb and right precordial leads (with a shift in the transitional zone to the left), and (*c*) variations in the P-waves consisting of pacemaker changes ascribed to vagal effects. Although the mechanism of these changes is unknown, it was suggested that they were due to the development of pulmonary hypertension as a result of hypoxia.

In 1960 Penalzoa and his group (126) reported studies made on 540 normal children, 350 at sea level and 190 at Morococha; the ages ranged from newborn to fourteen years. In the newborn, both groups showed the same electrical activity of the heart. Within a few weeks, however, the children at altitude showed an accentuated right AQRS deviation. It was noted, also, that the T-loop shifted to a forward position and the T-wave became positive in the right precordial leads. A moderate degree of ventricular hypertrophy was noted. (For a discussion effect of hypoxia on electrocardiographic tracings in acclimatized subjects see chap. x.)

CARDIAC DILATATION

Studies on man.—It was reported by clinicians several decades ago that hypoxia may cause cardiac dilatation. In 1917 Kaufmann and Meyer (86) clinically studied the hearts of soldiers who had returned from campaigns in mountainous districts and found these hearts greatly increased in size. Whitney (163) in 1918, working at Mineola, subjected ten medical officers to hypoxia by use of the rebreather. Five showed noticeable cardiac dilatation, as ascertained by percussion—one at a simulated altitude corresponding to 14,000 feet (4,270 meters), one at 16,000 feet (4,875 meters), two at 18,000 feet (5,485 meters), and one at 20,000 feet (6,095 meters). LeWald and Turrell (97) in 1920, working with aviators and using the X ray, could find no pronounced cardiac dilatation. On the Peruvian Expedition in 1922, Barcroft *et al.* (10), using the X ray at 14,000 feet (4,270 meters), found no cardiac enlargement and in several instances found the heart smaller than at sea level. Somervell (149) in 1925 reported that all the men who went higher than 27,000 feet (8,230 meters) on the Mount Everest Expedition had dilated hearts, recovery from which required one to three weeks.

Keys *et al.* (88) in 1942 pointed out that critical data on man on the size of the heart during hypoxia were absent or extremely meager. They subjected twenty-seven normal young men to various degrees of hypoxia and made roentgen-kymographic measurements of the heart. The pO_2 corresponded to simulated altitudes from 18,000 feet (5,485 meters) to 28,000 feet (8,535 meters). The exposures lasted from ten to forty-eight minutes. These workers found no cardiac dilatation. Their findings were in accord with those reported by LeWald and Turrell and with those of Barcroft.

It should be remembered that Kaufmann and Meyer and also Somervell reported on men who had been exposed previously to severe physical exercise. It should be recognized, however, that Keys and his associates were able to control their experiments most carefully.

Graybiel *et al.* (61) in 1950 studied the changes in heart size in man during partial acclimatization to simulated altitudes. Four healthy young subjects were exposed to simulated altitudes in a decompression chamber over a period of one month. The heart size was studied teleroentgenographically at frequent intervals. The subjects after the third week were able to remain at 22,500 feet (6,855 meters). The heart was found to decrease slightly in size. This was thought to be the result of decreased cardiac filling or smaller stroke volume or both. The authors felt that their results did not support the opinion frequently expressed that the heart readily dilates in healthy subjects exposed to hypoxia.

Pugh and Ward (127) reported observations made on one of the

Mount Everest Expeditions at a camp situated at an altitude of 21,200 feet (6,460 meters). Physical examinations were made on several men within an hour of their arrival from a hard climb. No evidence of cardiac dilatation was found.

It has been shown by a number of workers that people living at high altitudes may show cardiac hypertrophy, especially of the right ventricle. Assuming that hypertrophy is usually preceded by dilatation, it is not unreasonable to conclude that cardiac dilatation is also present in these instances.

In summary, it appears that cardiac dilatation at high altitudes is rarely seen in the normal human individual. More work should probably be done on individuals who were subjected to severe exercise at high altitudes.

Studies on animals.—There is no question that some animals show a significant cardiac dilatation when subjected to effective degrees of hypoxia. This has been shown by a number of workers (65, 82, 138, 152, 158, 159). A few of the investigators reported that under some conditions the heart was smaller during hypoxia. Probable explanations of this are that the cardiac rate was increased considerably above the normal (108) or, as suggested by Graybiel *et al.* (61), there was a decreased cardiac filling or a smaller stroke volume.

Explosive decompression and cardiac dilatation.—In 1949 Dowling and Gelfan (36) reported work on monkeys explosively decompressed to as high as 75,000 feet (22,860 meters). Roentgenograms showed dilatation of the monkeys' hearts during and after the decompression. These workers felt that the dilatation resulted from hypoxia rather than from pressure changes. Burch and Kemph and their co-workers (20, 87) found that dogs explosively decompressed showed a tremendous cardiac dilatation. They felt that the dilatation was secondary to the great change in pressure. Stickney, Northup, and Van Liere (152), studying cardiac hypertrophy in rats, found that these animals when subjected to explosive decompression also showed a significant cardiac dilatation, as manifested by the X ray.

In summary, since Starling and his co-workers (150) have shown that the energy of contraction is a function of the length of the muscle fiber, it is not illogical to interpret moderate cardiac dilatations at high altitudes as adaptive mechanisms. The fact that there is an increased cardiac output under hypoxic conditions also favors this view. There is good reason to believe, however, that in the normal heart there is an increased cardiac output under hypoxic conditions before noticeable cardiac dilatation may be manifested.

Pronounced dilatation (such as seen in the terminal stage of acute hypoxia) is known, however, to reduce greatly the efficiency of the heart. It is not unlikely that even moderate cardiac dilatation produced by acute hypoxia is a signal of distress.

THE SPLEEN

It was shown by Schafer and Moore (146) as early as 1896 that hypoxia causes the spleen of the dog to contract. In 1925 Barcroft and his associates (11) showed that, upon contraction, the spleen of the dog was capable of throwing a large number of red blood cells into the circulation. In the cat it was estimated that approximately one-sixth of the blood volume, or one-third of the number of red blood cells, can be expelled by the spleen. The immediate rise in hemoglobin and number of red blood cells at high altitudes observed by various workers has been attributed, in part, to the contractions of the spleen.

Blood stores in the body.—The question arises whether, through its organs or other means, the body can accumulate or store red blood cells. Krogh's (93) work on capillary circulation suggests the possibility that certain areas of the body store considerable numbers of red blood cells in dormant capillaries. Perhaps the capillaries of the skin or the muscles have such stores. When the proper stimulus arises, these stored erythrocytes in the dormant capillaries may augment somewhat the red blood cell count. Some proof of this has been offered.

Some investigators feel there is considerable evidence that reserves of blood may exist in the body (58, 84, 161). On the other hand, Parson and his co-workers (123) emphasize that there is no evidence of reserves of blood or blood cells subject to emergency mobilization in man. They quote the work of Ebert and Stead (41), of Kaltrieder *et al.* (84), of Ross and Chapin (133), and of Nylin (120). Parson *et al.* (123) gave subcutaneous injections of adrenaline in amounts sufficient to evoke good clinical responses but found no uniform or significant changes in the plasma or red cell volume. They concluded that if sympathetic stimulation or adrenaline influence any reservoirs, the effect must be very slight and of no significance. Their results, therefore, differ from those of other workers. This lack of uniformity in results of various workers probably can be partially explained by differences in method used in determining plasma volume. The work of Parson and his associates implies, of course, that the spleen of man does not serve as an important emergency reservoir; this would apply in conditions of hypoxia.

Contractions of spleen of various animals.—During the last decade or so considerable evidence has been produced to show that the spleen of the dog is relatively resistant to hypoxia and that contractions occur only when arterial saturation is low.

In 1949 Kramer and Luft (91) studied the response of the spleen to hypoxia in twenty dogs under light sodium pentobarbital anesthesia. The spleen was exposed and its weight recorded by an electric balance. When acute hypoxia was produced by breathing pure nitrogen, the spleen did not lose weight until the arterial oxygen saturation approached zero. However, when hypoxia was produced by use of the rebreather, the spleen began contracting when the arterial oxygen saturation dropped below 40 per cent (an extreme degree of hypoxia). Shortly before failure of respiration and after the asphyxial rise in blood pressure, the spleen weight dropped noticeably, and there was a rise in circulating hemoglobin concentration.

The same authors (92) two years later reported further studies on barbitalized dogs, and again acute hypoxia was induced. They observed that the spleen stores consist almost entirely of packed red blood cells and, further, that the hemoglobin content in the splenic vein showed rapid changes in the final stages of hypoxia, with peak values twice as high as in arterial blood. They concluded that in the critical phase of hypoxia the spleen of the dog releases large amounts of red blood cells with relatively high oxygen content into the portal venous system.

It appears, then, that the spleen in both man and dog is relatively resistant to hypoxia. Other animals like the cat and mouse do not share this resistance.

Hypoxia in splenectomized animals.—There is experimental evidence that some animals deprived of their spleen are less resistant to hypoxia. In 1951 Smith and Brown (148), studying the effects of acute decompression upon splenectomized cats, reported that they were less resistant to low oxygen tension (3.5 per cent oxygen) than normal animals. They showed further that acute decompression increased the hematocrit in normal animals but not in the splenectomized cats. De Franciscis (33) in 1955 placed splenectomized monkeys in a decompression chamber and found a marked decrease of their ceiling level as compared to animals with intact spleens.

Quantitative participation of the spleen and the bone marrow.— Cook and Alafi (27) in 1956, in an attempt to determine quantitatively the participation of the spleen and bone marrow separately during chronic hypoxia, subjected normal and splenectomized mice to hypoxia. The animals were kept at a simulated altitude of 15,000 feet (4,570 meters) for a period of thirty to fifty-eight days. At various intervals red blood cell counts and hematocrit determinations were made. It was observed that about two-fifths of the increase in red blood cells could be traced to tonic contraction of the spleen and the remaining three-fifths to the production of red blood cells by the red bone marrow.

In summary, more work is needed to determine the role the spleen plays at altitude in both man and animals. In this connection the effect of exercise on the spleen under conditions of oxygen want, too, should be investigated. It is possible that some of the observations made on the spleen at altitude were due to the effects of exercise as well as to hypoxia.

REFERENCES

1. ABRAMSON, D. I.; FIERST, S. M.; and FLACHS, K. 1943. *Amer. Heart J.,* **25:** 609.
2. ABRAMSON, D. I.; LANDT, H.; and BENJAMIN, J. E. 1941. *Proc. Soc. Exp. Biol. Med.,* **48:** 214.
3. ————. 1943. *Arch. Intern. Med.,* **71:** 583.
4. ALBERS, C., and USINGER, W. 1956. *Pflueger Arch. Ges. Physiol.,* **263:** 201.
5. ALVERYD, A., and BRODY, S. 1948. *Acta Physiol. Scand.,* **15:** 140.
6. ASMUSSEN, E., and CHIODI, H. 1941. *Amer. J. Physiol.,* **132:** 426.
7. BAGDONAS, A. B., *et al.* 1961. *Amer. Heart. J.,* **61:** 206.
8. BAINBRIDGE, F. A. 1919. *Physiology of Muscle Exercises,* p. 165. London: Longmans, Green & Co.
9. BARCROFT, J. 1925. *The Respiratory Function of the Blood,* Part I, "Lessons from High Altitudes," p. 111. Cambridge: Cambridge University Press.
10. BARCROFT, J., *et al.* 1923. *Proc. Roy. Soc., London,* B, **211:** 351.
11. BARCROFT, J., *et al.* 1925. *J. Physiol.,* **60:** 443.
12. BARTELS, H., *et al.* 1955. *Pflueger Arch. Ges. Physiol.,* **261:** 99.
13. BERNE, R. M. 1961. *Fed. Proc.,* **20:** 101.
14. BERNE, R. M.; BLACKMAN, J. R.; and GARDNER, T. H. 1957. *J. Clin. Invest.,* **36:** 1101.
15. BERNTHAL, T. G. 1930. *Amer. J. Physiol.,* **95:** 446.
16. BERNTHAL, T.; GREENE, W., Jr.; and REVZIN, A. M. 1951. *Proc. Soc. Exp. Biol. Med.,* **76:** 121.
17. BIDDULPH, C., *et al.* Sept., 1960. *USAF Sch. Aerospace Med.* (School of Aviation Medicine, Brooks Air Force Base, Texas), 60–83.

18. BLACK, J. E., and RODDIE, I. C. 1958. *J. Physiol.*, 143: 226.
19. BOGUE, J. Y.; CHANG, I.; and GREGORY, R. A. 1937–38. *Quart. J. Exp. Physiol.*, 27: 319.
20. BURCH, B. H., *et al.* 1952. *J. Aviat. Med.*, 23: 159.
21. BUZZARD, J. A., *et al.* 1956. *Proc. Soc. Exp. Biol. Med.*, 93: 156.
22. CASE, R. E.; BERGLUND, E.; and SARNOFF, S. T. 1954. *Fed. Proc.*, 13: 24.
———. 1955. *Amer. J. Med.*, 18: 397.
23. CHIODI, H., *et al.* 1941. *Amer. J. Physiol.*, 134: 683.
24. CHRISTENSEN, E. H. 1937. *Scand. Arch. Physiol.*, 76: 75.
25. COFFMAN, J. D.; LEWIS, F. B.; and GREGG, D. E. 1960. *Circulat. Res.*, 8: 649.
26. CONN, H. L., Jr. 1956. *Amer. J. Physiol.*, 184: 548.
27. COOK, S. F., and ALAFI, M. H. 1956. *Amer. J. Physiol.*, 186: 372.
28. CORDIER, D., and DESSAUX, G. 1951. *C. R. Soc. Biol. (Par.)*, 145: 727.
29. CORNBLATH, M.; MORGAN, H. E.; and RANDLE, J. 1961. *Fed. Proc.*, 20: 85.
30. CRAIG, F. N., and BEECHER, H. K. 1943. *J. Gen. Physiol.*, 26: 467.
31. DALY, M. B., and SCOTT, M. J. 1958. *J. Physiol.*, 144: 148.
32. DARIAN, SMITH, I. 1955. *Aust. J. Exp. Biol. Med. Sci.*, 33: 515.
33. DE FRANCISCIS, P. 1955. *Rev. Med. Aero.*, 18: 655.
34. DILL, D. B. 1938. *Life, Heat and Altitude*, p. 186. Cambridge, Mass.: Harvard University Press.
35. DOI, Y. 1921. *J. Physiol.*, 55: 43.
36. DOWLING, R., and GELFAN, S. 1949. *Fed. Proc.*, 8: 36.
37. DOYLE, J. T.; WILSON, S. J.; and WARREN, J. V. 1952. *Circulation*, 5: 263.
38. DREYER, N. B. 1926. *Canad. Med. Ass. J.*, 16: 26.
39. DRIPPS, R. D., and COMROE, J. H., Jr. 1947. *Amer. J. Physiol.*, 149: 277.
40. DURIG, A. 1909. *Physiologische Ergebnisse der im Jahr 1906 durchgeführten Monta Rosa Expedition*, Wien.
41. EBERT, R. V., and STEAD, E. A. 1941. *Amer. J. Med. Sci.*, 201: 655.
42. ECKSTEIN, J. W., and HORSLEY, A. W. 1960. *J. Lab. Clin. Med.*, 56: 847.
43. EULER, U. S., v., and LILJESTRAND, G. 1942. *Acta Physiol. Scand.*, 4: 34.
44. EYSTER, J. A. E., and MEEK, W. J. 1914. *Heart*, 119: 227.
45. FEINBERG, H.; GEROLA, A.; and KATZ, L. N. 1957. *Fed. Proc.*, 16: 36.
46. FISCHER, A.; TAKACS, L.; and MOLNAR, G. 1960. *Acta Med. Acad. Sci. Hung.*, 16: 61.
47. FISHMAN, A. P. 1961. *Physiol. Rev.*, 41: 214.
48. FORBER, V., and EVANS, G. T. 1943. *Proc. Soc. Exp. Biol. Med.*, 54: 1.
49. FORD, M. L., *et al.* 1940. *Proc. Soc. Exp. Biol. Med.*, 45: 353.
50. FRANZBLAU, S. A., *et al.* 1951. *Amer. J. Physiol. (Proc.)*, 167: 785.

51. FREEMAN, N. E.; SHAW, J. L.; and SNYDER, J. C. 1936. *J. Clin. Invest.*, **15:** 651.
52. FRITTS, H. W., *et al.* 1958. *J. Clin. Invest.*, **37:** 99.
53. GALDSTON, M., and STEELE, J. M. 1950. *J. Appl. Physiol.*, **3:** 229.
54. GANGLOFF, E. C., *et al.* 1960. *Fed. Proc.*, **19:** 110.
55. GELLHORN, E. 1937. *Ann. Intern. Med.*, **10:** 1267.
———. 1937. *Sigma Xi Quart.*, **25:** 156.
56. GELLHORN, E., and LAMBERT, E. H. 1939. *The Vasomotor System in Anoxia and Asphyxia.* Urbana, Ill.: University of Illinois Press.
57. GELLHORN, E., and STECK, I. E. 1938. *Amer. J. Physiol.*, **124:** 735.
58. GLICKMAN, N., *et al.* 1941. *Amer. J. Physiol.*, **134:** 165.
59. GOMORI, P., *et al.* 1960. *Acta Med. Acad. Sci. Hung.*, **16:** 93.
60. GOTT, V. L. 1961. *Fed. Proc.*, **20:** 127.
61. GRAYBIEL, A.; PATTERSON, J. L.; and HOUSTON, C. S. 1950. *Circulation*, **1:** 991.
62. GREEN, C. W., and GILBERT, N. C. 1921. *Arch. Intern. Med.*, **27:** 517.
63. ———. 1922. *Amer. J. Physiol.*, **60:** 155.
64. GREEN, H. D., and WEGRIA, R. 1942. *Amer. J. Physiol.*, **135:** 271.
65. GREMELS, H., and STARLING, E. H. 1926. *J. Physiol.*, **61:** 297.
66. GROLLMAN, A. 1930. *Amer. J. Physiol.*, **93:** 19.
67. ———. 1932. *Cardiac Output in Man in Health and Disease.* Springfield, Mo.: Thomas.
68. HACKEL, D. B., and CLOWES, G. H. H. 1956. *Amer. J. Physiol.*, **186:** 111.
69. HACKEL, D. B.; GOODALE, W. T.; and KLEINERMAN, J. 1954. *Circulat. Res.*, **2:** 169.
70. ———. 1953. *Fed. Proc.*, **12:** 59.
71. HALDANE, J. S.; KELLAS, A. S.; and KENNAWAY, E. L. 1919. *J. Physiol.*, **53:** 181.
72. HARRIS, A. S., and MATLOCK, W. P. 1947. *Amer. J. Physiol.*, **150:** 493.
73. HARRIS, A. S., and RANDALL, W. C. 1944. *Amer. J. Physiol.*, **142:** 452.
74. HARRISON, T. R., and BLALOCK, A. 1927. *Amer. J. Physiol.*, **80:** 169.
75. HARRISON, T. R., *et al.* 1927. *Amer. J. Physiol.*, **83:** 284.
76. HARRISON, T. R., *et al. Ibid.*, 275.
77. HASSELBALCH, K. A., and LINDHARD, J. 1911. *Scand. Arch. Physiol.*, **25:** 387.
78. HATCHER, J. D., *et al.* 1954. *Circulat. Res.*, **2:** 449.
79. HEMINGWAY, A. W. 1944. *J. Aviat. Med.*, **15:** 298.
80. HERBST, P., and MANIGOLD, K. 1936. *Arbeitsphysiol.*, **9:** 166.
81. HILTON, R., and EICHOLTZ, F. 1925. *J. Physiol.*, **59:** 413.
82. JARISCH, A., and WASTL, H. 1926. *J. Physiol.*, **61:** 583.
83. JOCHIM, K. 1940. *Blood, Heart and Circulation*, p. 97. Lancaster, Pa.: Science Press.
84. KALTREIDER, N. L.; MENEELY, R.; and ALLEN, J. D. 1942. *J. Clin. Invest.*, **21:** 339.

85. KATZ, L. N.; HAMBERGER, W. W.; and SCHULTZ, W. J. 1934. *Amer. Heart J.*, 9: 771.
86. KAUFMANN, R., and MEYER, H. H. 1917. *Med. Klin.*, 13: 1155.
87. KEMPH, J. P., *et al.* 1950. *Amer. J. Physiol.*, 163: 725.
88. KEYS, A.; STAPP, J. P.; and VIOLANTO, H. 1942. *Amer. J. Physiol.*, 138: 763.
89. KISCH, F. 1926. *Klin. Wschr.*, 5: 1227.
90. KLEIN, R. L., and EVANS, M. L. 1961. *Amer. J. Physiol.*, 200: 735.
91. KRAMER, K., and LUFT, U. C. 1949. *Fed. Proc.*, 8: 88.
92. ———. 1951. *Amer. J. Physiol.*, 165: 215.
93. KROGH, A. 1929. *The Anatomy and Physiology of the Capillaries.* New Haven, Conn.: Yale University Press.
94. KUHN, H. 1913. *Uber die Funktion des Herzen im Hochgebirge: Inaugural Dissertation, Halle.* (See *Z. Physiol.*, 27: 1357, 1913.)
95. LEMLEY, J. M., and MENEELY, G. R. 1952. *Amer. J. Physiol.*, 169: 61.
96. LEVY, R. L.; BARACH, A. L.; and BRUENN, H. G. 1938. *Amer. Heart J.*, 15: 187.
97. LEWALD, L. T., and TURRELL, A. H. 1920. *Amer. J. Roentgenol.*, 7: 67.
98. LITWIN, J., and AVIADO, D. M. 1960. *Circulat. Res.*, 8: 585.
99. LOWRY, O. H., *et al.* 1942. *Proc. Soc. Exp. Biol. Med.*, 46: 670.
100. LUFT, U. C. *In:* H. G. ARMSTRONG (ed.). *Aerospace Medicine*, p. 130. Baltimore: Williams & Wilkins, Co., 1961.
101. LUTZ, B. R., and SCHNEIDER, E. C. 1919. *Amer. J. Physiol.*, 50: 280, 228, and 327.
102. MASINI, V.; BUSNENGO, E.; and MARTINI, G. 1953. *Rev. Med. Aero.*, 16: 15.
103. MATHES, K., and MALIKIOSES, X. 1936. *Deutsch. Arch. Klin. Med.*, 179: 500.
104. ———. 1937. *Luftfahrtmedizin*, 1: 259.
105. MATHISON, G. C. 1910. *Heart*, 2: 54.
106. ———. 1910. *J. Physiol.*, 41: 416.
107. McFARLAND, R. A. 1937. *J. Comp. Psychol.*, 23: 181.
108. MEEK, W. J. 1924. *Amer. J. Physiol.*, 70: 385.
109. MERRICK, A. W. 1954. *Amer. J. Physiol.*, 176: 83.
110. MERRICK, A. W., and MEYER, D. K. 1954. *Amer. J. Physiol.*, 177: 441.
111. ———. 1954. *Fed. Proc.*, 13: 99.
112. MERRIL, J. M., *et al.* 1957. *Amer. J. Physiol.*, 190: 522.
113. MEYER, D. K., and PURDY, F. A. 1961. *Amer. J. Physiol.*, 200: 860.
114. MICHAL, G., *et al.* 1958. *Amer. J. Physiol.*, 195: 417.
115. MINUT-SOROKYTINA, O. P.; RAYEVA, N. B.; and LEMAZHIKHINA, B. M. 1948. *Fiziol. Zh. SSSR*, 34: 269.
116. MOSS, A. J. 1960. *Amer. Heart J.*, 59: 412.
117. MYERS, J. D. 1951. *Amer. J. Med.*, 11: 248.
118. NAHAS, G. G., *et al.* 1954. *Amer. J. Physiol.*, 177: 13.
119. NAHAS, G. G., *et al.* 1954. *J. Appl. Physiol.*, 6: 467.

120. NYLIN, G. 1946. *Acta Cardiol.*, 1: 225.
121. OLSEN, N. S.; RUDOLPH, G. G.; and GOLLAN, F. 1955. *Fed. Proc.*, 14: 108.
122. OPITZ, E. 1941. *Ergebn. Physiol.*, 44: 315.
123. PARSON, W., *et al.* 1948. *Amer. J. Physiol.*, 155: 239.
124. PATTERSON, J. W., and STARLING, E. H. 1914. *J. Physiol.*, 48: 357.
125. PENALOZA, D., *et al.* 1958. *Amer. Heart J.*, 56: 493.
126. ————. 1960. *Ibid.*, 59: 111.
127. PUGH, L. G. C., and WARD, M. P. 1956. *Lancet*, 271: 1115.
128. RABINOWITZ, M., *et al.* 1954. *Fed. Proc.*, 13: 114.
129. RAHN, H., and OTIS, A. B. 1947. *Amer. J. Physiol.*, 150: 202.
130. REEVES, J. L. Feb. 1961. *USAF Sch. Aerospace Med.* (School of Aviation Medicine, Brooks Air Force Base, Texas), 61–37.
131. RESNIK, M. H. 1925. *J. Clin. Invest.*, 2: 93, 117, and 125.
132. RODRIQUEZ, M. I. 1961. *Fed. Proc.*, 20: 124.
133. ROSS, J. F., and CHAPIN, M. A. 1942. *J. Clin. Invest.*, 21: 640.
134. ROTHSCHILD, M. A., and KISSIN, M. 1925. *Amer. Heart J.*, 8: 745.
135. ROTTA, A. 1947. *Amer. Heart J.*, 33: 669.
136. ROTTA, A., *et al.* 1956. *J. Appl. Physiol.*, 9: 328.
137. ROTTA, A.; MIRANDA, A.; and CHAVES, R., cited by HURTADO. November, 1949. "International Symposium on High Altitude Biology." Unpublished abstract, Lima.
138. SANDS, J., and DEGRAFF, A. C. 1925. *Amer. J. Physiol.*, 74: 416.
139. SCARBOROUGH, W. R., *et al.* 1951. *Circulation*, 4: 190.
140. SCHNEIDER, E. C. 1913. *Amer. J. Physiol.*, 32: 295.
141. ————. 1918. *J.A.M.A.*, 61: 1384.
142. ————. 1921. *Physiol. Rev.*, 1: 631.
143. SCHNEIDER, E. C.; SISCO, D. L.; and CHELEY, G. E. 1916. *Amer. J. Physiol.*, 40: 380.
144. SCHNEIDER, E. C., and TRUESDELL, D. 1921. *Amer. J. Physiol.*, 55: 223.
145. ————. 1924. *Ibid.*, 71: 90.
146. SCHAFER, E. A., and MOORE, B. 1896. *J. Physiol.*, 20: 1.
147. SIMONSON, E. 1960. *Fed. Proc.*, 19: 92.
148. SMITH, D. C., and BROWN, F. S. 1951. *Amer. J. Physiol.*, 164: 752.
149. SOMERVELL, T. H. 1925. *J. Physiol.*, 60: 282.
150. STARLING, E. H. 1918. "The Law of the Heart." Linacre Lecture, London.
151. STARR, I., and MCMICHAEL, M. J. 1948. *J. Appl. Physiol.*, 1: 430.
152. STICKNEY, J. C.; NORTHUP, D. W.; and VAN LIERE, E. J. 1956. *Circulat. Res.*, 4: 217.
153. STRUGHOLD, H. 1930. *Amer. J. Physiol.*, 94: 641.
154. SUNAHARA, F. A., and BECK, L. 1954. *Amer. J. Physiol.*, 179: 139.
155. SUNAHARA, F. A., and GIRLING, F. 1958. *Fed. Proc.*, 17: 158.
156. SUNDSTROEM, E. S. 1919. *Univ. Calif. Publ. Physiol.*, 5: 71, 87, 105, 113, 121, 133, 149, 159.

157. SZEKERES, L.; LENARD, G.; and SOTI, J. 1958. *Arch. Int. Pharmacodyn.*, **115:** 141.
158. TAKEUCHI, H. 1930. *Amer. J. Physiol.*, **94:** 641.
159. VAN LIERE, E. J. 1927. *Amer. J. Physiol.*, **82:** 727.
160. VAN LIERE, E. J., and CRISLER, G. R. 1933. *Amer. J. Physiol.*, **105:** 469.
161. WATSON, C. J., and PAINE, J. R. 1943. *Amer. J. Med. Sci.*, **205:** 493.
162. WHITEHORN, W. V.; EDELMANN, A.; and HITCHCOCK, F. A. 1946. *Amer. J. Physiol.*, **146:** 61.
163. WHITNEY, J. L. 1918. *J.A.M.A.*, **71:** 1382.
———. 1913. *Manual of Med. Res. Lab.* (Mineola, N.Y.) Washington, D.C.: U.S. Govt. Printing Office.
164. WIGGERS, C. J. 1941. *Ann. Intern. Med.*, **14:** 1237.
165. ———. 1954. *Circulat. Res.*, **2:** 278.
166. ———. 1959. *Reminiscences and Adventures in Circulation Research*, p. 313 *et seq.* New York: Grune and Stratton.
167. WIGGERS, C. J., and KATZ, L. N. 1928. *Amer. J. Physiol.*, **85:** 229.
168. WINBURG, M. M. 1955. *Fed. Proc.*, **14:** 394.
169. ———. 1956. *Amer. J. Physiol.*, **187:** 135.
170. WRIGHT, S. 1961. *Applied Physiology* (10th ed.), p. 136. New York: Oxford University Press.

CHAPTER VI

EFFECT OF HYPOXIA ON BLOOD PRESSURE

ACUTE EFFECTS ON ARTERIAL PRESSURE

A series of papers (31, 42, 48, 67, 69) dealing with circulatory responses to oxygen deficiency, as experienced during short exposures in connection with aviation physiology, was published during the years 1918–21. In the main these reports showed that in a rapid ascent to 15,000 feet (4,570 meters) or even 20,000 feet (6,095 meters), if the subjects were well compensated to the lower pO_2 and the psychic factor were not active, the systolic blood pressure remained practically unchanged. Occasionally, however, a slight rise of 10–15 mm. Hg was found. The diastolic pressure, too, remained practically unaffected up to an altitude of 15,000 feet (4,570 meters). If higher altitudes were attained, the diastolic pressure slowly decreased by about 10–15 mm. Hg. If, however, the compensation to the lowered partial pressure of oxygen was inadequate, the subject was likely to faint. This oncoming syncope could be predicted by the fall both in systolic and diastolic pressure. Schneider and Truesdell (69) have described in detail the various types of circulatory reaction.

McFarland (49) in 1937 reported that in ascents made by train from sea level to an altitude of 14,890 feet (4,540 meters) only three of seven subjects showed a slight rise in systolic and diastolic basal blood pressure. In the standing position only two showed a slight rise. In rapid ascent by airplane to 15,000 feet (4,570 meters), there was a slight rise in systolic blood pressure in three of the four subjects with no change in the diastolic pressure. One individual, however, showed an increase of 27 mm. Hg in the systolic pressure and a 10 mm. Hg rise in diastolic pressure. In the latter subject a psychic factor might have been at work.

More recent work on man (17, 25, 39, 79) has shown that even a moderately severe grade of hypoxia has little significant effect on blood pressure. These findings corroborate, for the most part, the early observations of Schneider and his co-workers previously mentioned.

It should be pointed out that in the dog hypoxia is more apt to produce slight elevations in systolic blood pressure (3, 33, 57).

It is of interest that Graybiel (30) in 1941 and Von Tavel (78) in 1943 confirmed the observation made by Schneider and his co-workers in 1919, namely, that the diastolic pressure tends to decrease as the systolic levels rise. Comroe and Dripps (11) feel that this fall in diastolic pressure is a significant factor in the regulation of the circulation during hypoxia. They call attention to the work of Abramson et al. (1), who showed that breathing 10 per cent oxygen caused a definite increase in the rate of blood flow through the leg and forearm in the normal individual. Comroe and Dripps point out that the circulatory response to hypoxia is similar to that following the subcutaneous injection of epinephrine, namely, cardiac stimulation with a decreased peripheral resistance.

Cause of blood pressure rise during severe acute hypoxia.—Although it has been shown that moderately severe hypoxia up to a simulated altitude of about 15,000 feet (4,570 meters) as a rule produces no significant changes in blood pressure, it is known that more severe grades of hypoxia produce a rise in arterial pressure. This phenomenon is frequently and erroneously spoken of as "an asphyxial rise." It will be recalled that the term *asphyxia* should be used only when there is an actual increase in the carbon dioxide content in the blood and in the tissues; if there is no accumulation of carbon dioxide during oxygen want, the condition is termed *hypoxia*. (See p. 5.)

In 1930 it was shown by Heymans et al. (35), working with dogs, that inhalation of nitrogen usually caused rise of blood pressure in the intact animal; but if the nerves to the carotid sinuses were severed and the vagi, too, were cut, hypoxia produced by inhalation of nitrogen caused a fall of blood pressure. In 1932 Selladurai and Wright (71) reported that after complete elimination of the chemoreceptor nerves, however, oxygen deficiency produced a variable effect on the blood pressure. Von Euler and Liljestrand (21) in 1936, working with intact anesthetized dogs, found that 8.5 per cent oxygen caused a slight rise in blood pressure but that after denervation of the carotid sinus the same degree of hypoxia caused a fall. These authors felt that complete denervation had not been performed in the experiments reported by Selladurai and Wright. Brewer (9) in 1937 found that nitrogen inhalation in an animal which had its sinus denervated produced a fall in blood pressure, thus confirming work reported by previous investigators. Bernthal (8) in 1938 recognized the importance of controlling respirations, as well as other experimental procedures, when working on reflexes from the carotid sinuses. He reported that if the chemoreceptors in the carotid bodies were stimulated either by hypoxia or by carbon dioxide excess, a vasoconstrictor reflex was produced; stimulation by hypoxia, however, gave the most effective result.

Gellhorn and Lambert (28) also felt that, in determining the role of the chemoreceptors in blood-pressure reactions to oxygen deficiency and carbon dioxide excess, respiration should be rigidly controlled. Extensive experiments were performed on dogs (for details the reader is referred to their monograph [28]). They concluded that ". . . oxygen deficiency causes a rise of blood pressure only by action on the carotid and aortic bodies, which in turn send afferent impulses to the vasomotor centers through the cartoid sinus nerves and the aortic nerves. . . ." They further pointed out that the vasomotor center actually was depressed by oxygen want after denervation of the chemoreceptors and that in this regard it behaved much like the respiratory center during oxygen want.

Cause of blood pressure fall during oxygen want after denervation of the chemoreceptors.—Gellhorn and Lambert (28) have offered three possible reasons for the fall of blood pressure caused by oxygen want after denervation of the chemoreceptors: (*a*) a depression of vasomotor tone, (*b*) a decrease in cardiac output, and (*c*) a peripheral vasodilatation. These authors felt that under the conditions of their own experiments the first factor was the cause for the reversal of blood pressure. It should be pointed out that the second cause, a decrease in cardiac output, is active only during severe degrees of hypoxia.

Effect of small amounts of carbon dioxide on blood pressure during acute hypoxia.—Raab (61) in 1931, working with decerebrate cats, showed that the combined action of carbon dioxide and low oxygen tension has a potentiating effect on the rise in blood pressure. Gellhorn (27) and Lambert and Gellhorn (41) confirmed Raab's work a few years later and showed, furthermore, that the potentiating effect of carbon dioxide and oxygen deficiency on the vasomotor center persisted after bilateral elimination of the carotid sinus. In their experiments they used 3–4 per cent carbon dioxide during the administration of the hypoxia and observed a noticeable effect on the blood pressure. These workers believed that this potentiating effect on the vasomotor center by relatively small amounts of carbon dioxide was beneficial to the organism during hypoxia.

VENOUS PRESSURE

Schneider and Sisco (68) in 1914 found that normal, healthy young men had a normal venous pressure at 6,000 feet (1,830 meters). On Pike's Peak (14,100 feet—4,300 meters), however, a fall between 20 and 87 per cent occurred in the venous pressure; the fall took place slowly, and in some of the subjects it was not manifested until they had been at a reduced pressure for a half-day or more.

Later work in 1924 by Schneider and Truesdell (70), again using man as a subject but using the rebreather method to induce hypoxia, corroborated the earlier work. They reported a fall in venous pressure beginning at about 16 per cent oxygen, which corresponds approximately to an altitude of 7,000 feet (2,130 meters); this became more pronounced between 12 and 10 per cent oxygen. They attributed the decrease in venous pressure, at least in part, to a dilatation of the splanchnic blood vessels.

In the studies reported on Pike's Peak no cases were seen in which the fall of venous pressure interfered with adequate filling of the heart or decreased cardiac efficiency. Studies reported on cardiac output during moderate degrees of hypoxia appear to corroborate these findings, namely, that if there is a decrease in venous pressure produced by hypoxia, it does not interfere with adequate cardiac filling.

Sands and DeGraff (66) in studying the effect of progressive hypoxia on the heart and circulation found that up to the crisis (which occurred at 9 per cent oxygen) there was a slight tendency for the effective venous pressure (i.e., the difference between intrathoracic and intra-auricular pressure) to decrease. When the crisis was reached, however, the effective venous pressure began to rise until it reached high levels. The elevation of effective venous pressure was the most definite criterion for the beginning of the crisis.

In 1943 Ershler et al. (20) studied the venous pressure in nineteen young, healthy males subjected to acute progressive hypoxia induced by rebreathing. The results were variable. Four subjects showed a progressive decrease, and seven fainted during the experiment; the venous pressure rose precipitously just before syncope. These latter findings are in accord with those reported by Sands and De Graff (66).

Nahas et al. (54) in 1954 subjected non-narcotized dogs to 8 per cent oxygen in nitrogen gas mixture. There was no significant change in effective pressures in the superior or inferior venae cavae. The investigators did observe, however, increases of 2.3 mm. Hg and 1.4 mm.

Hg in the venule and small vein pressures, respectively, of the dogs' forelegs.

More experimental laboratory studies are needed on the effect of hypoxia on venous blood pressure in various areas of the body of both man and animals.

CAPILLARY BLOOD PRESSURE

It has been shown by Lombard that the average capillary will disappear at a pressure between 35 and 45 mm. Hg; the most compressible ones will disappear at a pressure of 15–25; and the most resisting ones, at 60–70. It was found on Pike's Peak (14,100 feet—4,300 meters) that the capillary pressure in some subjects was slightly lower than at an altitude of 6,000 feet (1,830 meters) , while in others no difference could be observed (2) .

Liebesny (46) in 1922 reported that when persons travel from a low altitude to places of considerable height, certain alterations in the blood flow through the capillaries take place. Instead of the capillaries being homogeneously filled and the blood streaming through them rapidly, as occurs at low levels, the flow becomes impeded; and the vessels, owing to the apparent agglutination or sedimentation, present a beaded appearance. In 1924 Schneider and Truesdell (70) , working with human beings and using the rebreather method to induce hypoxia, came to the conclusion that capillary blood pressure very often is not affected by hypoxia but that in cases of extreme anoxic hypoxia the flow of blood through capillaries is gradually retarded and the blood passes from a homogeneous to a granular state. Their observations during extreme hypoxic conditions agree with those made by Liebesny.

Krogh (40) , in his book on the capillaries, mentions that he observed capillary dilatation during hypoxia. Vanotti (77) in 1931 also reported definite dilatation in capillary loops in the skin at high altitudes.

The conclusion which may be drawn from experimental evidence, then, is that hypoxia does not cause a rise in capillary pressure.

HEMORRHAGES AT HIGH ALTITUDES

A rather prevalent impression is that even at moderately high altitudes bleeding from the nose, mouth, lungs, and stomach often occurs.

This is probably a popular fallacy; the number of people who suffer from hemorrhages under these conditions has been greatly exaggerated. Major Hingston (36), medical officer of the 1924 Mount Everest Expedition, reported that none of the members suffered from hemorrhages. If hemorrhages do occur, they cannot be explained as being due to increased capillary pressure or, for that matter, to increased arterial pressure, except perhaps in cases of mountain sickness.

PULMONARY CIRCULATION

It was shown by Von Euler and Liljestrand (22) in 1946 that anoxic hypoxia produced pulmonary hypertension in animals, and in the following year Motley *et al.* (51) found this to be also true in man.

During the past decade or so a great deal of work has been reported on the effect of hypoxia on the circulation through the lungs. Indeed, a large number of workers have found that hypoxia increases pulmonary vascular resistance. A number of observations have been made on man (12, 16, 17, 23, 24, 37, 51, 65, 72, 73, 79), but most of the work has been done on dogs (5, 6, 7, 10, 13, 29, 32, 38, 43, 44, 45, 50, 52, 53, 55, 56, 57, 60, 62, 63, 64, 74, 75, 76, 80). The rabbit has also been used (14, 34), and several studies have been made on the isolated lung of the cat (18, 19, 47, 58, 59). Space does not permit a detailed discussion of the many papers published on this subject. Suffice it to say that nearly all the workers found that hypoxia increased pulmonary pressure, although in a few instances indeterminate results were reported.

Many different and often ingenious techniques were used, various anesthetic agents employed, and different drugs administered throughout the course of some of the experiments. This may account, in part, for the somewhat variable experimental results obtained by some of the workers.

Part of the interest in pulmonary hypertension no doubt is due to the prevalence of diseases which cause this condition, such as chronic lung diseases and cardiac disorders, especially mitral stenosis and left ventricular failure. It is not in the province of this monograph, however, to discuss these clinical conditions.

Cause of pulmonary hypertension during acute hypoxia.—This is still not thoroughly understood. A number of possible mechanisms are suggested in the literature. In evaluating factors which appear to be responsible for pulmonary hypertension during hypoxia, extreme care must be taken in drawing conclusions. Fishman (23) has written that, ". . . once hypoxia affects the systemic circulation it becomes difficult to distinguish between the direct action of hypoxia on the pulmonary circulation and the indirect effects operating from afar by way of nerves, hormones and displacements of blood from the systemic circulation."

It is well established that cardiac output is generally increased during effective degrees of hypoxia (see chap. v, p. 81). Some workers hold that this factor could largely explain the increase in pulmonary pressure. On the other hand, this has been questioned by others who have either controlled cardiac output or have not observed an increase in the output of the heart during the course of their experiments.

A number of workers (12, 18, 22, 32, 74) have suggested that hypoxia originates the pulmonary hypertension through a vasoconstrictor effect. There is some question, however, which vessels are constricted; for example, Hall (32) and Wiggers and his collaborators (80) feel that hypoxia must exert its action on the vessels peripheral to pulmonary alveolar capillaries. Rivera-Estrada *et al.* (63) have suggested that there is evidence of arteriolar dilatation associated with increased post-capillary vascular resistance.

Other factors may be mentioned as possible causes of pulmonary hypertension during acute hypoxia. Altered alveolar carbon dioxide tension may play a part, although it is felt that this factor has not as yet been well elucidated. There is a divergence of opinion regarding the distensibility of the pulmonary vascular bed. Cournand (12) has called attention to the large capacity and deformability of the arteriolar pre-capillary and capillary bed, whereas others (15) feel that the pulmonary bed is relatively indistensible. In this connection, Fritts *et al.* (26) produced interesting evidence that thoracic blood volume is not appreciably affected by hypoxia. Fishman (23) has emphasized that it is most difficult to find out exactly what happens to pulmonary blood volume during acute hypoxia.

Recently Aviado (4) has critically reviewed the action of acute hypoxia on the pulmonary circulation. He has summarized the present views as follows:

1. There is general agreement that pulmonary artery pressure rises during hypoxia but that increased left atrial pressure does not occur. Further, the increased cardiac output which is known to occur could contribute to the pulmonary hypertension but may actually cause a decrease in the calculated pulmonary vascular resistance. (There is no general agreement with the latter statement.)

2. There is strong evidence, but not entire agreement, that hypoxia, by sympathetic stimulation, causes constriction of the lung ves-

sels (probably due to chemoreceptors). Furthermore, hypoxia, by increasing discharge from the adrenal medulla, causes cardiac stimulation, increases venous return, and also produces pulmonary constriction.

3. Whether hypoxia causes direct constriction or dilatation of pulmonary vessels is still controversial. The exact site of action is unknown. The participation of arteries, capillaries, veins, a-v anastomoses, and bronchial vessels in bringing about the hypoxic responses of calculated pulmonary resistance and of estimated pulmonary blood volume remains to be elucidated.

The authors feel that, on the whole, this is a fair summary of present knowledge of the effect of acute hypoxia on pulmonary pressure.

Pulmonary hypertension during mountain sickness.—Patients afflicted with chronic mountain sickness showed a marked increase in pulmonary pressures. Rotta *et al.* (65) have pointed out that this might be accounted for by the fact that in this condition an abnormal degree of polycythemia is present, there is a low arterial oxygen saturation, and a noticeable increase in cardiac output.

(For a discussion of pulmonary circulation in residents at high altitude see chap. x.)

REFERENCES

1. ABRAMSON, D. I.; LANDT, H.; and BENJAMIN, J. E. 1943. *Arch. Intern. Med.,* **71:** 583.
2. *Air Service Medical,* p. 150. Washington, D.C.: U.S. Govt. Printing Office, 1919.
3. ALBERS, C., and USINGER, W. 1956. *Pflueger Arch. Ges. Physiol.,* **263:** 201.
4. AVIADO, D. M., JR. 1960. *Pharm. Rev.,* **12:** 159.
5. AVIADO, D. M., JR., *et al.* 1954. *Fed. Proc.,* **13:** 4.
6. AVIADO, D. M., JR.; LING, J. S.; and SCHMIDT, C. F. 1957. *Amer. J. Physiol.,* **189:** 253.
7. BEARD, E. F.; BELL, A. L. L., JR.; and HOWELL, T. W. August, 1953. *USAF Sch. Aviat. Med.,* Project No. 21–1204,0001, Report No. 1.
8. BERNTHAL, T. 1938. *Amer. J. Physiol.,* **121:** 1.
9. BREWER, N. R. 1937. *Amer. J. Physiol.,* **120:** 91.
10. BORST, H. G., *et al.* 1957. *Amer. J. Physiol.,* **191:** 446.
11. COMROE, J. H., JR., and DRIPPS, R. D., JR. 1945. *Ann. Rev. Physiol.,* **7:** 653.
12. COURNAND, A. 1950. *Circulation,* **2:** 641.
13. DALY, I. DE BURGH, and DALY, M. DE BURGH. 1959. *J. Physiol.,* **148:** 201.

14. DIRKEN, M. N. J., and HEEMSTRA, H. 1948. *Quart. J. Exp. Physiol.,* 34: 193.
15. DOYLE, J. T., *et al.* 1951. *J. Clin. Invest.,* 30: 345.
16. DOYLE, J. T., *et al.* 1951. *Fed. Proc.,* 10: 37.
17. ———. 1952. *Circulation,* 5: 263.
18. DUKE, H. N. 1951. *Quart. J. Exp. Physiol.,* 36: 75.
19. ———. 1954. *J. Physiol.,* 125: 373.
20. ERSHLER, I.; KOSSMAN, C. E.; and WHITE, M. S. 1943. *Amer. J. Physiol.,* 138: 593.
21. EULER, U. S., VON, and LILJESTRAND, G. 1936. *Scand. Arch. Physiol.,* 74: 101.
22. ———. 1946. *Acta Physiol. Scand.,* 12: 301.
23. FISHMAN, A. P. 1961. *Physiol. Rev.,* 41: 214.
24. FISHMAN, A. P.; HIMMELSTEIN, A.; and COURNAND, A. 1955. *Fed. Proc.,* 14: 48.
25. FISHMAN, A. P., *et al.* 1952. *J. Clin. Invest.,* 31: 770.
26. FRITTS, H. W., JR., *et al.* 1960. *Circulation,* 22: 216.
27. GELLHORN, E. 1937. *Ann. Intern. Med.,* 10: 1267.
———. 1937. *Sigma Xi Quart.,* 25: 156.
28. GELLHORN, E., and LAMBERT, E. H. 1939. *The Vasomotor System in Anoxia and Asphyxia.* Urbana, Ill.: University of Illinois Press.
29. GORLIN, R., and LEWIS, B. M. 1952. *Fed. Proc.,* 11: 57.
30. GRAYBIEL, A. 1941. *J. Aviat. Med.,* 12: 183.
31. GREENE, C. W. 1919. *Amer. J. Physiol.,* 49: 118.
32. HALL, P. W., III. 1953. *Circulat. Res.,* 1: 238.
33. HARRISON, T. R., and BLALOCK, A. 1927. *Amer. J. Physiol.,* 80: 169.
34. HEEMSTRA, H. 1954. *Quart. J. Exp. Physiol.,* 39: 83.
35. HEYMANS, C.; BOUCKAERT, J. J.; and DAUTREBANDE, L. 1930. *Arch. Int. Pharmacodyn.,* 39: 400.
36. HINGSTON, R. W. G. 1925. *Geog. J.,* 65: 4.
———, cited by J. BARCROFT, 1925. *The Respiratory Function of the Blood,* Part I, "Lessons from High Altitudes," p. 181. Cambridge: Cambridge University Press.
37. HULTGREN, H., and SPICKARD, W. 1960. *Stanford Med. Bull.,* 18: 76.
38. HURLIMANN, A., and WIGGERS, C. J. 1953. *Circulat. Res.,* 1: 230.
39. KEYS, A.; STAPP, J. P.; and VIOLANTE, A. 1943. *Amer. J. Physiol.,* 138: 763.
40. KROGH, A. 1929. *The Anatomy and Physiology of the Capillaries.* New Haven, Conn.: Yale University Press.
41. LAMBERT, E. H., and GELLHORN, E. 1937. *Proc. Soc. Exp. Biol. Med.,* 36: 169.
42. LE WALD, L. T., and TURRELL, G. H. 1920. *Amer. J. Roentgenol.,* 7: 67.
43. LEWIS, B. M., and GORLIN, R. 1952. *Amer. J. Physiol.,* 170: 574.
44. ———. 1952. *Fed. Proc.,* 11: 93.
45. LEWIS, B. M.; GORLIN, R.; and HOUSSAY, H. E. J. 1953. *Fed. Proc.,* 12: 87.

46. Liebesny, P. 1922. *Med. Wschr.,* No. 18.
47. Liljestrand, G. 1958. *Acta Physiol. Scand.,* **44:** 216.
48. Lutz, B. R., and Schneider, E. C. 1919. *Amer. J. Physiol.,* **50:** 280, 228, and 327.
49. McFarland, R. A. 1937. *J. Comp. Psychol.,* **23:** 181.
50. McGregor, M., *et al.* 1955. *Amer. J. Physiol.,* **183:** 643P.
51. Motely, H. L., *et al.* 1947. *Amer. J. Physiol.,* **150:** 315.
52. Nahas, G. G. 1956. *J. Appl. Physiol.,* **9:** 65.
53. ———. *Ibid.,* 352.
54. Nahas, G. G.; Josse, J. W.; and Muchow, G. C. 1954. *Amer. J. Physiol.,* **177:** 315.
55. Nahas, G. G., *et al.* 1951. *Amer. J. Physiol.* (Proc.) , **167:** 812.
56. Nahas, G. G.; Mather, G. W.; and Kitchell, R. L. 1953. *Fed. Proc.,* **12:** 102.
57. Nahas, G. G., *et al.* 1954. *J. Appl. Physiol.,* **6:** 467.
58. Nisell, O. I. 1950. *Acta Physiol. Scand.,* **21** (Suppl.) : 73.
59. ———. 1951. *Acta Physiol. Scand.,* **23:** 85.
60. Peters, R. M., and Roos, A. 1952. *Amer. J. Physiol.,* **171:** 250.
61. Raab, W. 1931. *Arch. Intern. Med.,* **47:** 727.
62. Rahn, H., and Bahnson, H. T. 1953. *J. Appl. Physiol.,* **6:** 105.
63. Rivera-Estrada, C., *et al.* 1958. *Circulat. Res.,* **6:** 10.
64. Robbard, S., and Harasawa, M. 1959. *Amer. Heart J.,* **57:** 232.
65. Rotta, A., *et al.* 1956. *J. Appl. Physiol.,* **9:** 328.
66. Sands, J., and De Graff, A. C. 1925. *Amer. J. Physiol.,* **74:** 416.
67. Schneider, E. C. 1918. *J.A.M.A.,* **61:** 1384.
68. Schneider, E. C., and Sisco, D. L. 1914. *Amer. J. Physiol.,* **34:** 7 and 29.
69. Schneider, E. C., and Truesdell, D. 1921. *Amer. J. Physiol.,* **55:** 223.
70. ———. 1924. *Ibid.,* **71:** 90.
71. Selladurai, S., and Wright, S. 1932–33. *Quart. J. Exp. Physiol.,* **22:** 233.
72. Siebens, A. A.; Smith, R. E.; and Storey, C. F. 1954. *Fed. Proc.,* **13:** 137.
73. ———. 1955. *Amer. J. Physiol.,* **180:** 428.
74. Stroud, R. C., and Conn, H. L., Jr. 1954. *Amer. J. Physiol.,* **179:** 119.
75. Stroud, R. C., and Rahn, H. 1953. *Amer. J. Physiol.,* **172:** 211.
76. Thilenius, O. G.; Hoffer, P. B.; and Fitzgerald, R. S. 1961. *Fed. Proc.,* **20:** 104.
77. Vanotti, A. 1931. *Klin. Wschr.,* **10:** 253.
78. Von Tavel, F. 1943. *Helv. Physiol. Pharmacol. Acta,* **1:** 1.
79. Westcott, R. N., *et al.* 1951. *J. Clin. Invest.,* **30:** 957.
80. Wiggers, C. J.; Hurlimann, A.; and Hall, P. W., III. 1953. *Science,* **117:** 473.

CHAPTER VII

EFFECT OF HYPOXIA ON LYMPH AND ON VESSEL PERMEABILITY

EFFECT ON LYMPH

The effect of hypoxia on the composition and circulation of the lymph has engaged the attention of a number of workers. Drinker and Field (6) in their monograph mention the effects of asphyxia and of carbon dioxide on lymph flow. They emphasize the importance of recognizing the fact that, when lymph is collected from the thoracic duct, any factor which causes an increase in breathing augments lymph flow. The increase in breathing produces a rise in intra-abdominal pressure during inspiration and suction of lymph into the thorax.

These authors point out that, since hypoxia increases capillary permeability, it produces a condition which is presumably favorable to augmenting an increase in the flow of lymph. The general consensus now is, however, that hypoxia within physiologic limits has little, if any, effect on capillary permeability.

Although recognizing that increasing carbon dioxide produces dilatation of arterioles and capillaries, Drinker and Field are not confident that carbon dioxide actually increases lymph flow, since it greatly stimulates breathing. They subjected two dogs to 7 per cent carbon dioxide and observed an increase in the flow of lymph from vessels in the leg; but, since there was an increase in breathing, they suggested that the experiments should be repeated on curarized dogs and the breathing controlled artificially.

A pronounced stagnant hypoxia may produce an increased filtration of lymph from blood capillaries and so cause an edema. Drinker and Field (7) called attention to the fact that it is quite difficult to produce an edema by venous stasis. If a widespread venous thrombosis is produced, however, an edema rich in protein appears. They interpreted this to mean that, in order to produce edema in the presence of a normal blood flow, the circulation must be obstructed sufficiently to produce asphyxial damage to the capillary endothelium. This

117

means, of course, that not only is hypoxia present, but asphyxia as well.

Maurer (18) in 1941, working with dogs and using a rebreather, reported studies on the effect of decreased blood oxygen and increased blood carbon dioxide on the flow and composition of cervical and cardiac lymph. He found that increased lymph production began when the arterial oxygen saturation reached 75 per cent, corresponding to an approximate altitude of about 17,000 feet (5,200 meters), and that the greatest production took place at an arterial saturation of 52.5 per cent, approximately 20,000 feet altitude (6,100 meters).

Since the increased flow of lymph persisted even after exposure to pure oxygen, and since erythrocytes appeared in the lymph, Maurer felt that the hypoxia damaged the cardiac blood capillaries. The increased passage of protein from the blood stream into the lymph indicated that low blood oxygen and increased carbon dioxide caused an increase in capillary permeability, so that there was a loss of fluid and protein from the circulating blood.

In a subsequent paper Maurer (19) reported the effects of carbon monoxide on the flow and composition of lymph. Dogs and cats under pentobarbital anesthesia were exposed to 0.5 per cent carbon monoxide. An average increase of flow of cervical lymph 2.42 times the control flow was observed. Since the increase in lymph production began when the average oxygen saturation was 61 per cent, the author pointed out that the results obtained compared favorably with those observed when the animals were subjected to anoxic hypoxia. He suggested further that this confirmed the belief that carbon monoxide is, of itself, nontoxic and that it acts only through its ability to reduce oxygen-carrying capacity. All physiologists, however, would not concur in this belief. The reader is referred to the discussion concerning the question of histotoxic action of carbon monoxide (p. 28).

Warren and Drinker (28) in 1942 subjected curarized dogs, which were kept alive by artificial respiration, to 8.6 per cent of oxygen in nitrogen. As soon as the animal began to breathe the low oxygen mixture, the flow of lymph from the lungs increased. They found that this flow constantly increased to a level of hypoxia as low as 4.4 per cent oxygen. When the animals were ventilated with pure oxygen, the lymph flow returned to normal almost immediately. The authors stated that no permanent damage was done to the blood capillaries.

In a subsequent study, published the same year, Warren and Drinker and their colleagues (29) subjected dogs to progressive, severe hypoxia under artificial respiration. When 10 per cent oxygen was administered, a sudden increase in the flow of lung lymph occurred which ceased promptly when ventilation with air was used. The authors concluded that when sufficient oxygen is not available, lung capillaries become abnormally permeable. The action is reversible if the period of hypoxia is not too prolonged.

Since it is generally accepted that capillaries are quite resistant to hypoxia, it is difficult to understand the results obtained by Drinker and his colleagues. Drinker has pointed out, however, that he and his colleagues reached the inescapable conclusion that pulmonary capillaries are peculiarly susceptible to oxygen lack as a cause of increased permeability. Besides Drinker and his collaborators, other workers (2, 18) have considered the pulmonary capillaries to be especially vulnerable to oxygen want. This has, however, been challenged by Korner (13), who feels that there is only slight evidence for supposing that the capillaries of the lung are more susceptible to damage by hypoxia than capillaries in other regions of the body.

In summary, it may be stated that, because capillaries, on the whole, are resistant to hypoxia, edema is not easily produced by oxygen want. There is evidence that at a simulated altitude of 17,000 feet (5,182 meters) and over there may be an increased lymph production. Carbon monoxide (if the oxygen saturation is 61 per cent or less) may also cause an increase in lymph production. Marked stagnant hypoxia causes filtration of lymph. There is considerable evidence that the capillaries in the lungs are especially susceptible to anoxic hypoxia, although this has been challenged.

VESSEL PERMEABILITY

In the brief discussion of hypoxia and permeability in this monograph, no attempt will be made to discuss in detail the effect of hypoxia on cell permeability. The reader is referred to the volume of Gellhorn and Regnier (8) and to the reviews of Collander (3), Hober (11), Osterhout (22), Toerell (26), Wilbrandt (31), and others. Most of these reviews mention, in one way or another, the effect of oxygen want on the permeability of the cell.

The works of Bainbridge (1) on the permeability of the visceral capillaries, Starr (24) on the kidney, Landis (15, 16) on the capillary, Magee and Macleod (17) on the intestine, and Van Liere and his co-workers (27) on the gastrointestinal tract indicate the role hypoxia, in this connection, may play in physiologic functions.

Bainbridge (1) in 1906, in explaining some of the factors concerning the flow of post-mortem lymph, suggested that lack of oxygen in-

creased the permeability of visceral capillaries. The glomerular fil-
trate in a kidney with normal circulation is relatively protein free, as
shown by Wearn and Richards (30). However, Starr (24) in 1926
showed that, if the blood is stopped or even a reduction made in its
rate of flow, a transient albuminuria not accompanied by any visible
pathologic change is produced.

Landis (14) in 1928 reported the effects of oxygen, high tensions of
carbon dioxide, and increased hydrogen-ion concentration on capillary permeability in single capillaries of the frog mesentery. He produced oxygen lack by compressing the mesenteric artery and vein,
thereby producing a stagnant hypoxia, and found that after a three-
minute period the permeability was so increased that the fluid in the
capillary filtered through the walls at approximately four times its
normal rate. Not only the fluid, but the protein as well, passed
through the capillary wall, so that the effective osmotic pressure of the
plasma was reduced to one-half its normal value. The capillary wall
recovered its impermeability as soon as the circulation was allowed to
return.

The capillary permeability to fluid was slightly increased when the
mesentery was exposed to Ringer's solution completely saturated with
carbon dioxide, but it remained normally permeable to protein; one-
half saturation of carbon dioxide had no effect.

Within physiologic limits an increase in hydrogen-ion concentration had practically no effect on capillary permeability, which proved
that it was oxygen lack, and not the change of pH, which produced
the variation in tissue permeability.

In 1934 Landis (15) made further studies on capillary permeability. He reported that an increased carbon dioxide content has no effect on capillary permeability until a pH of 4 is reached; this degree
of hydrogen-ion concentration produces gross damage to the tissues.
In another report in 1946, Landis emphasized that mild degrees of
hypoxia had little effect on the capillaries of the frog's mesentery.
Severe degrees, however, increased capillary permeability both to
plasma and to fluid. He cautioned that these findings probably cannot
be applied to mild clinical hypoxia (16).

Maurer (18, 19), working on capillary permeability in dogs, studied the effect of hypoxia on the rate of flow and protein content of
cervical lymph. Lymph flow increased steadily with progressive hypoxia as low as 7 volumes per cent oxygen content. Warren and
Drinker (28), employing essentially the same technique, found that
the lung lymph constantly increased to a level of hypoxia as low as 4.4
volume per cent oxygen. Pochin (23) also demonstrated, by occlud-

ing the blood vessels at the base of the rabbit's ear for from two to twenty-four hours, that graded hypoxemia caused an increase in capillary permeability. He noted an increase in the thickness of the ear in proportion to the time of occlusion.

Several investigators have utilized the procedure of producing venous congestion of the upper extremities of human beings. Mc-Michael and Morris (20) found no increase in swelling of the arm at 9.5 volume per cent oxygen. Henry *et al.* (10) observed that at 15 or 20 per cent arterial saturation (4 to 6 volumes per cent content) a significant loss of protein occurred. Stead and Warren (25), working with patients with chronic emphysema in which the blood was 50 to 60 per cent saturated, could find no signs of protein "leakage."

Henry *et al.* (10) studied capillary permeability in human beings, using the cuff technique of Landis. Four individuals were subjected to a simulated altitude between 18,000 feet (5,485 meters) and 20,000 feet (6,095 meters). No significant differences between these four and the controls were observed.

In 1947 Hopps and Lewis (12), studying the effect of hypoxia on capillary permeability, subjected guinea pigs for thirty minutes to 6.4 per cent oxygen, corresponding to a simulated altitude of about 30,-000 feet (9,145 meters). This severe grade of hypoxia did not facilitate the passage of antibody globulin or serum albumin through vascular endothelium, and no significant alterations in the quantity of plasma protein were observed.

Nairn (21) in 1951 perfused the femoral artery in a series of dogs which had been subjected to an oxygen saturation of about 50 per cent for six to seven hours. The hypoxic, perfused limb did not develop edema. In another series of dogs, edema was produced by various methods; hypoxia had no effect on the edema produced, nor did it reduce the rate of reabsorption of edema fluid. The author concluded that capillary hypoxia plays no part in the production of edema.

In the same year Di Pasquale and Schiller (4) studied the effect of hypoxia on edema formation in the perfused, isolated hind limb of the rat. They came to the conclusion that the critical hypoxic level affecting capillary permeability lies between 2.6 and 5.5 volumes per cent oxygen content.

In 1954 Hendley and Schiller (9) studied changes in capillary permeability during hypoxia by perfusion experiments on isolated hind-legs of rats. These investigators employed what they termed severe hypoxia (0 to 2 volumes per cent oxygen) and mild hypoxia (5 to 10 volumes per cent oxygen). They studied the relationships between flow, pressure, and rate of edema formation. It was concluded that hypoxia over a wide physiological range does not alter capillary permeability. However, at a critical oxygen content (less than 5 volumes per cent oxygen), they observed an abrupt increase in capillary permeability.

It should be mentioned that a number of investigators (2, 5, 18, 28, 29) have considered pulmonary capillaries more vulnerable to oxygen lack than capillaries elsewhere in the body. This has been challenged by Korner (13), who feels that definitive proof of this is lacking.

In summary, there is apparent consensus that hypoxia within physiologic range has little, if any, effect on capillary permeability. There is considerable proof that capillary permeability to fluid and protein does not increase unless the venous pO_2 falls below 10–12 mm. Hg pressure. It is possible that the capillaries in the lungs are somewhat more susceptible to oxygen lack, although this, too, has been questioned.

REFERENCES

1. BAINBRIDGE, F. A. 1906. *J. Physiol.*, **34**: 275.
2. BEZNAK, A., and LILJESTRAND, G. 1949. *Acta Physiol. Scand.*, **19**: 170.
3. COLLANDER, R. 1937. *Ann. Rev. Biochem.*, **6**: 1.
4. DI PASQUALE, E. L., and SCHILLER, A. A. 1951. *Proc. Soc. Exp. Biol. Med.*, **78**: 567.
5. DRINKER, C. K. 1945. *Pulmonary Edema and Inflammation.* Cambridge, Mass.: Harvard University Press.
6. DRINKER, C. K., and FIELD, M. E. 1933. *Lymphatics, Lymph, and Tissue Fluid*, p. 164. Baltimore: Williams & Wilkins Co.
7. ———. *Ibid.*, p. 178.
8. GELLHORN, E., and REGNIER, J. 1936. *La Perméabilité en physiologie et en pathologie générale.* Paris: Masson & Co.
9. HENDLEY, E. E., and SCHILLER, A. A. 1954. *Amer. J. Physiol.*, **179**: 216.
10. HENRY, J. P.; GOODMAN, J.; and MEEHAN, J. 1947. *J. Clin. Invest.*, **26**: 1119.
11. HOBER, R. 1936. *Physiol. Rev.*, **16**: 62.
12. HOPPS, H. C., and LEWIS, J. H. 1947. *Amer. J. Pathol.*, **23**: 829.
13. KORNER, P. I. 1959. *Physiol. Rev.*, **39**: 687.
14. LANDIS, E. M. 1928. *Amer. J. Physiol.*, **83**: 528.
15. ———. 1934. *Physiol. Rev.*, **14**: 404.
16. ———. 1946. *Ann. N.Y. Acad. Sci.*, **46**: 713.
17. MAGEE, H. F., and MACLEOD, J. J. R. 1929. *Amer. J. Physiol.*, **90**: 442.
18. MAURER, F. W. 1941. *Amer. J. Physiol.*, **131**: 331.
19. ———. *Ibid.*, **133**: 170.

20. McMichael, J., and Morris, K. M. 1936. *J. Physiol.*, **87**: 74.
21. Nairn, R. C. 1951. *J. Path. Bact.*, **63**: 213.
22. Osterhout, W. J. V. 1936. *Physiol. Rev.*, **16**: 216.
23. Pochin, E. E. 1939–1942. *Clin. Sci.*, **4**: 341.
24. Starr, I. 1926. *J. Exp. Med.*, **63**: 31.
25. Stead, E. H., and Warren, J. V. 1944. *J. Clin. Invest.*, **23**: 283.
26. Toerell, T. 1937. *Fortschr. Zool.*, **2**: 303.
27. Van Liere, E. J. 1941. *Physiol. Rev.*, **21**: 307.
28. Warren, M. F., and Drinker, C. K. 1942. *Amer. J. Physiol.*, **136**: 207.
29. Warren, M. F.; Peterson, D. K.; and Drinker, C. K. 1942. *Amer. J. Physiol.*, **137**: 641.
30. Wearn, J. T., and Richards, A. N. 1924. *Amer. J. Physiol.*, **71**: 209.
31. Wilbrandt, W. 1938. *Ergebn. Physiol.*, **40**: 204.

CHAPTER VIII

EFFECT OF HYPOXIA ON RESPIRATION

ANOXIC HYPOXIA

The first to report systematic observations of the effects of high altitude on respiration seems to have been Jourdanet (71), who worked in the mountainous districts of Mexico and whose works were published in 1875 and before. For later studies of the influence of hypoxia on respiration the reader may consult the monographs of Barcroft (5), Haldane (54), Haldane and Priestley (57), L. J. Henderson (61), Y. Henderson (62), Loewy (84), Loewy and Wittkower (85), Meakins and Davies (88), Means (89), Mosso (92), Van Liere (122), Verzar (125), Zuntz *et al.* (131), and the reviews of Haldane (55) and Schneider (111, 112).

The confusion among physiologists concerning the way in which hypoxia stimulates respiration cleared rather rapidly with the discovery of Heymans *et al.* in 1930 of the chemoreceptive reflexes of the carotid sinus region (62). Comroe's precise delineation of the function of the aortic chemoreceptors in 1939 served further to add to our understanding (19). Since these discoveries the idea has developed that the hyperpnea of anoxic or arterial hypoxia is almost completely due to reflexes from the carotid and aortic chemoreceptors.

CHANGES IN COMPOSITION OF ALVEOLAR AIR

During mild or moderate hypoxia the metabolic rate is not altered, and the production of carbon dioxide is unchanged. But the resulting hyperpnea causes increased elimination of carbon dioxide from the lungs, and the concentration in the alveolar air gradually declines. As a result, the arterial carbon dioxide tension is reduced. The tissues in turn participate in this decline with the result that carbon dioxide tension and content fall generally until a new equilibrium is reached.

The hypoxic hyperpnea is beneficial and adaptive in that it elevates alveolar oxygen tension above what it otherwise would have been. This in turn permits higher arterial, and finally somewhat higher tissue, tensions. The elevated oxygen tension is a consequence of the increased ventilation of the lungs in displacing carbon dioxide.

This new equilibrium takes a definite period for its attainment and depends largely upon the degree of hypoxemia—the greater the altitude, for example, the longer the time. It has been customary to insist that at least an hour is needed, particularly for the higher altitudes.

Table 5, from the older literature, shows the way oxygen and carbon dioxide behave at specific locations above sea level. Since the values appear to be from partially acclimated persons, the data are actually out of place because in this chapter only acute phases of respiratory adaptation will be discussed. However, the table is included

TABLE 5

THE EFFECT OF ALTITUDE ON THE ALVEOLAR CARBON DIOXIDE
AND OXYGEN TENSION IN THE LUNG*

Place	Altitude (Meters and Feet)	Barometer (Mm. Hg)	Water Vapor (Mm. Hg)	Carbon Dioxide (Mm. Hg)	Oxygen (Mm. Hg)
Sea level..............	0	760	47	42	100
Colorado Springs......	1,800 6,000	620	47	36	79
Pike's Peak...........	4,300 14,000	460	47	28	53
North Col of Everest....	6,400 21,000	335	47	19	39
Summit of Everest......	9,100 29,000	240	47	15	24(?)

* Modified from Y. Henderson, *Adventures in Respiration* (Baltimore: Williams & Wilkins Co., 1938), p. 79.

to help identify the physiologic and barometric data with particular areas and thus lend concreteness.

The results of some modern studies made in the altitude chamber on eight subjects in acute exposure lasting one hour on the average are shown in Table 6. It will be noticed that as simulated altitude increases and ambient pressure decreases (and with it the tension of oxygen) the alveolar gas tensions decline. The fall in oxygen tension is due directly to its reduced pressure in the inspired air; that for carbon dioxide, as has been mentioned, is due to the increased pulmonary ventilation.

Alveolar equation.—The relationships of the tensions of oxygen and carbon dioxide in alveolar air at a given barometric pressure can be precisely determined by the use of the general alveolar equation, whose modern correct form was developed by Gray (50). The equation is based upon the premises (Dalton's Law) that the total pressure of the gases in alveolar air (the barometric pressure) is made up of the sum of the partial pressures (pO_2, pCO_2, pN_2, pH_2O) of the individual gases and that where three are known the other may be obtained by subtraction. In practice the pressure of water vapor is taken to be 47 mm. Hg, or that found in complete saturation at normal body temperature. The pressure of a respiratory quotient other than unity requires in most cases a correcting factor based upon the actual value of the quotient. Where atmospheric air is inspired, the relation is further simplified by assuming zero concentration of carbon dioxide.

TABLE 6

EFFECT OF REDUCED BAROMETRIC PRESSURES ON PULMONARY
FUNCTION AND HEART RATE IN MAN*

	Barometric Pressure (Mm. Hg)					
	748	483	412	379	349	321
	Altitude (Feet and Meters)					
	Ground Level	12,000 3,658	16,000 4,877	18,000 5,486	20,000 6,069	22,000 6,705
	Exposure Time (Minutes)					
	20	40–60	40–60	40–60	40–45	30
Alveolar pO_2 (mm. Hg)........	100.3	47.0	40.1	37.4	34.6	30.2
Alveolar pCO_2 (mm. Hg)......	37.6	36.6	30.8	27.3	24.7	24.3
Alveolar R.Q.................	0.83	0.82	0.86	0.90	0.86	0.95
Minute-volume (l/min)........	8.85	9.71	9.47	11.06	13.00	15.31
Respiratory rate (per min.).....	12	14	12	12	13	15
Tidal volume (ml.)............	715	694	789	922	1,000	1,021
Arterial O_2 saturation (%).....	98	85	80	77	76	64
O_2 consumption (ml/min)......	302	327	268	286	320	359
Heart rate (82 = 100%).......	100	103	103	108	107	124

*From H. Rahn and A. B. Otis, *Amer. J. Physiol.*, **150** (1947), 202.

While not strictly true, this assumption does not introduce any significant error. Here is an adaptation from Comroe *et al.* (20) of a current simple form of the equation for breathing air:

$$p_{A_{O_2}} = F_{I_{O_2}} (p_B - 47) - p_{A_{CO_2}} \left(F_{I_{O_2}} + \frac{1 - F_{I_{O_2}}}{R} \right)$$

where

$p_{A_{O_2}}$ = alveolar oxygen tension,

$F_{I_{O_2}}$ = fraction of oxygen in inspired air,

p_B = ambient barometric pressure,

$p_{A_{CO_2}}$ = alveolar carbon dioxide tension, and

R = the respiratory exchange ratio (equals the metabolic respiratory quotient or R.Q. at equilibrium).

Ventilation equation.—Since, as mentioned above, carbon dioxide production is not increased at moderate degrees of hypoxemia, the hyperpnea causes a lowering of alveolar carbon dioxide tension in exact proportion. Therefore, it has been possible to develop a ventilation equation which expresses this relationship. When there is no significant carbon dioxide in inspired air, an appropriate equation is (98):

$$\dot{V}_A = \frac{\dot{V}_{O_2} \times R \times 0.863}{p_{A_{CO_2}}},$$

where

$\dot{V}_A$ = alveolar ventilation in 1/min BTPS (body temperature, pressure, saturated) and

$\dot{V}_{O_2}$ = oxygen consumption in ml/min STPD (standard temperature, pressure, dry).

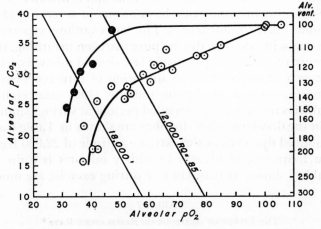

FIG. 8.—Alveolar gas composition in man acutely exposed to various altitudes (solid circles) and in man at altitude after partial and complete acclimatization (open circles). Scale of alveolar ventilation at right starts at 100 in arbitrary units for the resting ground-level value. (Modified from H. Rahn and A. B. Otis, *Amer. J. Physiol.*, **157** [1949], 445.)

Fenn carbon dioxide–oxygen diagram.—Fenn et al. (41) have devised a method of graphic portrayal of the changes in alveolar gases and ventilation under various conditions. The method referred to as the Fenn CO_2–O_2 diagram is based upon the equations given above. The pictorial representation gives vividness to the relationships. The data of Table 6 are reproduced on such a diagram in Figure 8. The upper line of the figure traces the average results for the acutely exposed man at several altitudes. For comparison, the lower line traces the averages obtained from acclimated and partially acclimated man as reported in the literature.

RESPIRATORY FREQUENCY

Although frequency of respiratory movements is not in itself an extremely fundamental measurement, we may nevertheless consider the results found by various workers. In the unanesthetized dog Swann (118) and Swann and Brucer (119) have found respiratory rate to double or better on pure nitrogen or severe hypoxia (breathing 2.43 per cent oxygen). These changes occurred within the short periods of one-half and one minute, respectively, after the onset of hypoxic breathing in the two types of experiments.

There is considerable difference of opinion concerning the threshold of low inspired oxygen tension for the appearance of rate changes in man (2, 37, 56, 64, 87). Since an increase in frequency may reveal merely anxiety in the subjects, which Lutz and Schneider (87) noted in their experiments, one must be cautious in accepting results obtained under such circumstances. The latter authors reported rather small increases in rate even during pure nitrogen breathing, the maximum occurring at the comparatively late time of thirty-six seconds on the average (range: 8–80) after initiation of nitrogen breathing.

The most recent studies of Rahn and Otis (100) using eight *experienced* subjects for relatively extended periods at various simulated altitudes in the decompression chamber are shown in Table 6 above. It will be noticed that even at the extreme altitude of 22,000 feet the increase in frequency of breaths for thirty minutes is quite modest.

As Table 7 shows, increases in rate during exercise are much more

TABLE 7

THE EFFECT OF ALTITUDE ON RESPIRATORY RATE*

	Sea Level	Pike's Peak (14,100 Feet)
In bed	16.8	17.3
Standing	17.0	20.0
Walking: 4 mph	17.2	29.0
Walking: 5 mph	20.0	36.0

*From E. C. Schneider, *Yale J. Biol. Med.*, 4 (1932), 537.

prominent at altitude than at sea level. This apparently reflects the response of the respiratory mechanism to a heightening spectrum of stimuli. The early response consists mainly of increased tidal volume; later there are rate increases. In this connection it is pertinent to call attention to the chemoreceptor-denervated animal which responds mainly with rate changes occurring after a relatively long latency (see below) .

DEPTH OF RESPIRATION

Since the minute-volume of pulmonary ventilation eventually increases with the increase in altitude (see below) , and rate changes, particularly in man at rest, are insignificant, one must conclude that it is the depth of respiration, i.e., tidal volume, that undergoes the preponderant change. Table 6 (above) includes the calculated average tidal volume at each simulated altitude. It can be seen that once the threshold has been passed, the deepening of breathing continues as the ambient pressure is reduced.

PULMONARY VENTILATION

In acute exposures in unacclimated man the increased rate of pulmonary ventilation does not usually begin until the alveolar oxygen tension has been reduced to 50 or 60 mm. Hg (Fig. 8 above) . This is roughly equivalent to 12,000 and 10,000 feet (3,700 and 3,000 meters) , respectively (12) . Beyond this threshold the increase appears to be proportional to altitude in a curvilinear manner. Table 6 also shows this phenomenon. This table and the figure fail to indicate the tremendous variation among different individuals in not only the threshold at which increased ventilation occurs but also in the degree of response beyond this point. Lutz and Schneider observed that in some the increase began at pressures comparable to altitudes of 3,000 and 4,000 feet (900 and 1,200 meters) or, as high as 89 mm. Hg oxygen tension (12) , while in an occasional person there was no response at all. It should be pointed out that the ventilation in question is stated in terms of ambient pressure, saturated with water vapor at body temperature (BTPS) .

CONTROL OF RESPIRATION

Respiratory center.[1]—In 1947 Davenport *et al.* (23) demonstrated the effect of hypoxia upon the respiratory center in three unanesthetized dogs whose carotid and aortic chemoreceptors had been denervated. There was a transient depression of ventilation which was followed by an increased effective alveolar ventilation due mainly to increased respiratory frequency. The depression could have been caused by the dissociation of oxygen from hemoglobin in arterial blood leading to an alkaline reaction, by the direct effect of hypoxia

[1] As used here respiratory center is loosely used to denote the associated neurons of the central nervous system upon whose particular co-ordinated activity the ventilation of the lungs depends.

upon the center, or by both. The authors suggested that the later and overpowering stimulation could have been centrally produced by chemical means. These experiments confirmed the earlier work of Gemmill *et al.* (47) upon the dog with only the carotid sinus region denervated.

The above experiments demonstrate that in the unanesthetized dog, with moderate hypoxia under careful laboratory supervision, the chemoreceptors may be dispensed with. The experiments also point up the central depression of respiration which accompanies hypoxia. This depression apparently summates with the activity of other centrally depressive agents as in anesthesia, extreme hypercapnia, or acidosis to cause a respiratory paralysis. The paralysis may be revealed by removal of chemoreceptor impulses either by the administration of pure oxygen or by denervating (34).

Carotid and aortic body chemoreceptive reflexes in experimental animals.—In the chemoreceptively intact animal, as has been seen above, the response to arterial hypoxia is a hyperpnea brought about mainly by increased depth of breathing. Since the 1930's it has been known that this is reflexly induced by stimulation of sensory receptors in the carotid and aortic bodies. Reduction of the arterial oxygen tension, rather than content, is the effective stimulus. Exactly how the low oxygen tension excites the chemoreceptive cell is not known. The cell is also excited by increased carbon dioxide tension and increased hydrogen-ion concentration. Since the cyanides are stimuli par excellence, perhaps metabolites of anaerobic metabolism within the cells are effective. De Castro (24), both from histologic observation and through experiment, concluded that the terminations of the chemoreceptive fibers of cranial nerves IX and X lie within the cytoplasm of the cell bodies. This and the evidence with ganglionic blocking agents (33, 91) seem to rule out the conception of a synaptic connection through the chemoreceptive cells functioning as ganglion cells. The claim that respiratory chemoreceptors occur in the abdominal region of mice and rats (66) needs confirmation.

Considerable work has been done in recent years upon the activity of the carotid chemoreceptors. In the anesthestized dog these are more important in respect to respiration than their aortic counterparts, which play the greater role in respect to circulation (19). A similar finding has been made in the chloralosed cat (49). Barcroft and Karvonen (7) concluded from the study of the respiratory response of sheep fetuses of varying ages that, although there were respiratory responses to cyanide midway through pregnancy, suggesting active chemoreflexes, at term such were held in abeyance as are other somatic reflexes at that time.

Threshold.—Several studies have been made to determine the threshold in arterial oxygen tension necessary to stimulate the chemoreceptors. In chloralosed cats prepared for recording chemoreceptive action potentials of the carotid sinus nerve Witzleb *et al.* (130) in 1955 found evidence for a threshold at 105 mm. Hg oxygen tension, which is about the eupneic level. Von Euler *et al.* (40) in similar, much earlier work found the threshold somewhat lower. The response curve as oxygen tension was lowered below the threshold seems more reasonable in the latter work, because its crescendo-like character more nearly follows the respiratory response curve. Alvarez-Buylla (1) has determined, particularly in the dog, that anesthesia (pentobarbital sodium, chloralose, urethane) may suppress the appearance of action potentials in such experiments. However, one would expect a lowered threshold of oxygen tension if anesthesia were a factor, so that the above thresholds occurring at eupneic levels of arterial oxygen tension must not have been too high in any circumstance.

In unanesthetized dogs Watt *et al.* (127) have found evidence of chemoreceptor activity in eupnea as indicated by decreased ventilation on respiring pure oxygen. Likewise Hornbein and Roos (68) found transient ventilatory stimulation at much higher oxygen tensions in cats during the response to two breaths of nitrogen gas than during steady-state exposures to hypoxia.

Gernandt (49) concluded from experiments on chloralosed cats that 36 per cent of the ventilation (under the necessarily abnormal experimental conditions) was controlled by chemoreceptive discharge as revealed by chemoreceptor inactivation with 0.5 N acetic acid. Of this, as determined by selective inactivation through the use of catheters, 23 per cent was the contribution from carotid, and 13 per cent, from aortic bodies. Since anesthesia depresses the respiratory center, the above chemoreceptive drive is probably exaggerated.

CHEMORECEPTOR REFLEXES IN MAN

Of course, experiments directly determining chemoreceptor activity in human subjects are impossible. However, recent indirect evidence with such subjects, suggests that chemoreceptive stimulation is at least present in eupnea. If in the latter state there is chemoreceptive activity, the continued breathing of pure oxygen might be expected to suppress it and lead to a decreased ventilation. This has not been observed, except initially (22, 35). The explanation has been that secondary stimulatory effects due to high oxygen tension cancel out the decreased chemoreceptive activity. Such stimulating effects are thought to arise as a result of various factors: increased saturation of hemoglobin in arterial blood causing increased hydrogen-ion concentration, reduced dissociated hemoglobin for carbon dioxide carriage in venous blood, decreased cerebral blood flow, irritation of respiratory membranes, increased irritability of the respiratory center, or baroceptor impulses secondary to circulatory changes (35, 75, 82, 116).

Loeschcke in 1953 (81) circumvented some of the above stimulatory effects by choosing an oxygen-nitrogen mixture in which the oxygen tension is only moderately high, as in 32 per cent oxygen in nitrogen. He found an 8 per cent reduction in ventilation volume in twenty subjects during the first minute. Dejours *et al.* in 1958 (25), using only three subjects, avoided the stimulatory effects by limiting the oxygen breathing to one breath and found reduced tidal volumes in subsequent breaths several seconds later. Stroud's more involved experiments have also been interpreted to demonstrate chemoreceptive activity during eupnea (117).

If one turns his attention from chemoreceptive activity in eupnea to look once more at the actual ventilation as hypoxia is increased (Table 6 and Fig. 8), one is struck by the paradox of inactivity until quite severe degrees of hypoxia are present. One must infer, from experiments on animals as well as those on human subjects, that chemoreceptive impulses must increase markedly as alveolar oxygen tension declines from its eupneic value of approximately 100 to 50–60 mm. Hg, where ventilatory increases have their threshold in the average subject. Georg and Sonne (48), using the oximeter in human subjects breathing air with decreasing oxygen tension, observed the decline in oxygen saturation of arterial blood well before any change in pulse or respiration. The absence of the early respiratory response has been ascribed to the alkaline reaction resulting from the increased dissociation of oxygen and hemoglobin in arterial blood (101) and to baroceptive changes secondary to circulatory phenomena (25). After hyperpnea has been established the resulting hypocapnia partially neutralizes the chemoreceptor drive (51).

Miller and Smull in 1955 (90) found no increased ventilation on breathing 12 per cent oxygen in nitrogen in either full-term or premature newborn infants. Older premature infants had about 40 per cent increased ventilation on the average. These findings suggest lowered chemoreceptor activity at birth, which is similar to the findings on sheep fetuses of Barcroft and Karvonen (7) noted above. However, Cross and Oppe, using 15 per cent oxygen mixtures, found evidence for greater activity in infants than in adults (22). It is possible that medullary depression with the 12 per cent mixtures masked any stimulation present in the experiments of Miller and Smull.

INTERACTION OF HYPERCAPNIA WITH HYPOXEMIA

The occurrence of pure hypoxemia other than at altitude is rather rare. Clinically, hypoxia is often associated with increased carbon dioxide tension as in drowning or emphysema. It has long been known that carbon dioxide is an excellent stimulus to respiration. Whether it stimulates as carbon dioxide per se, by its ability to form hydrogen ions, or both has long been debated. Recent evidence for receptors separately sensitive to carbon dioxide and hydrogen ion in the neighborhood of the respiratory center (39, 83) favors the last alternative. It has also been argued whether carbon dioxide controls respiration primarily through the central respiratory center or co-ordinately through the mediation of peripheral chemoreceptors and the center. That there is an optimum tension for the stimulant properties of carbon dioxide is now well recognized (51). Beyond about 65 mm. Hg, toxic phenomena increasingly appear, apparently interfering with the ability to respond to the stimulus.

Tschirgi and Gerard (121) found that the addition of carbon dioxide up to 35 per cent prolonged the gasping of rats placed in pure nitrogen gas. Since carbon dioxide is anesthetic in such concentration (51), it is tempting to ascribe its protective effect to that property in this instance.

Regardless of the manner or the locus of stimulation, we may ask whether the effect of carbon dioxide combined with oxygen lack is purely additive or, on the other hand, is it potentiating? Shock and Soley (116), using human subjects, found that the combination of hypercapnia and hypoxia produced with 2 per cent carbon dioxide and 17 per cent oxygen gave the same ventilation as the sum of the responses to the two gases separately. The same was true with 12 per cent oxygen mixtures. Hall has studied, in two groups of ten and fourteen young men (58, 59), the separate and combined responses of respiration to hypoxia and hypercapnia at stimulus levels other than those of Shock and Soley and has also found that the effects were simply additive.

On the other hand, Nielsen and Smith (94) and Lloyd *et al.* (80), with two and eight human subjects, respectively, in similar experiments, obtained results which indicated that there was potentiation—the combined stimuli gave greater responses than the sum of their separate effects. Other experiments along this line are those of Dill and Zamcheck (30). In these studies with intact subjects the addition or interaction of stimuli could have been at the respiratory center, peripherally, or both. Two investigations of the way hypoxia and hypercapnia act upon carotid chemoreceptors have been made on the isolated, perfused region in dogs. Winder (129) found evidence for simple additive effects, while Otey and Bernthal found potentiation (95). Obviously more work is necessary before we can decide whether there is addition or potentiation.

CHARACTER OF RESPIRATION AT REST AND IN MUSCULAR EXERCISE

It has been pointed out above that hyperpnea appears as a respiratory adaptation to decreased oxygen tension in the arterial blood. Even at higher altitudes increased ventilation is small compared to the maximum capacity attainable by the individual voluntarily or during muscular exercise. In the individual at rest exposed to hypoxia, the respiratory state cannot be characterized as dyspneic, denoting air hunger or difficulty in breathing. Moreover, Schneider (110) has noted: "All experiments in a low-pressure chamber and during airplane flights have shown that the increase in the ventilation of the lungs occurs so gradually and is so small in amount that the subject is unaware of the change. Some men have been carried so far that they have become unconscious, without feeling breathless at any time during the experiment."

However, when exercise is undertaken at altitude, reports on the character of breathing strongly suggest the common occurrence of dyspnea. Hingston (65), reporting the physiological difficulties in climbing Mount Everest, wrote: "But the very slightest exertion, such as the tying of a bootlace, the opening of a ration box, the getting into a sleeping bag, was associated with marked respiratory distress." He also gave Somervell's experience: "Somervell gives a record of his breathing at 27,000 feet. At that altitude he had to take 7, 8 or 10 complete respirations for every single step forward and even at that slow rate of progress he had to rest for a minute or two every 20–30 yards. At 28,000 feet Norton, in an hour's climb, ascended only about 80 feet."

Schneider and Clarke (114) reported their investigations upon a typical person working on a bicycle ergometer in a low-pressure chamber. They found that, regardless of the load between 2,000 and 6,000 foot-pounds per minute, the ventilation rate increased around 11 per cent above the sea-level value at 10,000 feet (3,000 meters); 23 per cent at 15,000 feet (4,600 meters); and 42 per cent at 20,000 feet (6,100 meters). Since at these altitudes the respiratory frequency increased 22, 27, and 47 per cent, respectively, all of the increase in minute-volume was due to an increase of the rate of breathing, with tidal volume either changing little or actually decreasing markedly at the lowest altitude.

These data also show, contrary to the interpretation of Schneider and Clark, that the linear relationship between load and pulmonary ventilation holds surprisingly well at altitudes as high as 20,000 feet and with loads between 2,000 and 6,000 foot-pounds per minute (114).

The interesting observation of Hornbein and Roos (67) on one subject, that increases of hematocrit by transfusion decreased the ventilation during exercise under 14 per cent oxygen, raises pertinent questions concerning respiratory control under these circumstances.

ABILITY TO HOLD THE BREATH

Schneider's amazing feat of holding the breath at altitude up to 16,000 feet (4,900 meters) as long as at sea level (110) has not been equaled by several teams of investigators using large numbers of subjects (14, 38, 96, 104). All have found that breath-holding times at simulated altitudes are shorter than at ground level. At various altitudes the time has been directly related to the oxygen tension of the inspired air (14, 104). The obvious conclusion—that oxygen tension is a factor here—cannot be ignored. In fact, a rough Gray's analysis of the total stimulus to breathe based on the alveolar gas tensions at the breaking points suggests that both carbon dioxide excess and oxygen lack are factors (96).

AFTEREFFECTS ON RESPIRATION IN ACUTE EXPOSURES

In the recovery from short exposures to high altitudes the alveolar carbon dioxide tension may increase to its normal value within a relatively brief time. For example, Lutz and Schneider (86) found, after thirty to ninety minutes at 15,000 feet (4,600 meters) simulated altitude, a recovery in some subjects within twenty minutes of the end of hypoxia; but Boycott and Haldane, after twenty hours at about 9,000 feet (2,700 meters), found no return by the end of two days (13).

PERIODIC BREATHING

Unacclimatized subjects at high altitudes often show a change in their breathing pattern. This was first described by Mosso (92). Respiration becomes irregular and resembles the Cheynes-Stokes type of breathing, although it differs from it in some respects. This irregularity most frequently occurs during sleep at night. It is caused by oxygen want, shown by the fact that the administration of oxygen abolishes it.

The breathing pattern shows much individual variation, but ordinarily the breaths occur in groups of three or four, each successive breath being deeper; and an apneic pause may follow the last one. Aviators flying at high altitudes may be troubled by this periodic breathing. Birley (11) reported a case in which it became so marked that the pilot had difficulty in controlling the airplane. Hingston (64) observed this in members of the Mount Everest Expedition and wrote: "I heard one member of the party breathing in this way as low as 12,000 feet, though as a rule, it seldom occurs when awake yet at the base camp I was conscious of this type of breathing before passing off to sleep. Illness at high altitudes markedly increased it."

When acclimatization becomes established, the tendency to periodic breathing disappears. Schneider (111) emphasizes the point that the onset of periodic breathing ordinarily is a pause in breathing, and he calls attention to the experiences of the members of the Anglo-American Expedition to Pike's Peak. The first few days, when they read gas burettes shaved, or performed any task which called for close attention, periodic breathing would manifest itself, since in tasks of this nature most people unconsciously hold their breath.

The pronounced individual variation in occurrence of periodic breathing was attributed by the Anglo-American Expedition to varying susceptibilities of the respiratory center. If the individual had a respiratory center responsive to hypoxia, he suffered from frequent attacks of periodic breathing, while the reverse was the case in a man whose breathing responded slowly to the change in altitude.

VITAL CAPACITY AND REST POSITION OF LUNG

That the vital capacity decreases early in acute exposures to reduced barometric pressures has been known for a long time. Bert in 1878 (10) reviewed the work of Vivenot published in 1868 in which the latter had observed the decrease in experiments conducted with the decompression chamber. Since that time numerous confirmations have been made (see 99, 120). According to Rahn and Hammond (99), few of the sources mention that corrections for water vapor and temperature were made for the spirometer volumes. Since the failure to do this could itself produce spurious decreases of vital capacity of the same order of magnitude as the true changes, the criticism is well taken. These workers studied the vital capacity in eighteen men in a low-pressure chamber at pressures simulating 10,000, 14,000, and 18,000 feet (3,000, 4,300, and 5,500 meters). Significant decreases of 2.4 and 3.8 per cent occurred at the higher two altitudes. The failure to find a change at 10,000 feet is similar to the findings of Schneider

(113). Another similarity in the two reports was the finding that the administration of pure oxygen at 18,000 feet could prevent or counteract the decrease in vital capacity. However, Rahn and Hammond were unable to prove that hypoxia was a factor because the administration of oxygen mixtures simulating the various altitudes failed to reveal a clear-cut reduction. Also, the prevention of significant hypoxia at simulated altitudes of 30,000 and 40,000 feet (9,100 and 12,000 meters) with the use of oxygen did not prevent a reduction in vital capacity of 4.3 and 7.2 per cent, respectively.

While expansion of gas in the abdominal viscera might be a factor at 30,000–40,000 feet, it does not seem an adequate reason for vital capacity reductions at 14,000–20,000 feet (99, 113, 123). Maximum expiratory pressures were found reduced in proportion to the degree of hypoxia (99), but under similar circumstances (breathing oxygen-nitrogen mixtures) the vital capacity was scarcely changed.

Verzar's theory (97,124), that under hypoxia there is an increased inspiratory muscle tonus which increases the volume of the lung at rest position, received some confirmation by Rahn and Hammond (99). There was a decrease in expiratory reserve volume nearly equal to the reduction in vital capacity in the hypoxia experiments with the oxygen mixtures. A later study (120) with four subjects on Mount Evans at 14,250 feet showed that expiratory reserve volumes increased during the first few days at altitude and that residual air volumes were well above sea-level values on the first day and fell off as the stay continued. (Similar studies have been made by Hurtado *et al.* [70].) In this study continuous positive pressure breathing was also tried in order to get rid of any excess blood that might be filling the pulmonary vessels and thus restricting lung volume. Since this maneuver did not alter the vital capacity measurements and since it should if engorgement were present (4), one must conclude that the theory of capillary dilatation to explain the vital capacity reduction does not seem applicable.

Further comments concerning the change in the rest position of the lung may be made. Both Greene in America and Verzar in Europe have devised for human subjects thoracic plethysmographs which are said to measure changes in the rest position. However, since these devices measure solely costal changes in chest volume and ignore the major diaphragmatic component (see Campbell [15]), we are of the opinion that they may fail to reveal a true picture of the overall changes. Furthermore, Greene (53), in a study of six persons rebreathing from a BMR apparatus, obtained positive results in only one person in spite of terminal oxygen percentages of 5, 6, 6, 7, 8, and

11. In the following citations body plethysmographs, used in animal experiments, were capable of recording the total or summed costal and abdominal components of respiration. Harris (60) found in anesthetized cats and dogs the hypoxic shift of mid-position after vagotomy reduced by two-thirds in cats and totally in dogs. Nicholson and Trimby have also observed the hypoxic shift in the anesthetized dog (93). Also, Peyser *et al.* (97) found in rabbits under urethane an increase in lung volume at mid-position which was inversely related to the inspired oxygen tensions. However, this correlation and that between ventilation rate and lung volume indicate the presence of a rather extreme variation. Finally, according to Verzar (126), the increase in lung volume is supposed to be adaptive by increasing the alveolar area for respiratory gas exchange. It supposedly reduces a normal physiologic atelectasis, or state of unopened alveoli.

EXCHANGE OF RESPIRATORY GASES IN THE LUNG

A recent excellent review by Forster (44) traces the development of the present concepts of the way in which the respiratory gases are exchanged in the lung. According to both Krogh (73) and Douglas and Haldane (31), Ludwig (44) prior to 1870 challenged the view that it occurred by diffusion alone and suggested that active secretion by the lung occurred. The crude methods available for blood-gas analyses in those days permitted the controversy to rage with Bohr and Haldane taking the secretion side and Krogh and Barcroft holding to diffusion. In 1910 Krogh (73), having accumulated excellent data with his microtonometric method which showed alveolar oxygen tensions always higher than arterial and carbon dioxide tensions about equal, could say confidently that the exchanges take place by diffusion alone. Haldane later retreated, holding that secretion was reserved for conditions of stress: low oxygen and exercise (31).

The secretion theory of oxygen received considerable support from observations made by the Anglo-American Pike's Peak Expedition. Douglas, Haldane, Henderson, and Schneider (32), using methods of Haldane and his co-workers, reported that, according to their computations, the oxygen pressure in the arterial blood, 88.3 mm. Hg, was 35.8 mm. higher than the normal resting alveolar oxygen pressure of 52.5. Dr. Marie Krogh (74) in 1915, however, made the work of these authors untenable by establishing a new diffusion coefficient for the passage of oxygen through a membrane. She showed, even in an unacclimatized body, that diffusion may take care of the oxygen requirement at rest to an altitude of 25,000 feet or 7,600 meters (barometric pressure of 290 mm. Hg), which is about as high as is compatible with life in an unacclimatized individual.

In 1920 Barcroft *et al.* (6) reinvestigated the tensions of oxygen in the blood under hypoxic conditions. By making an arterial puncture, blood was drawn directly from the radial artery of a man who had been kept at an oxygen pressure of 84 mm. Hg (altitude approximately 17,000 feet or 5,200 meters) for six days. The oxygen pressure of the blood was carefully measured by the most approved methods. The conclusion was reached that during both rest and work less oxygen was contained in arterial blood in vivo than in samples of the same blood exposed to alveolar air in vitro at body temperature.

The experiments performed by members of the expedition to the Peruvian Andes in the winter of 1921–22 at a height of 14,200 feet (4,330) meters) also showed that the arterial oxygen tension was somewhat lower than the alveolar. Experiments performed on dogs by the Greenes (52) also supported this view.

Work done in the Colorado Mountains by Dill *et al.* (28) in 1929 failed to support the secretion hypothesis, as did those experiments performed by Dill, Christensen, and Edwards (27) at very high altitudes in Chile in 1935. These workers all felt that the evidence fully confirmed Barcroft's conclusion that even at high altitudes oxygen passed into the blood by diffusion only.

Forster assumes that Haldane's difficulties lay in the subjective colorimetric titration method which he used to measure blood carboxyhemoglobin (44).

ALVEOLAR AIR–ARTERIAL BLOOD OXYGEN GRADIENT

Several studies have been made of the oxygen gradient between alveolar air and arterial blood during exposure of man to decreased ambient oxygen tension. An early report by Lilienthal *et al.* (79) pointed out that the gradient in normal man at rest, breathing air, was 8.9 mm. Hg; by calculation this was attributed largely to venous admixture. The gradient was slightly increased to 9.1 mm. Hg when average alveolar oxygen tension was reduced to 45.8 mm. Hg. Using Bohr's graphic integration method 1.1 mm. Hg of this was computed to be due to venous admixture, and 8 mm. Hg, or most of the gradient, due to a difference between end-pulmonary capillary blood and alveolar air. This is very similar to the value found by Dill and Penrod (29) by using the difference between total tension of arterial blood gases and the ambient pressure at an alveolar oxygen tension of 39 mm. Hg. Smaller values for the alveolar-arterial oxygen gradient in hypoxia have been reported by Schmidt (109) and Bartels and Rodewald (9) who found values of 1.3 and 4.4–4.7, respectively. For the dog (mostly anesthetized) Williams (128) reported negligible gradients in hypoxia.

Asmussen and Nielsen in 1960–61 (3) investigated the alveolar-arterial oxygen gradient on the basis of the difference in the actual oxygen content of arterial blood and the calculated, theoretical value if the blood were in equilibrium with alveolar air. They finally concluded that an oxygen gradient does exist during hypoxia in man but that with the above method a precise estimation can hardly be made.

DIFFUSING CAPACITY OF LUNG

An expression of the diffusing capacity of the lung is the number of milliliters of oxygen taken up per minute for each millimeter of mean pressure gradient between pulmonary capillary blood and alveolar oxygen tension. It is commonly measured with either carbon monoxide, including the original breath holding method introduced by Krogh (74), or by the use of oxygen at normal and moderately hypoxic levels. Riley et al. (102) have determined diffusing capacity of the lungs with oxygen at three different levels of alveolar oxygen tensions in each of three subjects. They concluded that, in producing arterial oxygen saturations in the range above 82 per cent, changes vitiating a valid estimation of pulmonary diffusing capacity were negligible. Similar relations were seen by Fishman et al. (42) on values obtained during bronchospirometry with one lung hypoxic. With severe degrees of hypoxia (arterial oxygen tension below 40 mm. Hg) in combination with exercise, Riley with other collaborators (103) discerned a direct effect of hypoxia in increasing the pulmonary diffusing capacity. Either increased capillary surface or higher pulmonary blood flow could theoretically account for this (44). Bartels et al. (8) likewise found greater values in hypoxia than under normal conditions, but their method left a critical uncertainty in the estimation.

Determinations of pulmonary diffusing capacity with carbon monoxide have shown increases as the alveolar oxygen tension is lowered (45, 46, 106, 107, 108). However, since the presence of oxygen affects the rate of uptake of carbon monoxide by the blood, it is difficult to say whether the increase is due to this or to improvements in capillary diffusing surface, blood flow, or a combination of these. Cander and Forster (16) attempted to separate out the oxygen effect on carbon monoxide uptake by using a prior conditioning period with various alveolar oxygen tensions before the breath holding with carbon monoxide and a different oxygen tension. No effect of the conditioning period could be seen, though the subsequent test procedure followed so close as to preclude any possible changes in capillary diffusing surface or blood flow. The tentative conclusion is, therefore, that apparent hypoxic increases in diffusing capacity are in part artifacts of the carbon monoxide method.

In summary, the recent experimentation with developing techniques has produced conflicting results concerning hypoxic effects on diffusion in the lung. At the moment one cannot discard the findings with the direct oxygen method, even though confirmation with the carbon monoxide method is wanting. If and when agreement should be found between the two methods under eupneic conditions, one may anticipate an understanding of the intricacies of hypoxic and other conditions.

HEMIC HYPOXIA

Since carbon monoxide in combination with hemoglobin temporarily prevents the uptake of oxygen by the carboxyhemoglobin, the result is a reduction in effective oxygen capacity or toxic hypoxia, a variety of hemic hypoxia. (See Table 1, p. 8.) Lilienthal *et al.* (77, 78), in their studies of the uptake of carbon monoxide in man, reported the subjective symptoms of hemic hypoxia due to this cause. No symptoms were noted until the carboxyhemoglobin exceeded 15 per cent of the oxygen capacity. Lilienthal writes: "From 15 to 25 per cent the symptoms consisted of mild to moderate post-orbital headache, 'giddiness' and slight dyspnea on standing erect or slight exertion and, on a few occasions, mild nausea." When carbon monoxide was given at altitude the two types of hypoxia apparently summated to make the symptoms "much more marked."

The above workers, as well as Forbes *et al.* (43), have shown that the initial uptake of carbon monoxide depends upon the tension of carbon monoxide in the inspired air and the ventilation rate. Improved techniques made their findings superior to earlier reports. The ventilation factor makes the relation applicable to rest or work at sea level or at altitudes above sea level.

CHARACTER OF PULMONARY VENTILATION

Theoretically, since in hemic hypoxia the oxygen tension of arterial blood is within normal limits while the subject is breathing air at sea level, one would not expect any increased ventilation due to reflexes from the chemoreceptors. Ample confirmation of this theory has been provided by several workers. Chiodi et al. (17), in man and in the anesthetized dog, found no hyperpnea with saturation of hemoglobin up to 52 per cent with carbon monoxide. Comroe and Schmidt (21) had earlier found that perfusion with blood treated with carbon monoxide of the carotid sinus region of anesthetized dogs failed to stimulate ventilation if the oxygen tension of the blood was kept high. Duke et al. (36), recording nerve action potentials from the carotid body in the anesthetized cat, found that reduction of oxygen content of the blood by means of spontaneous breathing of 1 or 2 per cent carbon monoxide did not stimulate the chemoreceptors. Hull (69) more recently, in anesthetized dogs with hemic hypoxia induced by hemodilution or by carbon monoxide, found no essential change in ventilation rate, but tidal volume decreased while rate of breathing increased.

On the other hand, Chiodi et al. (18) have observed increased ventilation ratios in three of four patients with severe anemia (hemoglobin content 4.5–8.7 g/100 ml). Landgren and Neil (76), recording the carotid or aortic body chemoreceptor discharge in anesthetized cats, also found slight hemorrhage (20 ml.) capable of increasing the discharge. Giving pure oxygen to breathe at the same time would reduce the discharge. It was postulated that the hemorrhage reduced the blood supply to the chemoreceptors by local vasoconstriction and caused stimulation in this way.

Position of Oxyhemoglobin Dissociation Curve

In a recent study by Rodman et al. (105) the right shift in the oxyhemoglobin dissociation curve in anemic patients was confirmed by use of an in vivo technique in twenty-three subjects. Moderate displacement was seen with hemoglobin contents between 9 and 6.5 g/100 ml; more marked shifts, below 6.5. This confirms the earlier work of Kennedy and Valtis (72) and of Dill et al. (26) by in vitro methods. Kennedy and Valtis have found by indirect means a decreased pH of the red blood cell which may explain the shift in part. In no case is there an acidosis of the serum in anemia, but rather an alkalosis. These points were originally made by Dill et al. (26). The practical value of the shift is that oxygen can be more readily unloaded in the tissue capillaries, and consequently tissue oxygen tension does not decrease as much as it otherwise would.

On the other hand, in carbon monoxide poisoning, that is, toxic hypoxia, there is a shift to the left of the oxyhemoglobin dissociation curve (107). This shift, unfortunately, severely increases the degree of tissue hypoxia for any given reduction in effective oxygen capacity, because oxygen unloading can occur only with more depressed oxygen tensions.

REFERENCES

1. ALVAREZ-BUYLLA, R. 1952. *Ciencia (Mexico)*, **12**: 129.
2. ARMSTRONG, H. G. 1939. *Principles and Practices of Aviation Medicine*, p. 251. Baltimore: Williams & Wilkins Co.
3. ASMUSSEN, E., and NIELSEN, M. 1960; 1961. *Acta Physiol. Scand.*, **50**: 153; **51**: 385.
4. BAHNSON, H. T. 1952. *J. Appl. Physiol.*, **5**: 273.
5. BARCROFT, J. 1925. *The Respiratory Function of the Blood*, Part I, "Lessons from High Altitudes." Cambridge: Cambridge University Press.
6. BARCROFT, J., *et al.* 1920. *J. Physiol.*, **53**: 450.
7. BARCROFT, J., and KARVONEN, M. J. 1948. *J. Physiol.*, **107**: 153.
8. BARTELS, H., *et al.* 1955. *Pflueger Arch. Ges. Physiol.*, **261**: 99.
9. BARTELS, H., and RODEWALD, G. 1953. *Pflueger Arch. Ges. Physiol.*, **258**: 163.
10. BERT, P. 1878. *La Pression barometrique*. Paris: Masson.
11. BIRLEY, J. L. 1918. *Repts. Air Med. Invest. Comm., London*, Nos. 2 and 3.
12. BOOTHBY, W. M., *et al. In: Handbook of Respiratory Physiology*, p. 39. USAF Sch. Aviat. Med., Sept., 1954.
13. BOYCOTT, A. E., and HALDANE, J. S. 1908. *J. Physiol.*, **37**: 355.
14. BROWN, E. B., JR. 1944. *Res. Rept., USN Air Training Base* (Pensacola).
15. CAMPBELL, E. J. M. 1958. *The Respiratory Muscles and the Mechanics of Breathing*. Chicago: The Year Book Publishers.
16. CANDER, L., and FORSTER, R. E. 1955. *Amer. J. Physiol.*, **183**: 601.
17. CHIODI, H., *et al.* 1941. *Amer. J. Physiol.*, **134**: 683.
18. CHIODI, H., *et al.* 1948. *J. Appl. Physiol.*, **1**: 148.
19. COMROE, J. H., JR. 1939. *Amer. J. Physiol.*, **127**: 176.
20. COMROE, J. H., JR., *et al.* 1955. *The Lung, Clinical Physiology and Pulmonary Function Tests*, p. 186. Chicago: The Year Book Publishers.
21. COMROE, J. H., JR., and SCHMIDT, C. F. 1938. *Amer. J. Physiol.*, **121**: 75.
22. CROSS, K. W., and OPPE, T. E. 1952. *J. Physiol.*, **117**: 38.
23. DAVENPORT, H. W., *et al.* 1947. *Amer. J. Physiol.*, **148**: 406.
24. DECASTRO, F. 1951. *Acta Physiol. Scand.*, **22**: 14.
25. DEJOURS, P., *et al.* 1958. *Rev. Franc. Etud. Clin. Biol.*, **3**: 105.
26. DILL, D. B., *et al.* 1928. *J. Biol. Chem.*, **78**: 191.

27. DILL, D. B.; CHRISTENSEN, E. H.; and EDWARDS, H. T. 1936. *Amer. J. Physiol.,* 115: 530.
28. DILL, D. B., *et al.* 1931. *J. Physiol.,* 71: 47.
29. DILL, D. B., and PENROD, K. E. 1948. *Amer. J. Physiol.,* 155: 433.
30. DILL, D. B., and ZAMCHECK, N. 1940. *Amer. J. Physiol.,* 129: 47.
31. DOUGLAS, C. G., and HALDANE, J. S. 1912. *J. Physiol.,* 44: 305.
32. DOUGLAS, C. G., *et al.* 1931. *Phil. Trans. Roy. Soc., London,* B, 103: 185.
33. DOUGLAS, W. W. 1952. *J. Physiol.,* 118: 373.
34. DRIPPS, R. D., and COMROE, J. H., JR. 1944. *Amer. J. Med. Sci.,* 208: 681.
35. ———. 1947. *Amer. J. Physiol.,* 149: 277.
36. DUKE, H. N.; GREEN, J. H.; and NEIL, E. 1952. *J. Physiol.,* 118: 520.
37. ELLIS, M. M. 1919. *Amer. J. Physiol.,* 50: 267.
38. ENGEL, G. L., *et al.* 1946. *J. Clin. Invest.,* 25: 729.
39. EULER, C. VON, and SODERBERG, U. 1952. *J. Physiol.,* 118: 555.
40. EULER, U. S. VON; LILJESTRAND, G.; and ZOTTERMAN, Y. 1939. *Scand. Arch. Physiol.,* 83: 132.
41. FENN, W. O.; RAHN, H.; and OTIS, A. B. 1946. *Amer. J. Physiol.,* 146: 637.
42. FISHMAN, A. P., *et al.* 1955. *J. Clin. Invest.,* 34: 637.
43. FORBES, W. H.; SARGENT, F.; and ROUGHTON, F. J. W. 1945. *Amer. J. Physiol.,* 143: 594.
44. FORSTER, R. E. 1957. *Physiol. Rev.,* 37: 391.
45. FORSTER, R. E., *et al.* 1954. *J. Clin. Invest.,* 33: 1135.
46. FORSTER, R. E., 1957. *J. Appl. Physiol.,* 11: 277.
47. GEMMILL, C. L.; GEILING, E. M. K.; and REEVES, D. L. 1934. *Amer. J. Physiol.,* 109: 709.
48. GEORG, J., and SONNE, L. M. 1948. *Acta Physiol. Scand.,* 16: 52.
49. GERNANDT, B. E. 1946. *Acta Physiol. Scand.,* (Suppl. 35) 11: 1.
50. GRAY, J. S. April 12, 1943. *AAF Sch. Aviat. Med. Proj. No. 131.*
51. GRAY, J. S. 1950. *Pulmonary Ventilation and its Physiological Regulation,* p. 30. Springfield: Thomas.
52. GREENE, C. W., and GREENE, C. H. 1922. *Amer. J. Physiol.* (Proc.) , 59: 442.
53. GREENE, J. A. 1933. *A. M. A. Arch. Intern. Med.,* 52: 447.
54. HALDANE, J. S. 1922. *Respiration.* New Haven, Conn.: Yale University Press.
55. HALDANE, J. S. 1927. *Physiol. Rev.,* 7: 363.
56. HALDANE, J. S., and POULTON, E. P. 1908. *J. Physiol.,* 37: 390.
57. HALDANE, J. S., and PRIESTLEY, J. G. 1935. *Respiration* (2d ed.) . New Haven, Conn.: Yale University Press.
58. HALL, F. G. 1951. *Proc. Soc. Exp. Biol. Med.,* 78: 580.
59. ———. 1953. *J. Appl. Physiol.,* 5: 603.
60. HARRIS, A. S. 1945. *Amer. J. Physiol.,* 143: 140.

61. HENDERSON, L. J. 1928. *Blood: A Study in General Physiology.* New Haven, Conn.: Yale University Press.
62. HENDERSON, Y. 1938. *Adventures in Respiration.* Baltimore: Williams & Wilkins Co.
63. HEYMANS, C.; BOUCHAERT, J. J.; and DAUTREBANDE, L. 1930. *Arch. Int. Pharmocodyn.,* **39:** 400.
64. HINGSTON, R. W. G. 1925. *Geog. J.,* **65:** 4.
65. HINGSTON, R. W. G., cited in J. BARCROFT. 1925. *The Respiratory Function of Blood,* Part I, "Lessons from High Altitudes." (Consult Appendix I.) Cambridge: Cambridge University Press.
66. HOLLINGSHEAD, W. H. 1946. *Amer. J. Physiol.,* **147:** 654.
67. HORNBEIN, T. F., and ROOS, A. 1958. *J. Appl. Physiol.,* **12:** 86.
68. HORNBEIN, T. F., and ROOS, A. 1960. *Fed. Proc.,* **19:** 374.
69. HULL, W. E. 1957. *Amer. J. Physiol.,* **190:** 361.
70. HURTADO, A.; KALTREIDER, N.; and McCANN, W. S. 1934. *Amer. J. Physiol.,* **109:** 626.
71. JOURDANET, D. 1875. *Influence de la pression de l'air sur la vie de l'homme.* Paris: G. Masson.
72. KENNEDY, A. C., and VALTIS, D. J. 1954. *J. Clin. Invest.,* **33:** 1372.
73. KROGH, A. 1910. *Skand. Arch. Physiol.,* **23:** 248.
74. KROGH, M. 1915. *J. Physiol.,* **49:** 271.
75. LAMBERTSEN, C. J. *et al.* 1957. *Fed. Proc.,* **16:** 76.
76. LANDGREN, S., and NEIL, E. 1951. *Acta Physiol. Scand.,* **23:** 158.
77. LILIENTHAL, J. L., JR., and PINE, M. B. 1946. *Amer. J. Physiol.,* **145:** 346.
78. LILIENTHAL, J. L., JR., *et al.* 1946. *Amer. J. Physiol.,* **145:** 351.
79. ———. 1946. *Amer. J. Physiol.,* **147:** 199.
80. LLOYD, B. B.; JUKES, M. G. M., and CUNNINGHAM, D. J. C. 1958. *Quart. J. Exp. Physiol.,* **43:** 214.
81. LOESCHCKE, G. C. 1953. *Pflueger Arch. Ges. Physiol.,* **257:** 349.
82. LOESCHCKE, H. H. 1949. *Pflueger Arch. Ges. Physiol.,* **251:** 211.
83. LOESCHCKE, H. H.; KOEPCHEN, H.; and GERTZ, K. H. 1958. *Pflueger Arch. Ges. Physiol.,* **266:** 569.
84. LOEWY, A., and MOERIKOFER, W. 1932. *Physiologie des Hohenklimas.* Berlin: J. Springer.
85. LOEWY, A., and WITTKOWER, E. 1937. *The Pathology of High Altitude Climate.* London: Oxford University Press.
86. LUTZ, B. R., and SCHNEIDER, E. C. 1919. *Amer. J. Physiol.,* **50:** 280.
87. ———. *Ibid.,* p. 327.
88. MEAKINS, J. C., and DAVIES, H. W. 1925. *Respiratory Function in Disease.* Edinburgh and London: Oliver & Boyd.
89. MEANS, J. H. 1924. *Dyspnoea.* Baltimore: Williams & Wilkins Co.
90. MILLER, H. C., and SMULL, N. W. 1955. *Pediatrics,* **16:** 93.
91. MOE, G. K.; CAPO, L. R.; and PERALTA, B. 1948. *Amer. J. Physiol.,* **153:** 601.

92. Mosso, A. 1899. *Life of Man in the High Alps.* London: Fisher.
93. Nicholson, H. C., and Trimby, R. H. 1942. *Amer. J. Physiol.*, 137: 136.
94. Nielson, M., and Smith, H. 1952. *Acta Physiol. Scand.*, 24: 293.
95. Otey, E. S., and Bernthal, T. 1960. *Fed. Proc.*, 19: 373.
96. Otis, A. B.; Rahn, H.; and Fenn, W. O. 1948. *Amer. J. Physiol.*, 152: 674.
97. Peyser, E.; Sass-Kortsak, A.; and Verzar, F. 1960. *Amer. J. Physiol.*, 163: 111.
98. Rahn, H., and Fenn, W. O. 1955. *A Graphical Analysis of the Respiratory Gas Exchange, The O_2—CO_2 Diagram*, p. 37. Washington, D.C.: The American Physiological Society.
99. Rahn, H., and Hammond, D. 1952. *J. Appl. Physiol.*, 4: 715.
100. Rahn, H., and Otis, A. B. 1947. *Amer. J. Physiol.*, 150: 202.
101. ———. 1949. *Amer. J. Physiol.*, 157: 445.
102. Riley, R. L.; Cournand, A.; and Donald, K. W. 1951. *J. Appl. Physiol.*, 4: 102.
103. Riley, R. L., et al. 1954. *J. Appl. Physiol.*, 6: 573.
104. Rodbard, S. 1947. *Amer. J. Physiol.*, 150: 142.
105. Rodman, T.; Close, H. P.; and Purcell, M. K. 1960. *Ann. Intern. Med.*, 52: 295.
106. Roughton, F. J. W. 1945. *Amer. J. Physiol.*, 143: 621.
107. ———. *In: Handbook of Respiratory Physiology*, p. 51. USAF Sch. Aviat. Med., Sept. 1954.
108. Roughton, F. J. W., and Forster, R. E. 1957. *J. Appl. Physiol.*, 11: 290.
109. Schmidt, C. F. *In:* P. Bard (ed.). *Medical Physiology*, p. 312. St. Louis: Mosby, 1956.
110. Schneider, E. C. 1932. *Yale J. Biol. Med.*, 4: 537.
111. *Ibid.*
112. Schneider, E. C. 1921. *Physiol. Rev.*, 1: 631.
113. ———. 1932. *Amer. J. Physiol.*, 110: 426.
114. Schneider, E. C., and Clarke, R. W. 1926. *Amer. J. Physiol.*, 75: 297.
115. Shock, N. W., and Soley, M. H. 1940. *Proc. Soc. Exp. Biol. Med.*, 44: 418.
116. ———. 1942. *Amer. J. Physiol.*, 137: 256.
117. Stroud, R. C. 1959. *J. Appl. Physiol.*, 14: 353.
118. Swann, H. G.; Dittmer, D. S.; and Grebe, R. M. 1958. *In: Handbook of Respiration*, p. 151. (Proj. 7158; Task 71801) WADC TR 58–352) .
119. Swann, H. G., and Brucer, M. 1949. *Texas Rep. Biol. Med.*, 7: 539.
120. Tenney, S. M., et al. 1953. *J. Appl. Physiol.*, 5: 607.
121. Tschirgi, R. D., and Gerard, R. W. 1947. *Amer. J. Physiol.*, 150: 358.

122. VAN LIERE, E. J. 1942. *Anoxia, Its Effect on the Body.* Chicago: University of Chicago Press.
123. VERZAR, F. 1933. *Schweiz. Med. Wschr.,* **63:** 17.
124. ———. 1933. *Pflueger Arch. Ges. Physiol.,* **232:** 322.
125. ———. 1945, 1948. *Hohenklima-Forschungen des Basler Physiologischen Institutes.* Basel: Schwabe.
126. VERZAR, F., and JEKER, L. 1936. *Pflueger Arch. Ges. Physiol.,* **238:** 379.
127. WATT, J. C.; DUMKE, P. R.; and COMROE, J. H., JR. 1943. *Amer. J. Physiol.,* **138:** 610.
128. WILLIAMS, M. H., JR. 1953. *Amer. J. Physiol.,* **173:** 77.
129. WINDER, C. V. 1942. *Amer. J. Physiol.,* **136:** 200.
130. WITZLEB, E., *et al.* 1955. *Pflueger Arch. Ges. Physiol.,* **261:** 211.
131. ZUNTZ, N., and LOEWY, A. 1906. *Hohenklima und Bergwanderungen.* Berlin: Bong & Co.

CHAPTER IX

MOUNTAIN SICKNESS AND ALTITUDE SICKNESS

MOUNTAIN SICKNESS

It has been known for a long time that ascent to a high altitude often produces illness; the typical symptoms are nausea, vomiting, headache, physical and mental depression, and gastrointestinal disturbances.

The symptoms of mountain sickness have been described in some detail by Mosso (34), Barcroft (3, 4), Haldane and Priestley (14), Monge (30, 31, 32, 33), Hurtado (23), and others writing on the physiology of high altitudes. This subject has also received considerable attention from various authors in treatises on mountaineering (10, 12, 15, 17). The reader is referred to these sources for many details of this interesting subject.

A considerable individual variation exists in the ability to withstand oxygen want, as has been emphasized repeatedly; this is especially true when applied to the possibility of suffering from mountain sickness. Some individuals are affected at a relatively low altitude, such as 7,000 or 8,000 feet (2,130 or 2,400 meters, respectively), while others are comparatively immune. It has been said that an elevation of 10,000 feet (3,050 meters) may produce symptoms in some subjects, while others may escape symptoms up to 14,000 feet (4,270 meters); very few, however, can venture to a height of 19,000 feet (5,790 meters) without showing marked symptoms of mountain sickness (1).

Mountain sickness may manifest itself suddenly when the subject has gone too far beyond his own critical line. An example of this is the mountain sickness which some tourists experience on Pike's Peak or that which is experienced by aviators in airplanes flying at high altitudes without the use of oxygen. On the other hand, mountain sickness may develop more slowly. The subject first experiences a feeling of exceptional well-being but soon shows signs of cyanosis and experiences some premonitory symptoms, such as a feeling of dizziness when stooping over. In a few hours a feeling of lassitude appears. Toward evening a headache may develop, followed by a restless and troubled sleep. On awakening in the morning he suffers from a bad frontal headache and shows the symptoms of acute mountain sickness, which have been listed earlier. There may be not only nausea and vomiting but other gastrointestinal disturbances; the tongue becomes furred, there is a loss of appetite, and diarrhea and abdominal pain sometimes develop. Some subjects complain of sensations of cold. In fact, the symptoms are very much like an acute attack of migraine. There may also be a tendency to periodic breathing, and at times hyperpnea accompanies physical exertion.

McFarland (29) in 1937 reported that the ten most commonly observed physiological changes in members of the International High Altitude Expedition to Chile, in order of frequency, were as follows: (*a*) shortness of breath on exertion and easy fatigability, (*b*) breathing irregularities, (*c*) cold extremities, (*d*) dry skin, (*e*) disturbed sleep, (*f*) gas in stomath or intestine, (*g*) headache, (*h*) sore throat, (*i*) irregular pulse, and (*j*) lassitude.

Interestingly enough, McFarland also pointed out that the following symptoms, which are frequently mentioned in the literature, seldom occurred: marked sensory impairment, nose bleeding, loss of appetite, nausea, tremors, and muscular impairment. It must be remembered, however, that the observations made by the members of this expedition were obtained from a small number of subjects (ten) and from a highly select group.

Barcroft (3) pointed out that after the acute symptoms of *soroche* (the South American term for acute mountain sickness) had subsided, cyanosis remained in some degree in members of his South American party. Other aftereffects of low oxygen want also manifested themselves, such as some retardation in mental processes, shown by repeated errors made in performing routine laboratory experiments and by difficulty in the use of the slide rule and logarithms. In fact, both the mental and the physical factors were impaired to some extent in all or nearly all members of the party.

Some relatively recent experiences in mountain sickness are of interest. Pugh and Ward (36) have reported observations on mountain sickness in groups of mountain climbers in the Himalayas in the early 1950's. They pointed out that although few people escape acute symptoms altogether, the fully developed picture of acute mountain sickness reported by Barcroft (3) in 1925, characterized by headache, irritability, nausea, vomiting, cyanosis, fever, tachycardia and dyspnea lasting one to three days, was rarely if ever observed. In the

Himalayas the principal effects above 18,000 feet (5,485 meters) were lassitude, retardation, anorexia, hyperpnea, and Cheynes-Stokes respiration. During exercise a heaviness of the limbs, breathlessness, and reduced endurance was noted.

High-altitude disease.—Monge[1] (30) in 1932 described what he termed "high-altitude disease," which subsequently has been called "Monge's disease." He classified this disease into two types: (*a*) the erythremic type, which he called "high-altitude erythremia," since the symptoms resembled those of Osler-Vaquez disease; and (*b*) the emphysematous type, in which the respiratory symptoms are more marked.

1. High-altitude erythremia: According to Monge, this type may appear in one of two forms: (*a*) the subacute type, which is mild; and (*b*) the chronic mountain sickness, which is severe.

a) Subacute type: This condition is not always preceded by a preliminary attack of acute mountain sickness. The symptoms may appear insidiously; there is first a feeling of generalized fatigue, which bears no relation to the amount of work performed. Common ailments are poorly resisted and convalescence unduly prolonged. Other symptoms are: cyanosis (produced by the least effort), cephalalgia, tendency to sleepiness, periodic type of breathing, and a marked congestion of the mucous membranes of the eyes, ears, and nose. Digestion is impaired, and the subject loses weight. If the patient continues to live in high altitudes, the symptoms often become worse; and nausea, vomiting, and dizziness appear, as well as troublesome paresthesias. The red blood cell count is generally about 7,000,-000 per cubic millimeter, and the hemoglobin is increased from 10 to 20 per cent. The disease may disappear spontaneously, which means that complete acclimatization has taken place. If this does not occur, the symptoms become aggravated, and the patient suffers from the second type, or chronic mountain sickness.

b) Chronic mountain sickness: This is a serious disease, and unless the afflicted subject moves to lower altitudes, he may die. The symptoms are, for the main part, similar to those already described under the subacute type, but they are more severe. The cyanosis, for example, may be so pronounced that the face is purple or almost black; the cephalalgia may be violent; the tendency to sleep is more marked; and, in severe cases, the subject may fall into a coma for several hours. In addition to the symptoms enumerated under the subacute type,

[1] The reader is referred to Monge's monograph, "La Enfermedad de los Andes," *An. de la Facultad de ciencias medicas* (Lima), 1932; and also to Monge's review, "Chronic Mountain Sickness," *Physiol. Rev.*, 23 (1943), 166.

there may be a clubbing of the fingers, and the hands often become large and engorged with blood. There is often aphonia and epistaxis. The dyspnea is profound, and the thorax becomes large and emphysematous. Bronchitis is frequently found, and considerable congestion of the lungs manifested; hemoptysis occurs and fever may be present. There also may be signs of cardiac insufficiency of the right heart.

The nervous and mental symptoms are extremely annoying; the patient complains of severe algesias and paresthesias, which may occur in almost any portion of the body. There may be an entire change in the personality. Monge gave an instance of an engineer who suffered crises of mental confusion at which times he made gross errors in drawing and in his mathematical computations. Often the subjects become indifferent and apathetic, and Monge cites an example of a subject who refused to go down to sea level and finally had to be taken down in a comatose condition. There is a marked polycythemia; the red blood cell count may vary from 7,000,000 to 12,000,000 per cubic millimeter. Hultgren and Spickard (19) have pointed out that chronic mountain sickness is essentially the hypoventilation syndrome occurring at high altitude.

As mentioned previously, in severe cases the patient will die unless he is taken down to sea level. If he remains at a low altitude for a while, he can return to the high regions again; but once the disease manifests itself, it is apt to recur with increasing severity, so that more frequent trips must be made to lower levels and longer sojourns made there. In some instances the subject can no longer reside at high altitudes. If he persists in remaining at high altitudes, death is caused from hemorrhage, pulmonary thrombosis, bronchopneumonia, or progressive cardiac insufficiency.

2. Emphysematous type: The pulmonary symptoms predominate in this type of mountain sickness, as previously mentioned. As a rule, the patient has a long history of bronchitis; dyspnea is the major symptom and is produced by the least effort. Cyanosis is pronounced, and sometimes there is hemoptysis. The thorax is globular in shape, and the vital capacity is diminished. There may be an insufficiency of the right heart and a clubbing of the fingers—in short, a rather characteristic picture of a chronic emphysematous condition.

It is seen that high-altitude disease produces protean manifestations. Monge points out that the predominance of any one symptom is probably a result of the fact that the particular organ involved suffers the most from oxygen want. Lastly, he feels that high-altitude sickness is a distinct nosographic entity, since all symptoms disappear as soon as the patient reaches sea level.

Chronic mountain sickness is seen less frequently today, probably because of improved methods of transportation and higher health standards of workers (19, 24). A patient who develops symptoms of chronic mountain sickness may now be moved immediately and rapidly to a lower elevation.

Cause of acute mountain sickness.—It was first pointed out by Paul Bert (5) that the essential cause of mountain sickness was the lowered partial pressure of oxygen in the lungs. His theory, however, was challenged by Langstaff and also by Mosso. Langstaff ascribed the symptoms of mountain sickness to a combination of physical fatigue and a poverty of diet. He wrote a treatise expounding his views, called *Mountain Sickness and Its Probable Causes* (London, 1906). Filippi (10) held virtually the same view.

Mosso (34), the Italian physiologist, thought that at high altitudes carbon dioxide left the body in some unknown manner and that this caused mountain sickness. This was called the "acapnia theory" and enjoyed wide acceptance for some time. In 1939 Dill, Edwards, and Robinson (9) produced some evidence which supported Mosso's original theory, namely, that the loss of carbon dioxide from the body at high altitudes played an important part in mountain sickness. These investigators allowed subjects to breathe, at a total pressure of 435 mm. Hg, a mixture containing enough oxygen to cause it to exert a partial pressure of about 90 mm. Hg. The arterial carbon dioxide tension was found to be lower than when the subjects breathed mixtures containing oxygen at a similar partial pressure but at sea level. Dill *et al.* felt that this could not be accounted for by the difference in pulmonary ventilation or in oxygen consumption but that carbon dioxide actually left the blood more rapidly at low barometric pressures, as first claimed by Mosso. One factor to which they ascribed the difference was the better mixing at low barometric pressures of the alveolar and dead-space air.

Neither Langstaff's nor Mosso's theory, however, is now generally accepted. The present concept is that the lowered partial pressure of oxygen in the lungs is the essential factor in the production of mountain sickness. This was the original view expressed by Paul Bert.

There are other factors which may play a part in the production of mountain sickness. One is the psychic element; it is hard to evaluate how important this is, but it probably plays a more significant role than is generally recognized. The sight or smell of food, for example, often produces nausea at high altitudes much as it does in passengers on board ship.

Any factor which lessens the blood supply to the brain may aid either in bringing on a bout of mountain sickness or in accentuating one already present. Exercise, which causes the blood to go to the muscles, and eating, which causes it to go to the splanchnic area, are thought capable of playing such a role. It should be stated, however, that some authors feel that these factors do not materially reduce the blood supply to the brain.

There are, moreover, more subtle, not thoroughly understood factors which may influence mountain sickness. A number of observers have noticed that mountain sickness varies in incidence from one locality to another even though these localities are at the same approximate altitudes. Zuntz (40) long ago pointed out that this was an important consideration. He made the statement that mountain sickness occurred at 9,840 feet (3,000 meters) in the Alps and the Caucasus; at 13,125 feet (4,000 meters) in the Andes; and at 16,405 feet (5,000 meters) in the Himalayas. Some authors would probably question the validity of this and would quote different experiences; but many writers nevertheless agree that the chance of suffering from mountain sickness varies in different localities, although the altitudes are approximately the same.

Still other factors have been mentioned from time to time which may influence either the severity of the attack of mountain sickness or its production; among these are wind, weather, the incidence of ice or snow on the rocks, or their barrenness. Pugh and Ward (36) have pointed out that the intense heat and glare on Himalayan glaciers at altitudes between 18,000 feet (5,485 meters) and 22,000 feet (6,705 meters) are considered by some to be almost as important a cause for headache and lassitude as the hypoxia. Other factors besides those mentioned may be found in the literature of mountaineering.

Although the main cause of mountain sickness, as has been emphasized, is the lowered partial pressure of oxygen in the lungs, some of the other factors mentioned cannot entirely be ignored. At any rate, there has not been, as yet, a complete and satisfactory explanation of its occurrence. It was postulated by Barcroft (3) that mountain sickness is produced by the effect of oxygen want on the brain. On the other hand, he at one time mentioned that vomiting is produced by lack of acid in the blood, which stimulates the vomiting center. On this account he urged the subject to engage in physical exercise to raise the acid content of the blood.

Haldane, Kellas, and Kennaway (13) have expressed the view that mountain sickness is probably due to a combination of hypoxia and alkalosis. They felt that if the kidneys were able to eliminate excess blood alkalies quickly, the subject's tolerance to high altitudes would be greater. Lenggenhager (26) in 1942 also reported that high altitude sickness is probably caused by a combination of oxygen deficiency and accompanying acute alkalosis.

Sundstroem (38) found in himself an alkalosis of the blood during an attack of mountain sickness; in the afternoon of the same day that his attack subsided, he found a normal hydrogen-ion concentration. He, too, felt it was likely that mountain sickness might be explained by the inability of the kidneys to respond quickly enough to the excess bases in the blood.

Pertinent, too, is the observation (7, 16, 35) that inhalation of proper dilutions of carbon dioxide reduces the symptoms of mountain sickness. This points to the theory that alkalosis may play an important part in its development. Barcroft also suggested long ago that the production of acid should be encouraged if an attack of mountain sickness seemed pending. On the other hand, the ingestion of ammonium chloride (see p. 353), which is known to produce an acidosis, has given rather disappointing results in combating the development of mountain sickness. The problem, therefore, is apparently not so simple.

In summary, the mechanisms actually responsible for acute mountain sickness are not, as yet, thoroughly understood. They are doubtless associated with chemical changes in the body brought about by the low oxygen pressure. A complete explanation of the cause of mountain sickness cannot be given until the exact nature of these changes is known.

Cause of chronic mountain sickness.—The cause for chronic mountain sickness is quite unknown. It has been suggested by Talbott and Dill (39) that the symptoms may be due to pathologic changes occurring in tissues which have been exposed to oxygen want for a long time. They also suggest that the abundant ultraviolet rays at high altitudes may be responsible for this condition.

Acute high-altitude pulmonary edema.—It was first pointed out by Hurtado (22) in 1937 that exposure to high altitude may produce an acute pulmonary edema. Since Hurtado's observations this syndrome has engaged the attention of a number of workers (18, 19, 20, 21, 25).

The newcomer to altitude who travels in a day or two to elevations of 10,000 feet (4,877 meters) or so may suffer from acute pulmonary edema from six to thirty-six hours after his arrival. The symptoms first noticed are a dry cough, dypsnea, or weakness on effort. The patient often complains of a feeling of pain or pressure over the lower substernal region. On occasion the patient experiences anorexia, nausea, and even vomiting. In grave conditions orthopnea and hemoptysis occur, and coma and death may follow. If, however, patients so afflicted receive bed care and are given oxygen before these grave symptoms appear, the majority recover rapidly and may be entirely well within two or three days.

Acute high-altitude pulmonary edema may also be seen in the acclimatized mountaineer. It is more apt to occur when such an individual has been residing at lower levels for a little time and returns to high elevations. Unless oxygen is administered, or unless he is transported to lower levels, such a person may die.

Sickness produced by types of hypoxia other than anoxic—While anoxic hypoxia produces what is generally understood to be "true mountain sickness," other types of hypoxia can produce symptoms which, in many ways, resemble it. In stagnant hypoxia, such as that produced by circulatory disturbances, the patient often experiences nausea and, in severe cases, vomiting. Intestinal disturbances are also manifested, and a feeling of lassitude and weakness, as well as a physical and mental depression, is exhibited.

In the hemic type of hypoxia, such as that found in pernicious anemia, disturbances similar to those described under stagnant hypoxia may occur. The anemia must be very severe, however, before grave symptoms appear. Later, when the nervous system becomes involved because of the lack of oxygen there may be great muscular weakness and inco-ordination. These symptoms, however, are the result of organic changes in the central nervous system; so, in this respect, they differ from those produced by the hypoxic type.

The symptoms of histotoxic hypoxia fall into a somewhat different category. Cyanide, of course, causes an intense stimulation of the respiratory center, and hypernea is the most noticeable symptom. Alcohol, which is generally considered a histotoxic agent, produces many of the symptoms observed in the hypoxic type. If taken in excess, nausea and vomiting result; this, however, is caused by local irritant action. It also produces headache, lassitude, and physical and mental depression.

ALTITUDE SICKNESS

General H. G. Armstrong (2) pointed out that Professor E. C. Schneider in 1918 suggested the term "altitude sickness"[2] be used to des-

[2] For a detailed discussion of altitude sickness the reader is referred to chapter 13 of General Armstrong's *Principles and Practices of Aviation Medicine* (3d ed.; Baltimore: Williams & Wilkins Co., 1952) ; and to chapter 9, by U. C. Luft, in *Aerospace Medicine*, edited by H. G. Armstrong (Baltimore: Williams & Wilkins Co., 1961). The authors of this monograph have drawn freely on these two chapters for the discussion concerning altitude sickness.

ignate illness produced by flights at high altitude, to differentiate it from mountain sickness. Altitude sickness is produced by breathing air containing a low partial pressure of oxygen and can be brought about by aircraft flights at high altitudes. Dr. Luft (27) has recently written that altitude sickness may be defined as a state of acute oxygen want resulting from reduced partial pressure of oxygen in the inspired air at altitude. Armstrong recognized two forms, acute and chronic.

The reader may question whether an actual distinction can be made between altitude sickness and mountain sickness. It may be pointed out, however, that in the former instance the rapid rate of ascent, about 1,000 feet (305 meters) per minute, is worthy of note; and furthermore, the individual presumably is not under the influence of exercise.

TABLE 8

SUBJECTIVE SYMPTOMS OCCURRING IN ORDER OF FREQUENCY DURING
FLIGHTS AT HIGH ALTITUDES*

12,000 Feet (3,660 Meters)	14,000 Feet (4,270 Meters)	16,000 Feet (4,875 Meters)
Sleepiness	Headache	Headache
Headache	Altered respiration	Altered respiration
Altered respiration	Sleepiness	Psychologic impairment
Lassitude	Psychologic impairment	Euphoria
Fatigue	Lassitude	Sleepiness
Psychologic impairment	Fatigue	Lassitude
Euphoria	Euphoria	Fatigue

* From H. G. Armstrong, *Principles and Practices of Aviation Medicine* (3d ed.; Baltimore: Williams & Wilkins Co., 1952), p. 201.

Acute altitude sickness.—It has been stated (2) that in young, healthy male adults the first significant changes which occur in the body from altitude disease are at about 9,000 feet (2,745 meters). At a rate of ascent of 1,000 feet per minute the subject will become unconscious at an altitude of approximately 25,000 feet (7,620 meters).

Subjective symptoms.—Table 8 gives the subjective symptoms which occur, in the order of their frequency.

Armstrong emphasizes the fact that it is not unusual for a person subjected to acute hypoxia to become unconscious without being aware of any change from the normal. Most individuals, however, experience mild subjective symptoms during an attack of altitude sickness. During aircraft ascent at a rate of climb of 200 feet (60 meters) per minute or at a rate of climb of 1,000 feet (305 meters) per minute, the first subjective symptoms are usually noted at about 10,000 feet (3,050 meters) or 12,000 feet (3,660 meters) altitude.

Individuals may respond differently to an exposure of 12,000 feet altitude or above. Some may complain of fatigue and mental depression and have a tendency to fall asleep. Others may become euphoric and engage in outbursts of hilarity and uncontrolled laughter; still others may become surly and even pugnacious. The subjects, of course, are totally unaware of their unnatural behavior. These symptoms may occur also during the ascent of a high mountain.

It has been pointed out by Armstrong that when hypoxia is induced suddenly, such as might occur from pressurized cabin failure, the subjective symptoms are much more pronounced than those described in Table 8. Under such circumstances the subject may become dizzy, see spots before his eyes, and have a disagreeable sensation of suffocation. If the altitude is not too great, the body brings into play certain compensatory mechanisms which help alleviate some of the acute symptoms.

It is extremely important to recognize, as emphasized by Armstrong, that in some instances the symptoms of altitude sickness are so mild that the subject is unaware of any danger. Indeed, the symptoms may be entirely absent, or worse, the subject feels euphoric. This is most unfortunate since a pilot, who is responsible for the lives of his passengers, might wreck his plane. It is a pity that altitude sickness does not manifest itself early by a painful, or at least a disagreeable, process. Fortunately pilots now are required to use oxygen masks if they fly above a certain elevation, and then, too, most passenger planes have pressurized cabins.

Objective symptoms.—The effects of acute hypoxia on the various organs of the body are responsible for the objective symptoms manifested in acute altitude sickness. These effects are considered in appropriate places throughout this monograph.

Aftereffects.—Armstrong states that prolonged passive exposure at altitudes less than 9,000 feet (2,745 meters) or momentary exposures up to 25,000 feet (7,620 meters) produce no uncomfortable aftereffects.

Distressing symptoms such as intractable headache, nausea, and vomiting may be produced by flying at altitudes of 15,000 feet (4,570 meters) to 18,000 feet (5,485 meters) for several hours. Other symptoms associated with acute hypoxia, particularly mental confusion and muscular weakness, may also occur. At great altitudes, 24,000 feet (6,095 meters) or over, these symptoms sometimes appear in the unacclimatized individual within fifteen to twenty minutes. When such severe symptoms are produced, they often last from as long as forty-eight to seventy-two hours.

At 25,000 feet (7,620 meters), death may occur within twenty or thirty minutes. Death from acute altitude sickness is probably always due to failure of the respiratory center; this may occur at altitudes as low as 16,000 feet (4,875 meters).

Luft (28) has divided the various subjective and objective manifestations of altitude sickness into four phases: (a) Indifferent phase (ground level to 10,000 feet—3,050 meters). There is no significant impairment at this altitude. (b) Compensatory phase (10,000–15,000 feet—3,050–4,570 meters, respectively). At this range the physiologic adjustments are able to compensate fairly well for the effects of the hypoxia. (c) Phase of distress (15,000–20,000 feet—4,570–6,100 meters, respectively). At these heights the compensatory mechanism becomes inadequate. (d) Critical phase (20,000–25,000 feet—6,100–7,620 meters, respectively). At these extreme altitudes there is loss of compensation and of position. Convulsions may occur, and respiration ceases followed by circulatory failure.

Chronic altitude sickness.—According to Armstrong, chronic altitude sickness is produced by repeated aircraft flights to high altitudes, so that the subject is exposed repeatedly to air which contains a low partial pressure of oxygen. It is thought that repeated exposures to rarefied air have a cumulative effect on the body. It was observed by a number of investigators (6, 8, 11) during the war of 1914–18 that airplane pilots who had made successive flights to high altitudes showed evidence of chronic fatigue, while those pilots who had used oxygen at high altitudes did not show these symptoms to such a marked degree.

Although it was understood, in a general way, that repeated exposures to high altitudes caused considerable disability in pilots, no well-controlled experiments were carried out on this problem until Armstrong (2) made a rather extensive study on the effect of repeated exposures to high altitudes in human beings. He subjected ten healthy college students to a simulated altitude of 12,000 feet (3,660 meters) in a steel chamber for twenty-seven consecutive days (except Sundays). They were divided into two groups; one was kept at this simulated altitude for four hours, and the other, for seven hours.

Subjective symptoms.—After the first few days the four-hour group complained during the exposure of mild headaches, which persisted for several hours afterward. Later in the course of the experiment, the headaches were less frequent; but the subjects complained of sleepiness, disinclination for activity of any sort, and physical fatigue. During the third week they complained of increasing irritability, nervousness, insomnia, and other symptoms referable to the central nervous system.

The seven-hour group showed symptoms generally similar to those of the four-hour group, but at the end of the first week of exposure they had additional complaints of mild attacks of nausea, anorexia, indigestion and vertigo. These latter symptoms were obviously like those of mountain sickness.

Objective symptoms.—The objective symptoms observed in the individuals who had been exposed to a simulated altitude of 12,000 feet (3,660 meters) varied in the two groups. The seven-hour group showed a slight loss in average body weight. The group also showed distinct signs of acclimatization, as seen by the red cell count and the rise in hemoglobin; the four-hour group did not show these signs. Armstrong felt that this difference was important since it indicated that probably no less than a seven-hour daily exposure is necessary to produce what they termed a positive acclimatization.

In this connection it must be recognized that an increased red cell count and a rise in hemoglobin are not the only signs of acclimatization. It is quite possible that the four-hour group also showed a certain amount of adaptation to altitude (see chap. x on acclimatization).

Certain psychological changes were also noted, such as mental sluggishness and a slight loss of muscular co-ordination. Other symptoms referable to the central nervous system were noted.

Finally, Armstrong has called attention to the fact that the symptoms of chronic altitude sickness somewhat resemble those of Addison's disease. He mentions that, although it has not been proved, the symptoms might possibly be due to adrenocortical insufficiency. Obviously more work is needed on this interesting problem. The researches of Selye (37) in this connection are, of course, of distinct interest.

REFERENCES

1. *Air Service Medical,* p. 138. Washington, D.C.: U.S. Govt. Printing Office, 1919.
2. ARMSTRONG, H. G. 1952. *Principles and Practices of Aviation Medicine* (3d ed.). Baltimore: Williams & Wilkins Co.
3. BARCROFT, J. 1925. *The Respiratory Function of the Blood,* Part I, "Lessons from High Altitudes." Cambridge: Cambridge University Press.
4. BARCROFT, J., et al. 1923. *Phil. Trans. Roy. Soc., London,* B, **211:** 351.
5. BERT, P. 1878. *La Pression barometrique.* Paris: Masson.

6. BIRLEY, J. 1920. *Brit. Privy Counc. Med. Res. Counc., Spec. Rept. Ser.*, No. 53, p. 5.

7. CHILDS, S. B.; HAMLIN, B. H.; and HENDERSON, Y. 1935. *Nature*, 135: 457.

8. CORBETT, C. D. W., and BAZETT, H. C. 1920. *Brit. Privy Counc., Med. Res. Counc., Spec. Rept. Ser.*, No. 53, p. 18.

9. DILL, D. B.; EDWARDS, H. T.; and ROBINSON, S. 1939. *J. Aviat. Med.*, 10: 3.

10. FILIPPI, F., DE. 1912. *Karakoram and Western Himalaya.* London: Constable & Co.

11. FLACK, M. 1920. *Brit. Privy Counc., Med. Res. Counc., Spec. Rept. Ser.*, No. 53, p. 93.

12. GREEN, R. 1934. *Everest 1933*, chap. ii. London: Hodder & Stoughton.

13. HALDANE, J. S.; KELLAS, A. S.; and KENNAWAY, E. L. 1919. *J. Physiol.*, 53: 181.

14. HALDANE, J. S., and PRIESTLEY, J. G. 1935. *Respiration* (2d ed.) . New Haven, Conn.: Yale University Press.

15. HARTMAN, A. H. 1935. *Verh. Deutsch. Ges. Inn. Med.*, 46: 48.

16. HASSELBALCH, K. A., and LINDHARD, J. 1915; 1916. *Biochem. Z.*, 68: 265, 295; 74: 1.

17. HINGSTON, R. W. G. 1925. *Geog. J.*, 65: 4.

18. HOUSTON, C. S. 1960. *New Engl. J. Med.* 263: 478.

19. HULTGREN, H., and SPICKARD, W. 1960. *Stanford Med. Bull.*, 18: 76.

20. HULTGREN, H. N., *et al.* 1961. *Medicine*, 40: 289.

21. HULTGREN, H. N.; SPICKARD, W. B.; and LOPEZ, C. 1962. *Brit. Heart J.*, 24: 95.

22. HURTADO, A. *Aspectos Fisiologicos y Patologicos de la Vida en la Altura. Imp.*, ed. S. A. Rimae. Lima.

23. ———. 1942. *J.A.M.A.*, 120: 1278.

24. ———. 1960. (Personal communication.)

25. ———. 1960. *Ann. Int. Med.*, 53: 247.

26. LENGGENHAGER, K. 1942. *Helv. Med. Acta*, 9: 269.

27. LUFT, U. C. *In:* H. G. ARMSTRONG (ed.) . 1961. *Aerospace Medicine*, p. 120. Baltimore: Williams and Wilkins Co.

28. ———. *Ibid.*, p. 135.

29. MCFARLAND, R. A. 1937. *J. Comp. Psychol.*, 24: 147.

30. MONGE, C. 1932. "La Enfermedad de los Andes," *An. Fac. Ciencias Med., Lima.*

31. ———. 1937. *Arch. Int. Med.*, 59: 32.

32. ———. 1942. *Science*, 95: 79.

33. ———. 1943. *Physiol. Rev.*, 23: 166.

34. MOSSO, A. 1899. *Life of Man in the High Alps.* London: Fisher.

35. MOSSO, A., and MORRO, G. 1903. *Arch. Ital. Biol.*, 39: 402.

36. PUGH, L. G. C., and WARD, M. P. 1956. *Lancet*, 271: 1115.

37. SELYE, H. 1946. *J. Clin. Endocr.*, 6: 117.

38. SUNDSTROEM, E. S. 1919. *Univ. Calif. Publ. Physiol.,* 5: 105.
39. TALBOTT, J. H., and DILL, D. B. 1936. *Amer. J. Med. Sci.,* 192: 626.
40. ZUNTZ, N., cited by J. BARCROFT. 1925. *The Respiratory Function of the Blood,* Part I, "Lessons from High Altitudes," p. 9. Cambridge: Cambridge University Press.

CHAPTER X

ACCLIMATIZATION TO HYPOXIA

The literature on acclimatization up through the 1930's was summarized by Van Liere in 1942 (253). Since then, pertinent articles have appeared by Monge (163–66), Houston and Riley (109–11), Langley and Clarke (138), Opitz (179), Verzar (262, 263), Stickney and Van Liere (229), and Hurtado (116, 122).

TERMINOLOGY

The term "acclimatization," in respect to hypoxia, apparently has meant different things to different people. Since the condition is not yet completely comprehended, this is understandable. In the first place it would seem well to recognize the suggested criteria of full acclimatization: maintenance of growth in young animals, maintenance of body weight in mature animals, no loss of appetite, a feeling of general well-being, and normal fertility (253, p. 151). Coupled with these should be the principle stated by Henderson: "There are as many acclimatizations as there are altitudes at which a man can live" (104). Complete acclimatization would then be the sum total of the long-term adjustments which the organism makes in attaining the standards defined above.

This chapter excludes detailed discussion of short-term adjustments to acute hypoxia. Except for possibly the newborn, short-term residents are necessarily on the road to complete acclimatization to some particular altitude. These are dealt with nevertheless in other chapters of this book. It has been the practice of many investigators to consider any measurable adjustment to chronic hypoxia as acclimatizing and to speak as though acclimatization had occurred in such instances. It is possible that complete adjustment to *some* degree of low oxygen tension had occurred, although proof has been generally lacking. In view of this practice, it seems necessary to distinguish between incomplete, or partial, and complete acclimatization. Only in the latter is there presumably the homeostasis characteristic of acclimatization as defined by Monge (164).

For the most part, this chapter will be limited to the adjustments which are more or less attained by the completely acclimated individual subjected to a prolonged state of reduced oxygen tension in the inspired air—chronic anoxic hypoxia. Such an environment exists naturally at altitudes above sea level but may be artificially produced by mixtures of oxygen and nitrogen at sea level or by means of decompression chambers. However, it should be noted that Fenn *et al.* (81) have indicated the theoretical impossibility of duplicating exactly the respiratory conditions at altitude with gas mixtures unless respiratory exchange ratio is 1.0. Much work has been done with the artificial methods, and furthermore, the use of intermittent rather than continuous exposures has come into rather common practice. In the course of this chapter it will be necessary to decide whether discontinuous exposure has a place in a consideration of acclimatization. Since so much has been reported in this area, it seems profitable to consider these contributions along with the studies of continuous exposure.

RESPIRATION

Alveolar air.—The alveolar air composition of sojourners and of a few permanent residents at various altitudes up to 22,800 feet (6,950 meters), as recorded in the literature prior to 1949, has been plotted on the Fenn carbon dioxide–oxygen diagram by Rahn and Otis (193). (See Fig. 8, p. 127.) Similar data on a group of twenty-two young men acutely exposed over the same range of altitudes plotted similarly have revealed two striking differences between the respiratory behavior of the sojourners and that of unacclimatized man. At a given altitude the alveolar carbon dioxide tension is always lower and the oxygen tension, higher in the sojourners. The second difference is that the alveolar carbon dioxide tension does not fall in the acute exposures until an alveolar oxygen tension between 50 and 60 mm. Hg is reached, while after "acclimatization" the fall begins at approximately the sea-level value of 100 mm. Hg.

Since the above work of Rahn and Otis, the study of Chiodi (46) has appeared comparing the respiratory characteristics of sojourners and residents at the high altitudes of 13,090 and 14,800 feet (3,990 and 4,515 meters). The residents were "in most cases Indians (pure or mixed) who had been born in the Andean altiplano and had lived" at the above altitudes "for periods ranging from 3 to 42 years." Pulmonary ventilation was significantly greater than the sea-level values in both groups of subjects at both high-altitude places. However, that of the native residents was less than that of the sojourners. One year of residence at this approximate altitude, as shown in a study of Rotta *et al.* (208), did not eliminate this difference. In harmony with the increased ventilation, the sojourners had lower alveolar carbon dioxide tensions and higher alveolar oxygen tensions than the residents. The plotting of these data on the Fenn carbon dioxide–oxygen diagram revealed that the points for the residents fell in between the two curves of Rahn and Otis but with more of them fitting the unacclimatized curve (46).

A closer look at the basis of the Rahn and Otis curve for sojourners and residents reveals that the curve is dominated by the sojourners and so should probably not be called the acclimatization curve. Furthermore, proof is lacking that sojourners eventually would acquire the respiratory characteristics of the residents or that the latter had gone through the stage of adaptation represented by the sojourners. It is possible, particularly since the residents were mainly of Indian origin, that the acclimatization of a race is featured here.

The lower alveolar carbon dioxide tension in the sojourners can be attributed to the greater ventilation rate in the partially acclimatized individual. Hetherington, Luft, and Ivy (105) have reported an increase to 121 per cent of the control values in a group of twenty-seven subjects at 10,200 feet (3,110 meters) for two weeks. This value lies between those of 113 per cent in acute exposures and 133 per cent in subjects chronically exposed to that altitude, as calculated from values reported in the literature. The calculated ventilation ratios in the study of Rahn revealed similar increases in ventilation in the sojourner group. Such increases can be readily ascribed to the return of the pH of the blood to normal by the reduction in alkaline reserve which characterizes the acclimatized state. In the latter there is no alkalotic inhibition of the respiratory center to counteract the chemoreceptor drive resulting from the hypoxemia.

That intermittent hypoxia may induce adaptive changes in respiration is an interesting possibility. Such an eventuality is an explanation for the fact that the respiratory data in a group of thirty-five jet pilots who were subject to presumably discontinuous exposures to altitude indicated early acclimatory changes when plotted on the Fenn diagram (214).

Respiratory response.—The absence of respiratory response in acute exposures before 50 to 60 mm. Hg alveolar oxygen tensions have been reached has been attributed to the alkalinity produced by the lowered saturation of the arterial blood. According to this suggestion, compensatory adjustment in the blood pH would have to occur before the hypoxic stimulus could effectively exert itself. This may be attained, apparently, within a few hours (29, 193). Dejours (64) has suggested that increased pressoreceptor activity secondary to hypoxic increase in blood pressure might also act to hold respiratory activity in check. Increased oxygen saturation, upon return to sea level, should work the opposite way. The acclimated individual at sea level has been observed to hyperventilate for a matter of days after the return. It has been implied that the extent of the hyperventilation depended upon the altitude and that on return to sea level it would be unchanged initially. However, increased oxygen saturation of the blood should cause a concomitant increase in acid reaction, which should bring about an even greater ventilation rate. Since an immediate compensation through loss of carbon dioxide in the lungs could be expected, the appearance of the extra ventilation might be so tenuous as to escape notice.

Adaptive benefits.—The increased ventilation that accompanies acclimatization is of obvious benefit to the organism since it elevates the oxygen tension of alveolar air above that of the unacclimatized organism and, of course, markedly above what it would have been without any change in ventilation. Of interest is the analysis of Houston and Riley (111) of the alteration of respiratory and oxygen transport factors during the acclimatization of four young men exposed continuously for a month at simulated altitudes up to 20,000 feet (6,100 meters). While the men were apparently never completely acclimated (193), the partial changes are nevertheless instructive. Whereas at sea level the gradient between inspired and alveolar air oxygen was 52 mm. Hg, that at 20,000 feet had been reduced to 26, or half, owing largely to the shape of the oxyhemoglobin dissociation curve and partly to increased pulmonary ventilation.

Hurtado (119) has reported a similar finding in residents at 14,900 feet (4,540 meters) compared with those at sea level. In the former work, the sea-level gradient between alveolar air and arterial blood for oxygen was found reduced from 5 to 2 mm. Hg. At 20,000 feet this gradient was judged to be due almost entirely to the diffusion resistance of the pulmonary membrane. The diffusion constant of the lung, as calculated, was found to be 70 as compared with 20 to 30 determined under normal conditions. It was suggested that the increased value at altitude is a result of increased effective perfusing surface produced by better perfusion of pulmonary capillaries as well as by the greater ventilation. The high value for the diffusion constant given above is similar to the maximum diffusing capacity of the lungs during muscular exercise found by Velasquez (261) in twelve native residents of 14,900 feet (4,540 meters).

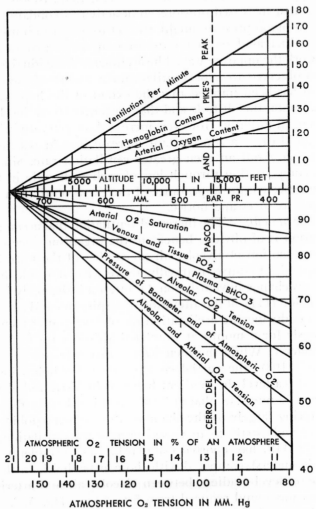

FIG. 9.—Effects of residence at high altitudes sufficiently long for acclimatization. Note that the values are plotted logarithmically. Ventilation and alveolar CO_2 tension change inversely in like proportion and both lag about 14 per cent behind barometric changes. The alveolar O_2 tension falls more rapidly than the barometer, because the lag of respiratory acceleration behind barometric fall permits a larger percentage of reduction to occur in the alveolar O_2 tension. (From J. P. Peters and D. D. Van Slyke, *Quantitative Clinical Chemistry* [Baltimore: Williams & Wilkins Co., 1932], I, 573.)

Blood gases.—The increased tension of oxygen in alveolar air is reflected as inferred above, in a better oxygen tension and saturation of arterial blood. The findings in studies of the blood of high-altitude residents of the Andes are consistent with the high alveolar values of acclimated subjects (45, 46, 117). Dill *et al.* (67) found similar values in members of the Andean Expedition (one to sixteen days after arrival, but some two and a half months after arrival above 9,220 feet [2,810 meters]) and residents at 17,500 feet (5,340 meters) in regard to arterial tensions of both oxygen and carbon dioxide. Apparently respiratory acclimatization becomes complete in a relatively short time. Arterial oxygen saturation rises from 84.4 per cent in rabbits recently brought to 5,900 feet (1,800 meters) to 88.3 per cent in those acclimatized (six months' residence) at that altitude (264).

Alveolar R.Q.—A depression of the alveolar respiratory quotient has been noted during a stay of some two to three weeks at 10,000 feet (3,000 meters), more or less. In one case it fell from 0.84 to 0.76 (193), and in another, from 0.80 to 0.75 (105). The average computed alveolar R.Q. of a miscellaneous group of acclimated subjects turned out to be 0.82 (193), but because of lack of standardization of conditions, probably too much significance should not be attached to this figure. The determining of the R.Q. in acclimated subjects under standard conditions would seem to be profitable, along with a continuation of the observations during the process of acclimatization. An interesting observation was that of Chiodi (46), who determined the fasting R.Q. in the acclimated residents and found 0.847 in those at 13,090 feet (3,990 meters) and 0.834 at 14,800 feet (4,515 meters). The sojourners under similar conditions had 0.826 at the lower and 0.795 at the higher altitude. Perhaps the early depression as adaptation proceeds reflects a deficiency in the marshaling of carbohydrate by the organism subjected to hypoxia.

SIZE AND SHAPE OF CHEST AT HIGH ALTITUDES

It has been reported by a number of observers that inhabitants of high altitudes have enlarged chests. It is generally conceded that this is true only for those who have grown up at high altitudes, although reports (102, 265) have been made in the literature that chest enlargement may occur after a prolonged sojourn at high altitudes. Rengger-Perlmann (200) reported that the male adults at Davos (5,120 feet—1,560 meters) had an increased circumference of their chests. Loewy and Marton (150) found also that the children of Davos showed an increase in chest circumference. Hurtado (115) measured the chest circumference of inhabitants between the ages of four and seventy-five at Morococha (14,900 feet—4,540 meters) and showed that from childhood on the chest was unusually developed. Barcroft *et al.* (19) showed, by means of the X ray, that in the Cholos living in the high Peruvian Andes the direction of the ribs was more horizontal than in lowlanders. The average value of the slope of the ribs in the members of Barcroft's party was 21°, while the average of the Cholos was only 13°. Barcroft mentioned that the chests of Peruvian laborers at an altitude of 14,200 feet (4,330 meters) were unusually broad and deep, and he wrote as follows: "Without laying too much stress on the shape, the above information may be summed up roughly by saying the native of five feet three inches has the chest of a man six feet" (19).

CHEST EXPANSION

Chest expansion is increased in inhabitants at high altitudes. It was observed by Loewy and Marton (150) in children at Davos, and by Rengger-Perlmann (200) in male adults in the same locality, that the chest expansion was greater than in those who lived at lower levels. Hurtado (115) obtained similar findings in Peruvian natives. He reported that the average difference between full inspiration and expiration in young adolescents was 3.5 inches; in adults, 3.2 inches; and in old people, 2.9 inches. By way of comparison, he considered the average chest expansion of a North American student, who was much taller and better developed physically than the natives, as 2.9 inches.

VITAL CAPACITY OF INHABITANTS AT HIGH ALTITUDES

The decrease in vital capacity noticed in unacclimatized subjects is only temporary, and most authors feel that there is an actual increase in vital capacity after acclimatization has taken place. It must be mentioned here, however, that Izquierdo (124) reported that the vital capacity of two hundred inhabitants at an altitude of 7,450 feet (2,270 meters) did not vary from the normal ranges, and Ocaranza (177) found no increase in vital capacity of men acclimatized to the valley of Mexico. Rengger-Perlmann (200), however, found an increase in the average vital capacity in thirty males at Davos (5,120 feet—1,560 meters). An average of 4.7 liters was reported, whereas, according to their height, normally the figure should have been 3.7 liters at sea level. Loewy and Marton (150) also found an increase in vital capacity of children at Davos.

Hurtado (114), working with Peruvian children, also concluded that the vital capacity was raised above the normal. He reported, further, that the vital capacity of the mountain inhabitants diminished with increasing age, as it does with those who live at sea level.

It must be remembered that high altitudes alone do not cause an increase in vital capacity, but physical training also increases it. An interesting study of the athletes at the Olympic Winter Games at Saint-Moritz showed that the physically trained lowlanders had about the same vital capacity as the Swiss highlanders (149).

Respiratory control.—Although the mechanism of respiratory control after complete acclimatization is not entirely understood, some outstanding characteristics are clearly evident. Douglas *et al.* (71) noted, after going down from a stay of several weeks on Pike's Peak (14,000 feet or 4,300 meters), the gradual increase over a number of days in alveolar carbon dioxide tension, which indicated a persistence of hyperventilation and its gradual decline. Recent observations (111, 117) have indicated the same thing. In fact, the mere hyperventilation under sea-level conditions for twenty-four hours has been found to persist in a diminished alkaline reserve with spontaneous hyperpnea following (35). After acclimatization to a given reduced oxygen tension, prompt removal to normal conditions is thought by some to be accompanied by the same alveolar ventilation as had occurred during hypoxia. If true, this would mean that chemoreceptor activity is no longer solely responsible for the maintenance of the hypoxic ventilation. It would mean that part of the control of respiration had been taken over by the medullary respiratory centers as the adaptation to hypoxia had been completed. Whether the change in alkaline reserve of blood and/or tissues is adequate of itself to permit this or whether there is in addition increased sensitivity of the centers to carbon dioxide is debated (13, 46, 47, 49, 96, 122, 128, 151, 188, 193, 194, 195).

Chemoreflexes.—There are a few studies which throw some light upon what happens to the chemoreflex drive during the process of acclimatization. Astrand (13), observing carotid chemoreceptor activity in anesthetized cats, found it present even after twenty-four hours of exposure to the simulated altitude of 13,300 feet (4,000 meters). Elevation of the altitude to 19,680 feet (6,000 meters) increased the activity, while pure oxygen reduced it essentially to zero. These results are contrary to the earlier findings of Bjurstedt (29) on the anesthetized dog in which he found diminution of chemoreceptor drive during eight-hour exposures to hypoxia.

Astrand (14), in work experiments upon man (mostly a single subject) before and after a four- to five-day exposure to 13,300 feet (4,000 meters) in a low pressure chamber, found that the decreased ventilation upon breathing pure oxygen persisted during the partial acclimatization, suggesting interruption of a chemoreceptor drive. Dejours et al. (64), in three human subjects at rest during the sixteenth to nineteenth days at 11,850 feet (3,613 meters) with the test using a single breath of pure oxygen, found evidence for similar interruption or reduction even in the resting state. The latter authors suggested that 50 per cent of the ventilating drive was due to chemoreceptor impulses, at their particular state of acclimatization. Chiodi (46, also 47), in the study of sojourners and residents at 13,087 and 14,809 feet referred to above, found ventilation unchanged in the residents upon breathing pure oxygen at altitude, while the decrease in the sojourners was modest: 11.8 per cent. Since the subjects of Astrand of Dejours et al. were sojourners, this would seem, at least, to play up again the fundamental differences between residents (acclimatized) and sojourners (partially acclimatized).

ACID-BASE BALANCE

Chronic hypoxia.—Dill et al. (68) have given a complete description of the physicochemistry of the blood of the acclimatized resident at 17,500 feet (5,340 meters). Serum electrolytes had one major change: bicarbonate content was at approximately two-thirds the sea-level value. The visiting party had a similar value (within 8 per cent), which is consistent with the view that respiratory acclimatization was nearing completion. Such individuals have a reduced capacity to neutralize fixed acids, the treatment of lactic being particularly interesting.

In the partially acclimated subjects of Houston and Riley (111), there was evidence that the alkaline reserve had fallen to approximately 75 per cent of the initial value. Other electrolyte findings were consistent with those of Dill et al.

Hurtado and Aste-Salazar (117) have made a complete study of the subject in residents at eight different altitudes from sea level to 15,940 feet (4,860 meters). A comparative study is rendered problematic by the low values they found in serum bicarbonate at sea level. However, the relative changes occurring with increasing altitudes were in line with those reported by Dill *et al.* In the native residents both groups found arterial serum pH's which were in the normal range, though in the lower half. The South American workers found the pH to decrease slightly with altitude. The more recent study of Chiodi (46, also 47), referred to above, found serum pH in residents at the two altitudes exactly at the sea-level average: 7.40. The sojourners in that study were still only partially acclimatized, their values being in the upper range of normal.

In the rabbit at 5,906 feet (1,800 meters) for six months (264) there was a reduction in alkaline reserve to 74 per cent of the control value. In mice (52) qualitatively similar changes occurred in the brief exposure of two weeks to 16,000–18,000 feet (4,900–5,500 meters). There was a marked reduction in the terminal pH (calculated). This was seen to a lesser extent in the Andean residents.

Intermittent hypoxia.—The changes in acid-base balance during repeated discontinuous exposures to hypoxia are pertinent to the question of the extent of acclimatization by such means. In rabbits, four hours per day, seven days per week for five weeks at 18,000 feet (5,500 meters), there was no change in carbon dioxide combining power nor in sodium or chloride ion concentration of blood serum, in spite of increased oxygen capacity of the blood (243). In a second group of rabbits exposed similarly to 25,000 (7,600 meters), there were slight reductions in the above components, but the exposures proved quite deleterious to survival and weight gain.

Boutwell and Ivy (32) and Burrill and Ivy (41) and their coworkers studied the excretion of fixed bases and the "acid metabolites," ammonia and phosphate, in the urine of human subjects exposed about one hour per day, three days a week for eight or nine weeks to 18,000 feet (5,500 meters). In the earlier study the hypoxia caused temporary rises in urinary sodium, potassium, and chloride ion excretion which were followed by compensatory reduction in these values, so that the 24-hour urine values were not altered. In the later study the excretion of both fixed bases and of "acid metabolites" in the 24-hour urine was increased (after an initial decrease) with the repeated exposures. As suggested by the workers of the later study, the results could be interpreted as indicative of a rebound acidosis following the period of acapnic alkalosis. It is puzzling why the two studies differed in regard to excretion of base. In the later study the *increase* in these urine values with continued exposure is baffling, because it suggests adaptation to discontinuous hypoxia.

ADRENAL CORTEX

On the basis of studies of the rat continuously exposed to 20,000 feet or to 25,000 feet (6,100 or 7,600 meters), there is evidence that supernormal involvement of the adrenal cortex requires rather severe degrees of hypoxia and that the change is only temporary (63, 244, 246). The same appears to be true of the dog (39), the guinea pig (237), and man (247). San Martin *et al.* (211) found urinary excretion of 17-ketosteroids and reducing corticosteroids in native residents at 14,900 feet (4,540 meters) no different from that of sea-level residents. Response to adrenocortical hormone in another study (232) showed no essential differences between the two groups. These negative findings lead to the viewpoint that the adrenal cortex has a noticeably heightened role mainly in the short-term adjustments to hypoxia. Further support for this view comes from the fact that the majority of reports concerning adrenocortical activation in hypoxia have to do with either the acute phases of continuous exposure, with discontinuous exposures, or with continuous exposure to fairly intolerable degrees of hypoxia (31, 40, 58, 61, 69, 86, 108, 136, 137, 138, 234, 242, 248).

There is evidence that the activation of the adrenal cortex in hypoxia is secondary to the associated hypocapnia, for the prevention of the latter by the addition of carbon dioxide to the inspired air failed to show the usual adrenocortical changes or the reaction secondary to excess liberation of adrenocortical hormones (98, 139, 140). It should be pointed out that it is difficult under these circumstances to control the degree of hypoxia. However, the observation that nephrectomy will prevent the adrenal cortical activation (140) would seem to argue for adrenocortical involvement secondary to acid-base changes. The latter finding makes it rather difficult to account for the report that discontinuous exposures of rats caused adrenal hypertrophy reaching a maximum after six weeks but regression of adrenal size and histologic signs of activation after that time, as though some adaptation to hypoxia had occurred (61). In the absence of data on acid-base changes in these rats, speculation is hardly profitable.

If hypocapnia is the specific stress activating the adrenal cortex during hypoxia, one would expect such activation to persist until the pH had returned to normal in the stage of complete respiratory adjustment. As has been mentioned above, such activation has been observed only in the acute phase. One might conclude that it is at such time that the demand for adrenocortical hormones is at a maximum and that the increased utilization of the hormone continues, but at rates which defy present methods of detection.

Acclimatization to high altitude seems to have no effect on other endocrine organs. Timiras *et al.* (244, 246) found in the rat born and reared at 12,470 feet (3,800 meters) no difference in the weights of other endocrine organs besides the adrenal—hypophysis, thyroid, testes—when compared to those of sea-level residents. Tappan and Reynafarje (237) found thyroid weights unchanged at altitude in guinea pigs but greater in animals recently moved there.

BLOOD GLUCOSE AND LIVER GLYCOGEN

Forbes (82) found little change in blood sugar level in partially ac-climated human subjects. Glucose tolerance was markedly increased at 17,500 feet, but only two normal subjects were studied. In rats con-tinuously exposed to low oxygen tension Sundstroem and Michaels (234; see also 245) found initial elevations of blood sugar within a third- to a half-day at simulated barometric pressures of 460 through 260 mm. Hg (13,300–26,000 feet—4,000–8,000 meters). These eleva-tions in the acute phase of hypoxia were presumably the result of emergency stimulation of the autonomic nervous system (80). Later in exposure the blood sugar fell to quite low values; the amount and time of occurrence seemed to depend more or less on the degree of stress. At certain times during the exposure to the higher simulated altitudes, glucose tolerance was found to be altered—either increased, decreased, or both at different times. The glucose changes subsequent to the initial change are generally thought to involve the adrenal cor-tex. However, Sayers (212) points out the possibility that the adrenal cortex may not induce the changes in carbohydrate metabolism char-acteristic of hypoxia but rather that the changes may be initiated by tissues whose functional activity requires the presence of cortical hormone. The latest viewpoint is that the activation of the adrenal cortex is triggered through the hypothalamopituitary system by even-tual decreases in blood levels of adrenocortical hormones but, also, by stress. The intermediary is, of course, adrenocorticotrophic hor-mone from the anterior pituitary.

Relatively recent studies (189, 190) of carbohydrate metabolism in natives at 14,900 feet (4,540 meters) have revealed low blood-glucose values, but response to intravenous glucose showed increased tolerance, if anything. Other related factors, such as pyruvic and lactic acids and potassium, did not appear different than those of sea-level residents, with the possible exception of inorganic phosphate. Rats born or long-resident at 12,470 feet (3,800 meters) have normal glycemia (245). In the above instances of hypoglycemia there is apparent inadequacy, temporary though it may be, of adjustment to the hypoxic stress.

In studies of discontinuous exposure to hypoxia, rats were found to have low fasting blood sugar and liver glycogen (204, 243) under relatively moderate degrees of stress. Boutwell *et al.* (31) and D'Angelo (62) could find no decided change in blood-sugar level or in glucose tolerance in human subjects under rather similar conditions. The difference in results may reflect a difference in the two species in response to fasting as much as to a more fundamental difference in adrenocortical function.

HEART AND CIRCULATION

Cardiac output.—In 1947, Rotta (207) reported an extensive investigation on native residents at 14,900 feet (4,540 meters) and at sea level. In a group of sixteen subjects at altitude in comparison with twenty at sea level, cardiac outputs (acetylene method) in liters per minute per square meter of body surface (cardiac index) were 2.42 and 2.23, respectively, indicating a slightly greater output (8.5 per cent) in the acclimated persons. Recent studies with the right heart catheterization technique have indicated no difference in normal resting cardiac output between the two groups (208, 210). This evidence limits the increased output to the short-term adaptation of the acute phase of hypoxic exposure, at least at rest. Christensen and Forbes (48), on the basis of indirect evidence, believed that the exercise cardiac output for the same grade of work was unchanged at altitude even for the incompletely acclimated individual.

In other studies made on native residents at 14,900 feet (4,540 meters) by Monge *et al.* (168) and by Theilen *et al.* (241), using the dye dilution technique, increases were found in cardiac index in the natives compared with normal adults at sea level. In the former study the increase was 53 per cent; and in the latter, 13. Since the right heart catheterization (direct Fick) method is such a straightforward method, one is tempted to discount, at least for the present, conflicting results produced by other methods.

Heart rate.—After a degree of acclimatization has been reached, hypoxia has not the same effect on the heart as it did before this took place. The early literature on this subject has been reviewed by Durig (75) and by Schneider and Sisco (217).

It is generally agreed by all workers that acclimatized inhabitants living at elevations from 8,000 (2,440 meters) to 9,500 feet (about 2,900 meters) show no altitude augmentation of heart rate. Barcroft (18) states that there is no evidence that altitude up to 14,000 feet (4,300 meters) quickens the pulse. Monge (169) observed that the Peruvian natives living at altitudes of 12,000 feet (3,700 meters) and 14,900 feet (4,540 meters) showed a tendency toward bradycardia; in over 12 per cent of those examined he found a resting pulse between forty and sixty beats per minute. At the latter altitude Rotta (207) in 1947 observed an average non-basal heart rate of 66.5 in 100 native residents. This is low compared to the general average for dwellers of the lowlands.

Studies of the effect of exercise on the heart rate after acclimatization are plagued by the variable of physical training, whether the comparison between sea level and altitude conditions is made on the same subjects or on different subjects. When made on the same subject the question of completeness of adaptation is a further problem. For studies on newcomers to high altitude conditions the reader is referred to the paper of Astrand and Astrand (15). Hurtado *et al.* (122) have studied the native residents of Morococha (14,900 feet— 4,540 meters) in comparison with natives at sea level. The impression is that heart rate in maximum exercise at altitude is considerably less after acclimatization.

Electrical activity.—Recent studies of Rotta and Lopez (209) and of Penaloza and collaborators (185–87) on the electrical activity of the heart have shown in a large number of subjects predominance of the right side. Rotta and Lopez studied the electrocardiogram of healthy men who had lived fifteen to thirty years at high altitudes (14,900 feet—4,540 meters). Although most of the subjects were Indians, the fourteen who were white or mixed had the same characteristics, indicating that race is presumably not a factor. Penaloza and his group followed the changes in a large number of infants and children up to fourteen years of age during the development of the adult pattern at the same high altitude. They also followed the changes in ten young, male residents of Lima at sea level during a year's stay at Morococha at 14,900 feet. In both groups at altitude evident right ventricular preponderance, presumably due to the right ventricular overload, was a characteristic feature. The changes of the ten newcomers were still incomplete, compared to native residents, after twelve months.

Arterial blood pressure.—Practically all investigators are agreed that people in normal health who live at high altitudes up to 14,000 feet (4,300 meters) or higher have no elevation of the blood pressure. Schneider and Hedblom (216) and Durig (75) have reviewed the early literature on this subject.

In 1947 Rotta (207), working with natives at altitude (14,900 feet —4,540 meters), found a low systolic blood pressure: 116 mm. Hg on the average.

Pulmonary circulation.—Rotta *et al.* (208) in 1956 reported studies on certain aspects of pulmonary circulation of residents and also some newcomers who lived at an altitude of 14,900 feet (4,540 meters). They found a moderate, but significant degree of pulmonary hypertension, which was more marked in the permanent than in the temporary dweller. It was still more marked in mountain sickness. Increased cardiac output was eliminated as a cause because this factor was not found in their subjects. Furthermore, they found that breathing oxygen did not alter the degree of pulmonary hypertension.

Rotta *et al.* also reported in this work that men at high altitudes have a marked dilatation of the vascular bed of the lungs. C. Monge, Jr., and his co-workers found that 19.4 per cent of the total blood volume was in the lungs of residents at this altitude, in contrast to 15.2 per cent at sea level (168).

Brisket disease in cattle is accompanied by pulmonary hypertension; the ailment is seen in those animals living at 8,000–12,000 feet (2,400–3,700 meters) (103, 269).

Cardiac hypertrophy in animals.—Strohl (230) in 1910 reported that the heart weight-body weight ratio of the alpine snowbird (*Lagopus alpinus* Nilss), which inhabits high altitudes, was much greater than that of its near relative, the moor snowbird (*Lagopus albus* Gmellin), which lives at lower levels. He concluded that the greater heart weight in the former was due to two factors, namely, a work hypertrophy and a specific adaptation to the rarefied atmospere.

Campbell (42) in 1932 found that mice exposed to chronic carbon monoxide poisoning for a period of nine months showed a definite cardiac hypertrophy. He thought this was brought about by the increase in viscosity of the blood owing to the increase in red blood cells.

In 1936 Van Liere (252) reported experimental work performed on guinea pigs that had been kept in a low-pressure chamber from 20 to 105 days at barometric pressures ranging from 446 to 380 mm. Hg, corresponding to simulated altitudes from 14,000 to 18,000 feet (4,270 to 5,490 meters). The average heart weight—body weight ratio in the animals increased 55.8 per cent above the normal. In 1943 Rotta (206) found heart weight in the guinea pig to vary with the altitude above 12,250 feet (3,730 meters), and at 14,900 feet

(4,540 meters) it was 30 per cent greater than at sea level. Tappan and Reynafarje (237) have recently found a more modest 11 per cent increase (**P:** <0.001) of heart weight-body weight ratio from 0.306 at sea level to 0.340 at 14,900 feet. In both the latter two studies the increases were seen in both newly acclimated and native animals. Histologically, the hypertrophy consisted of diminished numbers of cardiac capillaries, while the thickness of the muscle fibers increased as in clinical hypertrophy. Theoretically, such a change means a weakened heart. It is odd that in the guinea pig the state of the local circulation is at variance with the finding of increased vascularization of other tissues in other animals under similar circumstances. Finally, Valdivia (250) in 1957 exposed guinea pigs to a simulated altitude of 18,000 feet (5,500 meters). He found a progressive hypertrophy of the right ventricle for the first six weeks after which it reached a constant weight. No hypertrophy of the left ventricle was found. It was postulated that the right ventricular hypertrophy was due to pulmonary hypertension.

Moore and Price (170), on the other hand, found no changes in heart weight—body weight ratios in rats at 14,260 feet (4,350 meters) for two months. It is possible that the length of exposure was inadequate for Timiras *et al.* (246) have found cardiac hypertrophy in rats at 12,470 feet (3,800 meters) after ten months of continuous residence, as well as in those born and reared at that altitude.

Becker, in histological studies of cardiac muscle of puppies born at 20,000 feet (6,400 meters) simulated altitude, found evidence of hyperplasia (20).

Chronic discontinuous exposure to the severe stress of 25,000 feet (7,600 meters) simulated altitude was capable of increasing heart weights by 62 per cent in rats (6, 221, 255). However, since in these animals cardiac lesions were prevalent (6), it is rather obvious that a pathologic degree of hypoxia was involved. Dogs exposed approximately a third of the time to 18,000 feet (5,500 meters) for some twelve weeks had no changes in heart weight relative to body weight (257).

Cardiac hypertrophy in man.—In 1912 both Strohl (231) and Meyer (161), using the electrocardiographic method, found a hypertrophy of the right ventricle at high altitudes.

Gomez (88) in 1948 studied the transverse diameter of the heart by means of teleoroentgenograms of 480 inhabitants of Bogota, Colombia (altitude, 8,016 feet—2,440 meters), and found no cardiac enlargement. Furthermore, electrocardiographic studies showed no evidence of cardiac hypertrophy. Kerwin (129) in 1944, by means of roentgenologic studies of 273 natives living in Oroya, Peru (altitude, 12,000 feet—3,600 meters), found an increase of 11.5 per cent in the transverse diameter of the heart. In the same year Miranda and Rotta (162) measured the transverse diameter of the heart in 250 natives of Morococha, Peru (altitude, 14,900 feet—4,540 meters). They reported an average increase of 21 per cent (values ranged from 11 to 30 per cent).

Rotta (207), making studies on natives living at 14,900 feet (4,540 meters) above sea level, confirmed Kerwin's work. He took frontal X-ray films of 400 individuals and found an average increase in transverse diameter of 19.5 per cent in 69.5 per cent of cases. He also determined the frontal area and found an average increase in the cardiac silhouette of 21.3 per cent in 67 per cent of the cases.

Both authors have interpreted their results as indicative of cardiac hypertrophy, and Rotta has found that the right heart is rather frequently involved. This is explained by the elevated pulmonary arterial pressure. It would be difficult to account for hypertrophy in any other way, for cardiac output may not be elevated in the acclimatized. Increased red blood cell content has been discounted as a factor, because in the arterioles it is confined to the axial stream, and plasma is unchanged. Also, systemic blood pressure is reduced, if anything.

VASCULARIZATION

It has been noted that after a two-week stay at 9,800 feet (3,000 meters) the maximum capacity for work and the maximum oxygen consumption reach a peak which can never be attained by training at sea level (17). For example, the mean maximum oxygen consumption during exercise on the bicycle-ergometer in three trained subjects was determined before going to altitude, at 9,800 feet, and afterward. The findings were 3,750, 3,360, and 4,290 ml/min during the three periods, respectively. The improvement can not be attributed to increased cardiac output, blood hemoglobin, myoglobin, or entirely to increased pulmonary ventilation; so capillary flow in the muscles must have improved. Merino (158) has noted the marked vascularization of malar regions, conjunctivae, and oral mucosae of native residents at 14,900 feet (4,540 meters).

Morphologic evidence for the increased vascularization of other tissues has been found during chronic, discontinuous exposures to hypoxia. Merker (155) and Merker and Schneider (157), in the cerebral cortex of acclimated rats, found in the first work that the average diameter of capillaries changed from 1.96 to 3.9μ. This augmented vascularization has also been demonstrated in other tissues of altitude-acclimatized animals (through discontinuous exposures, more or less) : the fundus of the eye (112) and the pia mater (156) of the rabbit; the dental pulp and asodentin (180), the kidney (7,135) and the liver (157) of the rat; the brain, heart, and gastrocnemius muscle of the puppy born at 20,000 feet (6,100 meters) simulated altitude (21).

Hypertrophy (increased tortuosity and caliber), rather than hyperplasia, has been found to increase vascularization in the rabbit eye (181). In the rat exposed 120 days to 18,000 feet (5,500 meters) simulated altitude, Clark *et al.* (51) observed increased numbers of functioning capillaries in the heart and skeletal muscle. He used the method of injecting India ink into the anesthetized living animal. The length, number, and diameter of capillaries in the brain were also markedly increased in a study by Pawel *et al.* (184). Valdivia (251) found that guinea pigs native to 13,800 feet (4,200 meters) in the Peruvian Andes had considerably greater numbers of capillaries per unit of cross section area in skeletal muscle than those at sea level. In general then, hyperplasia as well as hypertrophy increase vascularization.

It may be noted in passing that increased vascularization throughout the body has been noted in cases of congenital heart diseases (173, 239). The result of such vascular extension is that diffusion distances for oxygen as well as for nutrients and metabolites are reduced, permitting, in particular, higher tensions of oxygen in cells and reduced concentrations of noxious humoral substances. It would seem that increased vascularization is one way in which the long-postulated tissue factor in acclimatization may, at least in part, manifest itself. Qualitative changes in tissue metabolism may be another way in which cells adapt themselves to oxygen deficiency, but such changes are thus far unknown.

BLOOD PICTURE

Hemoglobin.—Extensive studies on the blood of native residents at high altitudes in the Andes have been reported by Hurtado *et al.* (120), by Merino (158), and by Chiodi (45). The first-named authors summarized in the form of a graph (p. 47) their own and previously published findings concerning increases in hemoglobin concentration and decreases in arterial oxygen saturation in relation to altitude.

Hemoglobin concentration increases in curvilinear manner with altitude in residents at the various elevations from sea level to the highest altitudes studied (approximately 18,000 feet—5,500 meters), while arterial oxygen saturation decreases. The values reported by Chiodi, by Lawrence et al. (141), and by Reynafarje et al. (203) indicate reasonably close agreement with these generalizations. Increases in hemoglobin concentration have been observed in the blood of other species: hamsters at 20,000 feet (6,100 meters) for six weeks (50), albino mice at 15,000 feet (4,600 meters) for five weeks (267), guinea pigs moved to 14,900 feet (4,540 meters) or born and reared there (237), and rats moved to 12,500 feet (3,800 meters) or born and reared there (260). There can be no doubt that hemoglobin values generally increase during prolonged exposure to reduced oxygen tensions. However, the benefit to the organism accruing from the increase is theoretically rather slight (111).

On the other hand, there is experimental evidence that increases in hemoglobin or hematocrit add strikingly to hypoxic tolerance. Dorrance et al. (70) found that polycythemia induced with cobalt in rats increased the hypoxic work performance by 100 per cent, as compared with controls. In similar rats Van Liere et al. (254) found the threshold for hypoxic inhibition of the propulsive motility of the small intestine to be elevated from the range 14,000–18,000 feet (4,300–5,500 meters) to above 18,000 feet. Pace et al. (183) found that elevation of hematocrit from 46.2 to 58.3 per cent in human subjects by transfusion of erythrocytes conferred a tolerance equivalent to 5,200 feet (1,600 meters) in altitude, as judged by reduced pulse rate in exercise. If mice partially acclimated at one altitude are exposed to a higher altitude, their performance compared to that of ground-level controls is improved at a higher altitude (100). The improvement is reduced by bleeding, but not in proportion to the blood withdrawn, indicating the presence of other beneficial factors. Negative results have been reported in rats by Wetzig and D'Amour (266), but the test altitude of 40,000 feet (12,000 meters) seems unreasonably high.

The hemoglobin concentration of railroad personnel exposed daily to altitudes from sea level to 15,510 feet (4,740 meters) was found to be 18.07 g/100 ml blood (120) or like that of residents of about 10,000 feet (3,000 meters). Other workers have reported increases in human subjects during intermittent exposures to hypoxia (30, 36). Similar observations have been reported for monkeys (127), dogs (8, 33, 224, 228), rats (5, 55, 205), and guinea pigs (125).

The increase in total circulating hemoglobin found during prolonged exposure to hypoxia is much more impressive than the increase in the peripheral blood concentration (83, 120, 158, 196). For example, while hemoglobin concentration at 14,900 feet (4,540 meters) may increase to an average value of 20.76 g/100 ml blood representing a 30 per cent rise, total circulating hemoglobin may increase to an average value of 25.2 g/kg body weight, a 91 per cent rise over the value for comparable sea-level residents.

Oxygen capacity.—Increased hemoglobin concentration in the blood means simply that the capacity to hold oxygen is increased, and that, *pari passu.* As is well known, hemoglobin concentration may be determined quite reliably from oxygen capacity. In fact, this method was one of the two used by Hurtado *et al.* (120) referred to above. Chiodi (46) obtained an average value of 26.1 ml/100 ml blood in twenty-two residents at 14,800 feet (4,515 meters). This may be compared with the standard for North American adult males: 21.5 ml/100 ml (1). In the four human subjects of Houston and Riley (111), exposed for only about a month to simulated altitudes up to 22,000 feet (7,300 meters), increases in oxygen capacity were found of the same order of magnitude as those seen in the average resident at 14,900 feet (4,540 meters). Greater changes have been found in mice for two weeks at 16,000–18,000 feet (4,900–5,500 meters) in which oxygen capacity increased about 50 per cent (52).

Intermittent exposures to hypoxia have been found effective in increasing the oxygen capacity of the rabbit (243). Grant (93) found, also in the rabbit, that carotid chemoreceptor inactivation could magnify the increase by some 23–36 per cent. This was doubtless related to a more marked depression of arterial oxygen tension.

Oxyhemoglobin curve.—Aste-Salazar and Hurtado (12) have reported that the oxygen dissociation curve of hemoglobin in the blood or residents at 14,900 feet (4,540 meters) is shifted to the right. Part of the shift, at least, was considered to be evidence of reduced affinity of hemoglobin for oxygen. The presence of rather low values of blood pH has the practical effect of accentuating the shift. In any case, oxygen can be unloaded from hemoglobin more readily, with the result that the oxygen gradient from arterial blood is somewhat reduced as tissue oxygen is theoretically elevated. Chiodi (46) in his recent study at 13,090 and 14,800 feet (3,900 and 4,515 meters) found in five residents at each altitude very slight shifts to the right. These were of about the same order of magnitude as found by Keys *et al.* (130) for residents at 17,520 feet (5,340 meters). The sojourners of the latter study had a considerably larger average shift, a phenomenon which the authors suggested as possibly characteristic of partial acclimatization. A similar shift in the blood of rabbits during a six-month stay at 5,906 feet (1,800 meters) has been attributed to the compensated acidosis of acclimatization (264).

Erythrocytes.—Like oxygen capacity, the number of red cells (RBC's) per cubic millimeter of blood can be expected to parallel exactly the hemoglobin concentration, provided the amount of hemoglobin in each RBC remains unchanged. In the acute phase of hypoxia, the increase in RBC count may be a result of hemoconcentraton and/or mobilization from storage depots (10, 93, 120, 141). How soon and to what extent newly formed RBC's are added in increasing numbers is not exactly known; but Hurtado *et al.* (120) found a reticulocytosis definitely beginning the day after arrival of sea-level residents at high altitude, which might be interpreted, if findings (176) in the rabbit are applicable, as evidence of increased contribution from the bone marrow.

On theoretical grounds one would expect the reticulocytosis to disappear upon prolonged exposure to altitude when the total RBC volume reaches its final new and higher level. Normal life span of the RBC is assumed (see below). However, only in the study of Lawrence *et al.* (141) are comparable values seen at sea level and at 14,900 feet (4,540 meters). Hurtado *et al.* (120) and Merino (158) found about threefold, and Reynafarje *et al.* (203), about twofold increases at this altitude. Since the reticulocytes rather promptly disappear from blood on standing by "maturing" into the normal RBC's, freshly drawn blood must be used in making the smears; and standardization of the time factor is a necessity. Altland and Highman (8), in dogs discontinuously exposed up to 865 days, found percentages of reticulocytes essentially unchanged after the first week, in spite of dramatic increases in hematocrit, hemoglobin, and RBC's. Cook and Alafi (56), in comparing the response of splenectomized with normal mice exposed to 15,000 feet (4,600 meters) simulated altitude for a month or two, conclude that tonic contraction of the spleen is an important source of RBC's (about two-fifths of the total) in this species.

In residents at 12,240 and 14,900 feet (3,730 and 4,540 meters), mean corpuscular volume was found to be increased (120). Chiodi (45) failed to confirm this in his study of residents at 14,800 feet (4,515 meters). Since the value is a derived one involving the rather vague hematocrit plus a correction factor for shrinkage in one series (120), it seems that the question can be settled satisfactorily only with better methods of determination. A calculation from the data obtained in the two studies reveals a greater hemoglobin content in the RBC in the group studies by Hurtado *et al.* Both groups found white blood cell counts in the normal range, and both found an increase in percentage of lymphocytes in the differential count. The former workers found fragility of RBC's normal (so also in the intermittently exposed dog [224]) and blood viscosity increased at 12,240 feet to the remarkable value of 8.4 (sea-level value: 4.64). The latter worker found sedimentation rate decreased. In another species, the mouse, the RBC level increases notably at 15,000 feet (4,600 meters) (267).

As with hemoglobin, discontinuous exposure to hypoxia have been found to produce increases in the concentration of RBC's in man (36) and in lower animals (5, 8, 89, 93, 95, 125, 127, 205, 224, 228, 243).

As with increases in total circulating hemoglobin, the total RBC volume increases at altitude reflect more markedly the increased hemopoiesis under that condition. While the RBC count at 14,900 feet (4,540 meters) may be elevated (120) 20 per cent, the total RBC volume may be up 91 per cent. Lawrence *et al.* (141) in eleven, and Reynafarje *et al.* (203), in an undisclosed number of natives of 14,900 feet, using the newer radioactive tagged RBC technique found total RBC volume to be about 50 per cent above the comparable sea-level value. In dogs, Reissmann (196, 197) found increases up to 170 per cent of the ground level in the fifth week of exposure to 20,000 feet (6,100 meters) simulated altitude. Fryers, using Fe^{59} tagged RBC's in rats at 15,000 feet (4,600 meters) simulated altitude for ten days or more, found intermediate increases in total RBC volume (83).

Hematocrit.—In the acclimatized state the hematocrit reflects more roughly the accompanying hemopoietic changes. Such changes include the increase in RBC count and alterations, if any, in mean corpuscular, or in plasma, volume. For human beings at an altitude around 15,000 feet, a hematocrit reading of 60 per cent has been found (45, 120). In smaller groups of subjects, Merino (158) found a somewhat greater value; and Lawrence *et al.* (141), a somewhat smaller value. In the mouse such values may be attained in the surprisingly short time of two weeks (52); and in the rat, the higher value of 72.3 per cent in about five weeks at 15,000 feet (4,600 meters) followed by two weeks at 20,000 feet (6,100 meters) (83). Another study in the rat found 60 per cent after two and a half months at 12,500 feet (3,810 meters) and 63.1 per cent in those born and reared at that altitude (260). The increases in hematocrit (as well as in RBC) at fairly low altitudes may be so small as to make verification problematic (37, 85, 113, 144, 215, 240).

Discontinuous exposures to hypoxia are likewise capable of provoking increases in hematocrit (2, 5, 7, 8, 33, 93, 125, 127, 242, 243).

Altland and Highman (6) found the upper limit in rats to be approximately 80 per cent, an astounding figure. They also found that in order to maintain a relatively high hematocrit (55–75 per cent) the discontinuous exposures must be made at intervals of not less than two to three days. Such high hematocrits as have been experimentally produced reflect not only the height of the simulated altitude—25,000 feet (7,600 meters) or more—but also, doubtless, the failure of respiratory acclimatization under such conditions, which serves to render the hypoxic stress more severe than it otherwise would be.

Specific gravity.—In dogs the specific gravity of the blood was found to increase from 1.0569 to 1.0719 while hemoglobin increased 53 per cent during intermittent exposure to 18,000 feet (5,500 meters) simulated altitude (224).

Blood volume.—Hurtado et al. (120), in their studies of residents at high altitudes in which they used brilliant vital red for the determination of total blood and plasma volumes, found no essential change in plasma volume over the sea-level value. The total blood volume was greatly increased, reflecting therefore, for the most part, the greatly increased amount of formed elements—RBC's. However, on the basis of their use of the Evans blue method, one might conclude that total plasma volume decreased at the highest altitude (14,900 feet—4,540 meters). The latter finding is in agreement with the report of Merino (158) at the same altitude and with the use of brilliant vital red. The uncertainty, here, can be ascribed partly to difficulty with methods and partly to small experimental samples. Rotta (see 66) is said to have reported, and Lawrence et al. (141) with adequate methods has found, that at the latter altitude the increase in total blood volume is entirely RBC's, which confirms the viewpoint of Hurtado et al. Similar confirmations have been found in the fetal sheep at this altitude (192).

In the acute phase of hypoxic exposure in human subjects, decreases in total plasma volume, attributed to water loss, have been found (11, 141). A similar, but more persistent decrease is reported for the dog (196, 197), where total plasma volume fell gradually to a constant level, 75 per cent of the ground level. This is true also for the rat (83). By the use of a crude method, blood volume in rats has been found significantly elevated during discontinuous exposures to 18,000 feet (5,500 meters) simulated altitude (205).

Plasma protein.—The older conclusion (253), that plasma protein remains unchanged in the altitude-acclimated, person has been substantiated at the low altitude of 5,280 feet (1,610 meters) (113). Early increases during the acute phase have been attributed to hemoconcentration (11, 262).

With the use of discontinuous exposures in dogs, Thorn *et al.* (243) found no change in serum proteins, while Stickney *et al.* (224) found a progressive decrease during the experimental period (88 days).

PIGMENT METABOLISM

Bilirubinemia.—In human subjects residing at altitude, Merino (158) has made simultaneous studies of hematology, plasma bilirubin concentration, and urobilinogen excretion. As had been noted previously (120) and recently confirmed (203), the total bilirubin concentration of the plasma is doubled or better at 14,900 feet (4,540 meters). Fitzgerald *et al.* (see Verzar [262, p. 61]) found moderate increases in persons at 11,300 feet (3,450 meters) for three weeks. Merino found the excretion of urobilinogen to be increased to about the same extent as the total circulating hemoglobin, so that the hemolytic index (mg. daily urobilinogen excretion per 100 g. total hemoglobin) was essentially unchanged. This would appear to indicate that the rate of hemoglobin destruction relative to the circulating mass remains normal in acclimated subjects. A rather similar interpretation has been made by Reissmann *et al.* (198, 199) on the basis of bilirubin excretion in dogs with internal-type bile fistulae during exposure to simulated altitude for several months. Furthermore, evidence for unchanged longevity of the RBC produced in chronic hypoxia was found. Recent studies in human subjects have amply confirmed the fact that the RBC life span is not affected by changes in altitude either in ascent, at altitude, or in descent (25, 202, 203). This is true in the rat also (83).

The bilirubinemia in altitude residents (120, 158) has been attributed to defective liver function, secondary to the hypoxemic state and perhaps to other factors present in the acclimated person. Since bile pigment output relative to hemoglobin mass is unchanged, it would seem that liver function is not impaired, at least not in a simple way. Other factors must be involved, such as mass of hemoglobin disintegrating relative to total plasma volume, relation between plasma bilirubin concentration and excretory function of liver parenchyma, etc. A higher threshold for bilirubin excretion has been suggested (249).

Erythropoiesis.—Bile pigment studies during the development of polycythemia in chronic hypoxia as well as during its loss with return

to normal conditions are enlightening (158; 198; 199; 263, p. 65).
Reissman *et al.* (198, 199), with the dog, found definite increases of
pigment excretion during the acute phase of hypoxic exposure and
further pointed out that the data of Merino (158) on man could be
interpreted similarly. Reynafarje *et al.* (203) noticed the same thing
in their studies but concluded that since RBC life span is normal the
pigment must have some other source. The association of increased
pigment excretion with RBC formation has been recently postulated
in connection with other studies (97, 262, 263), but further work is
needed to substantiate the relationship and its meaning.

Decisive evidence for the production of new RBC's during chronic
hypoxia has been reported (73). The exact mechanism of this is still
uncertain, but erythropoietin appears definitely to play a part (91) in
the acute phase and probably in the chronic phase as well (159). Hypoxia in general, relative to the oxygen needs of the organism, results
in the appearance of the "hormone" in the plasma. The kidney may
play some role in its elaboration. The site of action of erythropoietin
is presumably the red bone marrow, where its stimulant activity is
exerted upon one or more of the developmental stages of the erythrocyte.

Merino and Reynafarje (160), in their studies of the bone marrow
of residents of 14,400 feet (4,390 meters) at Cerro de Pasco, Peru,
have observed a marked hyperplasia of erythroid elements. Oddly
enough, the hyperplasia in the newborn infant at 12,240 or 14,900
feet (3,730 or 4,540 meters) is no greater than that in the newborn
at sea level (201). In mitotic studies of bone marrow with the colchi-
cine technique, Grant (94) observed significant increases in the percentage of mitoses in erythroid elements after hemorrhage (anemic
hypoxia) or discontinuous exposure to 23,500 feet (7,160 meters)
simulated altitude.

During the early phase of loss of polycythemia on return of acclimated individuals to sea-level conditions (158, 198, 199), there is
reported to be an increased rate of hemoglobin destruction. Reynafarje *et al.* (203) found increased bile pigment excretion at this time
in two of six subjects but argued that since RBC life span is not altered
the pigment must have other sources than blood hemoglobin. In both
the dog (198, 199) and man (203), there is a reduced erythropoiesis
at this time.

In dogs intermittently exposed to hypoxia, the increased erythropoietic activity is associated with a marked increase in the splenic
weight relative to the body weight (257). The increase has been

found to persist for three months after the cessation of exposures, during the time of recession of the blood picture to that of ground level. The splenic enlargement is obviously related to the greater demands in the acclimatized state for blood storage and blood destruction. Splenic enlargement has been observed similarly in the guinea pig (125) but not in the rat for six weeks at 11,300 feet (3,450 meters) (263, p. 39).

OXYGEN CONSUMPTION

Recent studies confirm the previous conclusion (253) that resting oxidative metabolism is not changed in the acclimatized subject. This has been seen during acclimatization in mice (52), in rats (147, 148), and in human subjects (111; 262, p. 101). During adjustment in the acute phase of hypoxia, particularly of severe degree, there is a reduction of oxygen consumption which has been suggested as secondary to lowering in body temperature (84). The measurement of metabolism has been made (143) during acclimatization in which the subject breathed pure oxygen (partial pressure greater than at sea level). It would seem that such a procedure measures posthypoxic metabolism only. However, the finding is that the metabolic rate is unchanged in such circumstances, which at least rules out the presence of a hypoxic oxygen debt in the acclimated.

GROWTH

Early suggested criteria of the acclimated state are the continued growth in young animals and the maintenance of body weight in the mature. That such standards are reached in the Andean man has not been denied, although he tends to be of small stature and light body weight (114). In those studies of laboratory animals subjected to chronic hypoxia, normal growth has been observed under the moderate degree of hypoxia compatible with acclimatization (39, 170).

Body-weight loss has been commonly reported in studies of long discontinuous exposures (2, 4, 5, 65, 92, 243), particularly at simulated altitudes above 18,000 feet (5,500 meters). At this altitude with exposures of four hours per day, Thorn *et al.* (243) reported normal weight gain in rats, while Altland and co-workers (2, 7) found a 10 to 15 per cent retardation. Apparently rabbits tolerate poorly that degree of hypoxia, for their weight gain was reduced (243). Dogs have been found to withstand well exposures approximately twice as long per day to that degree of stress (227).

BLOOD HISTAMINE

Blood histamine has been found to increase in the dog mainly during the acute phase of exposure to chronic hypoxia (39). Although the level returns to the control value within eight days, spontaneous fluctuations persist which are not altered by histaminic blocking agents. Similar findings (74) have been observed in the guinea pig exposed to 19,700 feet (6,000 meters) simulated altitude in the low-pressure chamber except that about three weeks are required for the return to the control values. Since an antihistaminic agent blocked rises in plasma protein concentration and in leucocyte counts without preventing the rise in histamine during hypoxia, the possibility exists that histamine induced the change in protein and leucocytes.

MYOGLOBIN

The observation of Hurtado et al. (121) on the increased myoglobin concentration of skeletal muscle of dogs born and reared at altitude has not been confirmed in dogs intermittently (33), nor in hamsters (50) continuously, exposed. Confirmation has been observed in the guinea pig brought from sea level to 14,900 feet (4,540 meters) for an average of seventy-five days, but in animals reared at altitude the differences were not generally significant (237). Furthermore, in the rat, discontinuous exposures have been found either to have no effect (34) or to cause an actual decrease in myoglobin (191) in the skeletal muscles. In the former of the latter two studies, two to eight times more blood hemoglobin was found retained by the muscles of the experimental animals as compared with those of the controls. The amount retained varied with the hematocrit. Since the method used by Hurtado et al. depended upon ridding the muscles of contained blood hemoglobin by perfusion, which possibly may have been less effective in the acclimated dogs, it is possible that this is responsible for the discrepancy in the results. In rats chronically exposed to 12,500 feet (3,810 meters) altitude, Vaughan and Pace (260) found myoglobin concentration of the entire musculature to increase significantly, but individual muscles with the exception of the heart did not uniformly reflect this. In the work of Criscuolo and collaborators (57, 58) on rats chronically held at 20,000 feet (6,100 meters) simulated altitude, some confirmation of this was seen, particularly during the fourth to the sixth week of exposure. Quite oddly, however, continued exposure through the tenth week saw return to normal sea-level values; a similar situation was observed in rats reared at altitude. The latter evidence would seem to refute the suggestion (260) that intermittent exposure is an explanation for negative results. However, in groups of rats exercised on the treadmill at simulated altitude (50), greater (by 50 per cent) increases were seen than in the exercised controls at ground level. (See also 51, 260.) It is possible that hypoxia acts synergistically with muscular activity to cause myoglobin to increase. In the case of another active muscle, cardiac muscle, it has been less difficult to demonstrate an increase in myoglobin content during chronic hypoxia (50, 121, 191), though in the hamster no increase was seen. It is clear that more work is needed, especially on the influence of exercise plus hypoxia, before final answers to the problem of myoglobin increases during acclimatization can be given.

TISSUE RESPIRATION

Ullrick *et al.* (248) have compared the tissue respiration in control rats with those acclimated eleven weeks at 18,000 feet (5,500 meters) in a decompression chamber. With the Warburg technique no differences were found in brain, small intestine, liver, skeletal muscle, cardiac atrium, and cardiac ventricle. It is not surprising then to find few alterations in enzymes and metabolites in the tissues of guinea pigs which are native to high altitudes (14,000 feet—4,300 meters or above) (238) or in rats (58, 59) which have lived three months or more at 18,000 feet. Berry (26) has made extensive studies of tissue citrate in mice during and after three to four months at 20,000 feet (6,100 meters) simulated altitude. The decreases in the mouse could not be confirmed in a comparison between guinea pigs at sea level and those native to the Andean altiplano at 14,000 feet (4,300 meters) or higher (27).

Relatively short exposure to chronic hypoxia did not alter the cytochrome C value in regenerating liver (72) in the rat. No changes in skeletal muscle of rats or guinea pigs at 11,300 feet (3,440 meters) for six weeks were found (Tissieres in 263, p. 35). On the other hand, that of skeletal muscle of guinea pigs, during a much longer and more severe exposure, had increases of 16.5 per cent (65). In the rabbit discontinuously exposed, cytochrome C content of heart, tongue, kidney, and brain increased rather strikingly, while that of abdominal muscles remained unchanged, and that in lung and liver was decreased (101). It is not readily apparent how increased cytochrome C contents could be advantageous to an organism, for increased metabolic rate has been observed to be inimical to hypoxic tolerance. Nevertheless, further study is certainly in order for this important component of tissues.

Recent reports (66, 116, 122) on native residents (Indian miners) of the Andes maintain that these acclimated persons carry out their muscular activity with less production of lactate than sea-level men, both running on the treadmill in their native habitats. The earlier finding on the partially acclimated members of the International High Altitude Expedition to Chile (77) was that lactate levels, for a given amount of work, were equivalent to the sea-level values but that capacity for doing work and for accumulating greater lactate values was definitely limited in proportion to the altitude. But the recent studies (particularly that of Hurtado *et al.* [122]) report that the Indian miner has greater capacity than the man at sea level and that he accomplishes work with less expenditure of energy. Such accomplishments, if methodologic errors can be ruled out, may be due to tissue adjustments, encompassing perhaps increased vascularization, increased myoglobin and/or cytochrome, and adaptive mechanisms for energy liberation; but they could also conceivably be produced simply by the natural selection of a race or of individuals with unusually efficient muscular tissue.

KIDNEY

Becker *et al.* (23) have compared certain variables of kidney function of five native residents of 14,900 feet (4,540 meters) with the normal values given by Smith (220). Glomerular filtration rate was reduced about 11 per cent in the natives, and effective renal plasma and blood flows, 52 and 27 per cent, respectively; but filtration fraction was increased 89 per cent. The same authors have studied renal function in two anesthetized llamas native to 15,000 feet (4,600 meters) (22).

In the rat, discontinuous exposure to 15,000 feet simulated altitude results in an intense polyuria (219), and similar exposure to

25,000 feet (7,600 meters), in much greater urine volume. Less frequent intermittent exposures to varying simulated altitudes revealed that the extent of the polyuria was roughly proportional to the altitude (223). In acute exposures of longer duration no consistent evidence of polyuria has been seen (235), which suggests that it may be a characteristic limited to the first few hours of acute exposure. The possibility of increased insensible water loss at the expense of urine volume in the latter experiment makes it impossible to decide this point.

In the dog intermittently exposed to hypoxia, a striking increase in effective renal blood flow which accompanied lesser increases in glomerular filtration and filtration fraction was found (152, 153). There was a tendency for these values to return to the control values toward the end of the six-week period of the experiment. In the rat exposed intermittently to 15,000 feet (4,600 meters), a reduction in the polyuria with time has been reported (218). Such findings suggest adaptation, at least, but whether it is specifically toward the hypoxic condition is a moot point. A like series of exposures in the rat causes an increase in kidney weight and in hyperemia of the kidney (135, 218, 219, 242). Evidence of pathology in the kidney appears when the simulated altitude is as high as 25,000 feet (7,600 meters) (135, 242).

Discontinuous exposure in the human subject has been accompanied by increases in urine volume (also sodium, potassium, and chloride ions), but compensatory reductions have kept the twenty-four-hour values unchanged (41).

GASTROINTESTINAL TRACT

At a simulated altitude of 12,000 feet (3,700 meters), the stomach of dogs was found to take about 35 per cent longer to empty a standard, mixed meal (227). The cause of the delay was apparently related to the concomitant discharge over the autonomic nervous system in response to the stress. During some two to eight weeks of eight-hour daily exposures to this altitude, there was a gradual return of gastric emptying time toward the original control value. In the interval, changes had apparently occurred which may be viewed as acclimatizing and which apparently had reduced the vulnerability to untoward effects of the hypoxic stress. Elevation of the simulated altitude by a mere 4,000 feet then caused a reappearance of the gastric delay, which gradually disappeared, however, with continued intermittent exposure to the new altitude (see Fig. 10). Elevation of the altitude once again, to 18,000 feet, produced the same sequence of changes, except in this case adaptation appeared more slowly and, in all but one dog, failed to become complete. The experiment has illustrated the concept of Henderson (104) that there is an acclimatization for each altitude. It has also been interpreted to confirm the idea of a ceiling for acclimatization (44).

No alteration in small intestinal propulsive motility has been observed in response to hypoxia in the dog (256). In the rat, in which a reduction occurs under these circumstances, it has been possible

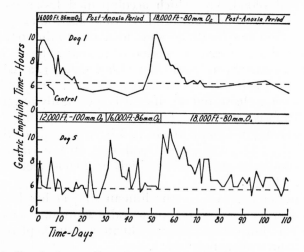

FIG. 10.—Acclimatization to discontinuous exposure to hypoxia. (*Amer. J. Physiol.*, **137** [1942], 160.)

through prolonged intermittent exposures to hypoxia to improve the propulsive motility, as revealed in a comparison with control rats at the severe degree of hypoxia found at 28,000 feet (8,500 meters) (259).

THE NERVOUS SYSTEM

A few reports on the nervous system in the acclimated subject have appeared since the monograph of Van Liere (253). A few weeks stay at moderate altitude (6,600 and 10,200 feet—2,010 and 3,110 meters) has been found to cause in man lengthening of the time of useful consciousness at an extreme altitude (26,200 and 25,000 feet—7,990 and 7,600 meters) (24, 105). Rabbits long subjected to discontinuous hypoxia have a longer latency between interruption of the circulation to the brain (by inflating a cuff at the neck) and loss of the corneal reflex (182).

The pathology of hypoxia has been evident in guinea pigs intermittently exposed for long periods to 30,000 feet (9,100 meters) simulated altitude. Loss of memory, as seen in the alternation maze test, and focal degeneration in the cerebellar vermis were found (126). Similar studies at 23,000 feet (7,000 meters) with the same animal revealed no changes in brain structure (270).

FERTILITY AND REPRODUCTION

In man.—In a translation of a monograph by Monge (166), the historical implications of acclimatization for a continent are reviewed. While fertility and reproduction were normal for the Indian native of the Andean highlands at 13,100 feet (4,000 meters), the colonial Spaniards waited for fifty-three years for their first birth. A capital was moved from Jauja (10,800 feet—3,300 meters) to Lima (sea level) because of the difficulties in adaptation, but one hundred years later Jauja was a flourishing city. In the ecologic interplay between a community and its hypoxic environment over the years, several factors may be operating. There is the acclimatization of the individual. There is the factor of natural selection—the unfit were compelled by nature of things to move away or, in case they did not, left no descendants—the individual capable of complete adjustment remained to pass his adaptability to the next generation. How much did the newcomers profit, in regard to perpetuity, by intermarriage with the already selected and acclimated native?

It is obvious that what has occurred in the case of man has occurred for every species which has successfully invaded an altitude region. Normal fertility (and reproduction) was mentioned as an acceptable criterion of the fully acclimated state.

In animals.—Up to 14,260 feet (4,350 meters), rats brought from near sea level can meet the fertility criterion (170). In this short-term study (60 days) reproduction was considered normal, in spite of cannibalism by mothers and subnormal growth due presumably to faulty lactation.[1] One might insist that adequate lactation and

---

[1] Stickney, Browne, and Van Liere (West Virginia Academy of Science Proceedings, **34:** 7, 196), working with goats over a four-year period, studied the effect on milk production of four hours' daily exposure to a simulated altitude of from 22,000 to 25,000 feet. Two goats showed but little reduction of milk output, but three of the animals showed a pronounced decrease (32–67 per cent). The authors concluded that there was a marked individual variation in the effect of hypoxia on the production of milk in goats. More work is needed on the effect of hypoxia on lactation.

proper maternal feelings toward the young properly belong to reproduction in the general sense and so question whether in the above
experiment the standard had been met.

In studies of the effect on rats of discontinuous exposures of one
hour per day at 18,000 feet (5,500 meters) was found to be innocuous
in respect to fertility and reproduction (175). Four-hour daily
exposures were found to reduce fertility, to decrease the seminal
vesicle/body weight ratio, and to produce abnormal gestation (5). At
25,000 feet (7,600 meters) (4) in rats similarly treated, complete
sterility in the male was seen, apparently resulting from the effect
of hypoxemia upon the primary sex organs. Failure in the female
was laid to general debility rather than to structural damage. Lack of
gonadotrophic hormone secretion does not occur under such circumstances (92). In these studies, in part carried on above the range
where acclimatization can occur, the pathologic effects of hypoxia
have been seen, while in no case has the observation of improvement
in reproductive physiology during continued exposure to hypoxia
been made. In other words, in none of them has there been an op-
portunity to observe the changes in reproductive physiology occurring
during the process of acclimatization. In sheep imported into the
high Andes, (76) improvement in semen quality of rams has been
noted during a month's residence.

THE ACCLIMATIZED INDIVIDUAL AT SEA LEVEL

Monge (166, 167) has held to the view that the acclimatized individual is at a disadvantage at sea level. This does not seem at all unreasonable. In support of the contention is cited the loss of battles in
South American history by the high-altitude residents when fought
in the lowlands and the present-day failure of athletes of the highlands to equal their high-altitude records at sea level. In both cases
there were uncontrolled variables, such as climatic conditions other
than barometric pressure and, in the case of the athletes, the factor of
competition. On the other hand, there is the finding that partial
adaptation, at any rate, to moderate altitudes improves sea-level exercise performance (17).

Continued residence of the altitude-acclimated individual at sea
level is accompanied by a return of all thus far measured adaptive
mechanisms and associated values to the normal range of sea-level
subjects (167). Respiratory modifications regress within days or
weeks (70, 111). The increased vascularization may apparently dis-

appear within two to three months (112). Values for oxygen capacity or related phenomena return to normal within weeks or months (2, 3, 7, 52, 120, 127, 158, 196, 199, 228, 243) in various species. A few observations have been made of the retention of a general adaptation for longer than six months (227, 258) and beyond the time of persistence of the above factors.

This brings up the question whether all the changes occurring during acclimatization are reversible. Since those studied thus far are known to be, the existence of any irreversible changes is largely speculative. The uncertainty could be resolved by determining whether any lasting benefits accrue from a bout of complete adaptation to chronic hypoxia. This might be approached by investigating whether the time required for a reacclimatization is altered in duration.

DOES INTERMITTENT EXPOSURE ACCLIMATIZE?

As we have seen in discussions of the various adaptations which the mammalian organism makes to chronic hypoxia, discontinuous exposure can result, with few exceptions, in similar qualitative, if not quantitative, changes. The failure, during intermittent exposures, in the long-term acclimatization (assumed on incomplete evidence) of respiration with its associated decline in alkaline reserve and concomitant increase in ventilation may simply mean that the effective altitude stress is correspondingly greater. This might mean only the alteration of thresholds. If the thus far overt or measurable adjustments to chronic hypoxia are beneficial, as most physiologists agree, their appearance during intermittent exposure could be expected to confer upon the individual acquiring them a corresponding resistance to hypoxic stress. This would be true only if the benefits were to outweigh the pathologic changes occurring at the same time. In the presence of adaptive changes, and in the absence of significant lesions, any superiority of acclimatization through continuous exposure may indicate the presence of hitherto unmeasured adaptive mechanisms.

Armstrong and Heim (9), as a result of their studies of the rabbit, concluded that intermittent exposures were not adaptive, but detrimental. Reynolds and Phillips (205) have made similar conclusions in respect to the rat exposed one hour per day for nine weeks to 18,000 feet (5,500 meters). The basis for their conclusion was the presence of lesions of heart, lungs, and stomach, and the inferior survival rate at 50,000 feet (15,000 meters), one week (but not immediately) after the end of the exposure period. The general physical condition and the rate of weight gain appeared normal. Under similar conditions Nelson and Burrill (175) have found reproduction and fertility unaltered. With two-hour daily exposures to both 18,000 and 26,000 feet (5,500 and 7,900 meters), Thorn et al. (242) found increased survival at 34,000 feet (10,000 meters), as compared with the controls. Such improvement was found to occur under conditions which produced no morphologic changes in the organs of the rats. Altland and Highman (6, 7), using longer daily exposures (four hours) in the same species, found cardiac and vascular lesions, reduced fertility and reproduction, and reduced weight gain in the males. Surprisingly enough, they found longevity unaffected in those rats returned permanently to normal barometric pressure after 540 days of age.

For the most part, discontinuous exposures of rats to higher altitudes are attended by high mortality, reproductive failure, and many pathologic changes (4, 60, 92, 106). However, such exposures may be accompanied by sufficient adjustment to reduce the untoward changes induced by hypoxia in certain organ systems (227, 259).

At 25,000 feet (7,600 meters) and above, the intermittently exposed rat fails completely to meet the normal reproduction criterion of complete acclimatization. At 18,000 feet (5,500 meters) the evidence is far from decisive. There is some reproductive shortcoming at the four-hour exposure duration and none for the one-hour exposure period. The two-hour period produces increased survival, either without lesions or at least at a time before they develop. It would seem that the survival test at 34,000 feet is more valid that at 50,000 feet, for the latter tests essentially anaerobic survival only. The presence of pathologic lesions even at the exposure rate of one hour per day is a factor to be considered. It is possible that the rat so exposed has acquired adaptation, perhaps fairly complete, to some degree of hypoxia, quite likely to that associated with a lower altitude than 18,000 feet. It is even more difficult to decide whether such an animal is as well adjusted for continuous exposure to hypoxia.

Similar studies on other species have been less complete. Guinea pigs, five hours per day at 23,000 feet (7,000 meters) (270), suffer no cerebral lesions, while at 30,000 feet (9,100 meters) (126) they suffer both cerebral lesions and impaired memory. In dogs, about eight hours per day at 12,000 to 18,000 feet (3,700 to 5,500 meters), gastric emptying reverts gradually toward normal (227). Four hours per day at 24,000 feet (7,300 meters) may be considered acclimatizing inasmuch as acute exposure to 28,000 feet (8,500 meters) in most cases eventually ceases to set off the emergency response (hyperglycemia) of the autonomic nervous system (258). Similar results, though not as regularly, have been seen in the sheep (225) and in the goat (226).

Several studies have been made of airplane pilots who are subjected to discontinuous hypoxia but to much less severe degrees than in the animal studies. Furthermore, exact degree and duration of stress are unknown in such studies. McFarland *et al.* (154) concluded that in their series "there appeared to be more evidence of acclimatization than of deterioration." Clinton and Thorn (54) found no evidence of increased hematopoiesis as did McFarland *et al.* but concluded that their series was normal. Hurtado and co-workers (118, 120), particularly in their second study, found some evidence of heightened erythropoiesis but concluded that on the whole there was no evidence that fliers develop compensatory adjustments to a constant and significant degree. The railroad personnel of the second study, daily subjected to altitudes up to 15,510 feet (4,740 meters), showed these changes to a greater degree. In the above studies on human subjects, the absence of clear-cut evidence of adaptation is not extraordinary in view of the mild nature of the hypoxic stress in general. It is possible that the adaptation was simply too small to be gauged by the means used to measure it. Such a means, as tolerance time, has revealed the superior adaptation of trained fliers as compared with non-fliers (30). The absence of signs of deterioration is significant for the hygiene of persons subjected to such conditions.

SUMMARY

Complete acclimatization to chronic exposure to low oxygen tension in the inspired air is characterized by an integrated series of adaptations involving the various organ-systems and tissues of the body, notably:

1. Increased ventilation of the lungs elevates appreciably the O_2 tension in the alveoli while simultaneously reducing the CO_2 tension. The adaptation is complete when alkaline reserve has been reduced so that blood pH is brought within the normal range. Respiratory control at this point is more completely based in the medullary respiratory centers, but the chemoreceptors still play a part.

2. The adrenal cortex may have a heightened activity in this state, but it is not apparent. Its chief role apparently has been discharged in the early adaptation of the acute phase of exposure while

acid-base balance was being adjusted and while increased demands were being made on carbohydrate metabolism.

3. While cardiac output may have been increased during the early adaptive process, output is not increased over the pre-exposure value in the completely adjusted organism either at rest or in exercise. There is possibly a minimal amount of cardiac hypertrophy involving mainly the right heart.

4. There is a tremendously increased vascularization of many tissues involving at least greater diameter and tortuosity of the smaller vessels. Improved diffusion of O_2, nutrients, and metabolites is visualized as the result of the hyperemia.

5. The O_2 carrying ability of the blood is markedly increased. There is experimental evidence that the value of the increase may be greater than formerly theorized. Oxygen is released from hemoglobin more readily either because of actually reduced affinity, reduced pH of the blood, or both. The end result is a gain in O_2 tension in the tissues. The evidence for altered size of the erythrocyte is conflicting. In the human being at least, since plasma volume is unchanged in the acclimated state, the increase in total blood volume reflects the increase in total O_2 capacity. The polycythemia is the result of an equilibrium between a heightened hematopoiesis and increased blood destruction (proportionate to total red cell mass) while the life of the red blood cell remains unaltered. The increased turnover in erythrocyte mass is associated with the bilirubinemia seen in the individual acclimated to rather high altitudes.

6. There is no evidence that the resting metabolic rate is changed.

7. Growth and body weight remain normal.

8. The question of increased muscle myoglobin content in the acclimated state remains in doubt. The possibility of increased cytochrome C content raises more questions than it answers.

9. The latest report that the acclimated subject has as great capacity for work as the sea-level resident and performs it more efficiently should be confirmed. If true, it points apparently to adjustments of a chemical nature.

10. As far as can be judged from incomplete evidence, there are alterations in renal physiology in acclimated man, but these do not prevent the effective functioning of the kidney.

11. On the basis of incomplete evidence, the gastrointestinal tract appears to maintain its normal function.

12. The findings of reduced performance in reaction time tests and of increased auditory threshold remain unchallenged. These and

the normal ability in the dotting test constitute our inventory of the higher responses of the nervous system. (See chap. xviii, p. 306.)

13. Normal fertility and reproductive powers remain cardinal criteria of the acclimated state.

Much of the work on intermittent exposure to reduced O_2 tensions has been carried out at levels which induce pathologic changes. Nevertheless, concomitant acclimatizing changes have been definitely found. They are probably never complete in the strict sense, but they doubtless elevate the ceiling altitude. The data from studies of human subjects definitely rule out deterioration as a result of discontinuous exposure to moderate altitudes.

ACCLIMATIZATION TO CARBON MONOXIDE

Man and animals may become acclimatized not only to air containing a low partial pressure of oxygen but also to air which contains small amounts of carbon monoxide. This is not unexpected, since it is thought that, for the main part, carbon monoxide produces a hemic type of hypoxia.

Acclimatization in animals.—The first systematic examination of acclimatization of animals to carbon monoxide was made by Nasmith and Graham (174) in 1906. These investigators found that guinea pigs kept continuously in a diluted carbon monoxide atmosphere showed an increase in the quantity of hemoglobin and in the number of RBC's. The blood, therefore, had increased its oxygen-carrying capacity. It has been shown by Campbell (43) that mice acclimatize slowly to atmospheres containing about 0.30 per cent carbon monoxide (30 parts per 10,000) and, further, that rabbits, rats, mice, and guinea pigs, after acclimatization produced by continuous exposure to carbon monoxide, could tolerate a much higher atmospheric concentration of carbon monoxide than they could when unacclimatized. Killick (132) in 1937, working with mice, showed that acclimatization occurred, in that there was an absence of positive signs of poisoning. Animals exposed for the first time to the atmosphere in which the acclimated mice lived, and which contained carbon monoxide, collapsed very soon.

Killick (134) has emphasized that animals develop a considerable degree of acclimatization to carbon monoxide; and, in summing up the results of the experimental work, she points out that many of them show an increased production of RBC's, a cardiac hypertrophy, an increase in the blood volume, and splenic enlargement. According to Killick, however, no evidence has been found indicating a change in the relative affinity of hemoglobin for carbon monoxide.

More recent studies in animals have confirmed the increase in oxygen capacity, hematocrit, RBC's, or hemoglobin concentration during chronic continuous or discontinuous exposure to atmospheres containing carbon monoxide (53, 90, 268). Gorbatow and Noro (90) found that, during forty-seven days of brief exposures of rats to 0.5 per cent carbon monoxide, RBC and hemoglobin concentrations reverted to original values after an initial elevation but tolerance remained increased nevertheless. New phenomena of adaptive nature have been found in dogs (145). On the other hand, Lewey and Drabkin (142) found, in dogs intermittently exposed to 0.01 per cent carbon monoxide (producing about 20 per cent carboxyhemoglobin, a saturation which had been deemed harmless to human beings) for eleven weeks, pathologic changes in cardiac muscle and in the brain. Definite shortcomings in acclimatization were also found by Suhrie and Miller (233) in rats discontinuously exposed to 0.04 per cent carbon monoxide. In comparison with controls, not only were there fewer litters, a smaller litter size, and lesser body weight at birth, but also the carbon monoxide exposed mothers refused to nurse their young.

Acclimatization in man.—It was pointed out as early as 1856 by Faure (79) that subjects whose work exposed them to carbon monoxide developed a certain amount of tolerance or acclimatization. Later writers (87, 178) also called attention to this phenomenon.

According to Killick (134), attempts to acclimatize human subjects to carbon monoxide have yielded conflicting results. In 1896 Haldane and Smith (99), who at that time were engaged in experiments which necessitated breathing a small amount of carbon monoxide, observed that after a certain length of time they became more resistant to it. In 1929 Sayers *et al.* (213) subjected individuals to repeated daily exposures to small amounts of automobile exhaust gas. The experiments extended over two months; the hemoglobin content of five of the six men increased; in four of the subjects there was an increase in the RBC count; the greatest increase in the amount of hemoglobin was 30 per cent; and in the RBC count, 1,000,000 per cubic millimeter. Killick (131) in 1936 reported somewhat similar studies on one human subject. She concluded that the subject developed a considerable degree of acclimatization, as evidenced by the symptoms experienced. She found, however, no increase in the number of RBC's nor in the hemoglobin. She pointed out that the exposures to carbon monoxide had not been very frequent. Killick in 1948 (133) repeated the studies on herself to determine whether specific activity of the pulmonary membrane, like excretion of carbon monoxide or prevention of its diffusion into the blood, actually occurred in acclimatization. Her confirmation of the original findings has been received by Lilienthal in his excellent review (146) with considerable skepticism as to the reliability of the method. He maintained, as well, his realistic conviction for the inert character of the pulmonary membranes.

ACCLIMATIZATION IN CONGENITAL HEART DISEASE

The patient with congenital cardiovascular defects in which there is shunting of large amounts of blood from the right heart to the left heart and thus bypassing of the lungs is subjected to hypoxia whose severity depends largely upon the magnitude of the shunt. Varying amounts of cyanosis may be present. Since the shunted blood contains venous amounts of carbon dioxide, the carbon dioxide tension in arterial blood may not be as low as it is in altitude hypoxia.

Respiratory factors.—In such patients pulmonary ventilation is increased presumably indirectly by stimulation of the respiratory center through chemoreceptors in carotid and aortic bodies because of the diminished oxygen saturation. Increases, if any, in hydrogen-ion concentration and/or in arterial carbon dioxide would be expected to stimulate the center directly. In 1941 Talbott *et al.* (236) reported the physiologic findings in one case of the tetralogy of Fallot and presented in addition those on other cases found in the literature.

Bing *et al.* studied a series of thirty patients with congenital heart defects in which the average arterial oxygen saturation was 75 per cent instead of the normal 95 per cent (28). The pulmonary ventilation was 4.87 liters per minute per square meter of body surface. Compared to a normal value of 2.82, this indicates a 70 per cent increase in minute-volume. More recently Husson and Otis (123) have reported a series of cyanotic congenital heart defects in forty-two patients. In their comparison of the respiratory characteristics of these subjects with those acclimatized to high altitude, they found, in spite of considerable scatter of points, many similarities in the two groups. However, the alveolar ventilation of the patients was generally not as great as in those at altitude. As the authors point out, it is interesting to speculate why the congenital heart patient does not attain as great a ventilation. In respect to oxygen, the benefit of increased ventilation is largely lost because of the shunt, for the arterial blood is nearly saturated anyway. Husson and Otis point out that the acidosis (frequently present) is beneficial, permitting unloading of oxygen from the blood at about 5 mm. higher oxygen tension than otherwise.

The work of the latter authors quite definitely indicates the presence of an acidosis, with reduced alkaline reserve and decreased pH as a general trend in the patients. Morse and Cassells (171), in a group of sixty patients with arterial oxygen saturations between 21 and 93 per cent, found pH of arterial serum below normal in one-third of the cases. They also observed a rough parallelism between the arterial unsaturation and the decrease in alkaline reserve and pH.

Systemic blood flow.—The determination of systemic blood flow is fraught with unusual difficulties in the congenital heart patient even with the classical Fick method. Because of the abnormalities in the structure of the heart, it is not always possible to obtain reliable samples of mixed venous blood. Furthermore, because of collaterals from the systemic circulation to the lung, not all blood leaving the heart will return by way of the venae cavae and right atrium.

Bing *et al.* (28), in the study referred to above, obtained an average systemic flow of 3.659 1/min/m^2; and Burchell *et al.* (38), a value of 3.70. The latter workers had twenty patients for subjects whose arterial oxygen saturation averaged 80.3 per cent. Both averages are somewhat higher than the 3.3 value Stead *et al.* (222) found for the composed normal subject. Theoretically, increased cardiac output should confer some benefit by keeping venous oxygen tensions from getting so low and thus not only sparing tissue oxygen tensions but also reducing the arterial oxygen saturation due to shunted blood.

Blood picture.—As in residents at high altitudes, congenital heart patients with cyanosis have increased oxygen capacities and hemoglobin concentrations. Bing *et al.* (28) obtained values of 29.9 ml oxygen/100 ml blood and 22.3 g/hemoglobin 100 ml blood, respectively. Burchell *et al.* (38) found an average capacity of 25.9. Ernsting and Shephard (78), in twenty-four patients, found 29.40 ml/100 ml oxygen capacity or 21.9 g/100 ml hemoglobin concentration. Husson and Otis (123) have plotted oxygen capacity and oxygen content of arterial blood against arterial oxygen saturation of high altitude subjects. They found a straight-line increase of oxygen capacity as saturation declined and a theoretical maximum oxygen content at 70.5 per cent saturation. When the values for their patients, many hypoxic because of right to left circulatory shunts, were treated in the same way, although much scatter was present, considerable similarity with the altitude dweller was noticed. Both Bing *et al.* (28) and Husson and

Otis (123) have pointed out the considerable gain to the congenital heart patient of increased oxygen capacity.

However, the shape of the normal hemoglobin dissociation curve is probably of most importance in keeping capillary oxygen tensions elevated in spite of reduced arterial tensions. This is true for the altitude dweller as well as the congenital heart patient. Whereas the normal arterial-capillary gradient may be 33 mm. Hg, the heart patient may unload the same amount of oxygen, other things being equal, with a 9.4 mm. gradient (28). Moreover, Morse *et al.* (172) found that in a group of twenty-five patients the oxyhemoglobin dissociation curve was significantly shifted to the right. The shift was particularly pronounced in those cases with stenosis of the pulmonary artery as an added complication of the defective circulation. This shift, of course, recalls the finding in subjects at high altitude (see p. 181) and, as in the latter subjects, is definitely beneficial and therefore adaptive.

Basal metabolism.—All the workers (38, 78, 107, 171) in the field have found basal metabolic rates to be in the normal range or increased, if anything (123), except Bing *et al.* (28), who found them rather generally below normal with an average value of −23. Obviously, reduced metabolic rate is not depended upon for adaptation, although the reduced physical activity of the more severely afflicted patients might be looked upon in this light.

Diffusing capacity.—Whether diffusing capacity of the lung is improved in these patients in a manner similar to the finding at high altitude (see p. 140) has not been widely determined. Auchincloss *et al.* (16) have studied sixteen patients with congenital cardiac defects, but arterial oxygen saturation was not particularly low in any of the patients. However, the diffusing capacity with the single breath carbon monoxide technique gave a value of 34 ml/min/mm Hg, which was higher than the value of 27 predicted upon the basis of studies on normal subjects. Such an adaptive mechanism might well be present in those patients having hypoxia as a further complication.

REFERENCES

1. ALBRITTON, E. C. 1952. *Standard Values in Blood.* Philadelphia: Saunders.
2. ALTLAND, P. D. 1949. *Fed. Proc.,* **8:** 3.
3. ———. 1949. *J. Aviat. Med.,* **20:** 186.

4. ALTLAND, P. D. 1949. *J. Exp. Zool.*, **110**: 1.
5. ———. 1949. *Physiol. Zool.*, **22**: 235.
6. ALTLAND, P. D., and HIGHMAN, B. 1951. *Amer. J. Physiol.*, **167**: 261.
7. ———. 1952. *Ibid.*, **168**: 345.
8. ———. 1957. *J. Aviat. Med.*, **28**: 253.
9. ARMSTRONG, H. G., and HEIM, J. W. 1938. *J. Aviat. Med.*, **9**: 92.
10. ASMUSSEN, E., and CONSOLAZIO, F. 1941. *Amer. J. Physiol.*, **132**: 555.
11. ASMUSSEN, E., and NIELSEN, M. 1945. *Acta Physiol. Scand.*, **9**: 75.
12. ASTE-SALAZAR, H., and HURTADO, A. 1944. *Amer. J. Physiol.*, **142**: 733.
13. ASTRAND, P. O. 1954. *Acta Physiol. Scand.*, **30**: 335.
14. ———. *Ibid.*, p. 343.
15. ASTRAND, P., and ASTRAND, I. 1958. *J. Appl. Physiol.*, **13**: 75.
16. AUCHINCLOSS, J. H., JR.; GILBERT, R.; and EICH, R. H. 1959. *Circulation*, **19**: 232.
17. BALKE, B. 1944. *Klin. Wschr.*, **23**: 223.
18. BARCROFT, J. 1925. *The Respiratory Function of the Blood*, Part I, "Lessons from High Altitudes," p. 111. Cambridge: Cambridge University Press.
19. BARCROFT, J., *et al.* 1923. *Phil. Trans. Roy. Soc., London*, B, **211**: 351.
20. BECKER, E. L. 1955. *Amer. J. Physiol.*, **183**: 203.
21. BECKER, E. L.; COOPER, R. G.; and HATAWAY, G. D. 1955. *J. Appl. Physiol.*, **8**: 166.
22. BECKER, E. L.; SCHILLING, J. A.; and HARVEY, R. B. 1955. *Amer. J. Physiol.*, **183**: 307.
23. ———. 1957. *J. Appl. Physiol.*, **10**: 79.
24. BENZINGER, T., and DÖRING, H. 1942. *Luftfahrtmedizin*, **7**: 141.
25. BERLIN, N. I.; REYNAFARJE, C.; and LAWRENCE, J. H. 1954. *J. Appl. Physiol.*, **7**: 271.
26. BERRY, L. J. 1957. *Proc. Soc. Exp. Biol. Med.*, **96**: 246.
27. BERRY, L. J.; FERRO, C. B.; and BOIT, C. K. Sept., 1957. *USAF Sch. Aviat. Med.*, 57–134.
28. BING, R. J., *et al.* 1948. *Bull. Johns Hopkins Hosp.*, **83**: 439.
29. BJURSTEDT, A. G. H. 1946. *Acta. Physiol. Scand.*, Suppl. 38, **12**: 1.
30. BLASIUS, W. 1948. *Z. Kreislaufforsch.*, **37**: 581.
31. BOUTWELL, J. H., *et al.* 1950. *J. Appl. Physiol.*, **2**: 388.
32. BOUTWELL, J. H.; FARMER, C. J.; and IVY, A. C. 1950. *J. Appl. Physiol.*, **2**: 381.
33. BOWEN, W. J., and EADS, H. J. 1949. *Amer. J. Physiol.*, **159**: 77.
34. BOWEN, W. J., and POEL, W. E. 1948. *Fed. Proc.*, **7**: 11.
35. BROWN, E. B., JR., *et al.* 1948. *J. Appl. Physiol.*, **1**: 333.
36. BRUEHL, W., and HANISCH, K. 1942. *Klin. Wschr.*, **21**: 253.
37. BUHLMANN, A., *et al.* 1951. *Schweiz. Med. Wschr.*, **81**: 80.
38. BURCHELL, H. B., *et al.* 1950. *Circulation*, **1**: 404.

39. BURKARDT, W. L., *et al.* 1951. *Amer. J. Physiol.* (Proc.), **167**: 772.
40. BURRILL, M. W., and IVY, A. C. 1950. *J. Appl. Physiol.*, **2**: 437.
41. BURRILL, M. W.; SMITH, F.; and IVY, A. C. 1945. *J. Biol. Chem.*, **157**: 297.
42. CAMPBELL, J. A. 1932. *J. Physiol.* (Proc.), **77**: 8*P*.
43. ———. 1932. *J. Physiol.*, **78**: 8.
44. ———. 1935. *Brit. J. Exp. Path.*, **16**: 39.
45. CHIODI, H. 1950. *J. Appl. Physiol.*, **2**: 431.
46. ———. 1957. *Ibid.*, **10**: 81.
47. CHIODI, H.; CALDERON, L. O.; and SUAREZ, J. R. 1952. *Ciencia Investigacion*, **8**: 466.
48. CHRISTENSEN, E. H., and FORBES, W. H. 1937. *Skand. Arch. Physiol.*, **76**: 75.
49. CHRISTENSEN, E. H. 1954. *Proc. Roy. Soc. London*, B, **143**: 8.
50. CLARK, R. T., JR.; CRISCUOLO, D.; and COULSON, C. K. 1952. *Fed. Proc.*, **11**: 25.
51. CLARK, R. T., JR., *et al.* 1953. *XIX Internat. Physiol. Cong.* (Montreal), p. 271.
52. CLARK, R. T., JR., and OTIS, A. B. 1952. *Amer. J. Physiol.*, **169**: 285.
53. CLARK, R. T., JR.; OTIS, A. B.; and LEUNG, S. W. 1949. *Amer. J. Physiol.* (Proc.), **159**: 564.
54. CLINTON, M., and THORN, G. 1943. *War Med.*, **4**: 363.
55. COHN, E. W., and D'AMOUR, F. E. 1951. *Amer. J. Physiol.*, **166**: 394.
56. COOK, S. F., and ALAFI, M. H. 1956. *Amer. J. Physiol.*, **186**: 369.
57. CRISCUOLO, D., and CLARK, R. T., JR., December, 1955. *USAF Sch. Aviat. Med.*, 55–84.
58. CRISCUOLO, D.; CLARK, R. T., JR.; and MEFFERD, R. B., JR. 1955. *Amer. J. Physiol.*, **180**: 215.
59. CRISCUOLO, D.; HALE, H. B.; and MEFFERD, R. B., JR. July, 1958. *USAF Sch. Aviat. Med.*, 58–94.
60. DALTON, A. J., *et al.* 1945. *J. Nat. Cancer Inst.*, **6**: 161.
61. ———. 1944. *Ibid.* **4**: 527.
62. D'ANGELO, S. A. 1946. *Amer. J. Physiol.*, **145**: 365.
63. DARROW, D. C., and SARASON, E. L. 1944. *J. Clin. Invest.*, **23**: 11.
64. DEJOURS, P., *et al.* 1959. *Rev. Franc. Etud. Clin. Biol.*, **4**: 115.
65. DELACHAUX, A. et BERSON, I. 1947. *Helv. Med. Acta*, **14**: 463.
66. DILL, D. B. 1950. *Science*, **111**: 19.
67. DILL, D. B.; CHRISTENSEN, E. H.; and EDWARDS, H. T. 1936. *Amer. J. Physiol.*, **115**: 530.
68. DILL, D. B.; TALBOTT, T. H.; and CONSOLAZIO, W. V. 1937. *J. Biol. Chem.*, **118**: 649.
69. DOHAN, F. C. 1942. *Proc. Soc. Exp. Biol. Med.*, **49**: 404.
70. DORRANCE, S. S., *et al.* 1943. *Amer. J. Physiol.*, **139**: 399.
71. DOUGLAS, C. G., *et al.* 1913. *Trans. Roy. Soc. London*, B, **203**: 185.
72. DRABKIN, D. L. 1947. *J. Biol. Chem.*, **171**: 409.

73. DRABKIN, D. L., and GRAYBIEL, A. 1951. *Fed. Proc.,* **10**: 177.
74. DUNER, H.; PERNOW, B.; and TRIBUKAIT, B. 1958. *Acta. Physiol. Scand.,* **44**: 365.
75. DURIG, A. 1909. *Physiologische Ergebnisse der im Jahr 1906 durchgeführten Monta Rosa Expedition.* Wien.
76. EASLEY, G. T. 1951. *J. Amer. Vet. Med. Ass.,* **119**: 278.
77. EDWARDS, H. T. 1936. *Amer. J. Physiol.,* **116**: 367.
78. ERNSTING, J., and SHEPHARD, R. J. 1951. *J. Physiol.,* **112**: 332.
79. FAURE. 1856. *Arch. Gen. Med.* (5th ser.) , **7**: 20.
80. FELDMAN, J.; CORTELL, R.; and GELLHORN, E. 1940. *Amer. J. Physiol.,* **131**: 281.
81. FENN, W. O.; RAHN, H.; and OTIS, A. B. 1946. *Amer. J. Physiol.,* **146**: 637.
82. FORBES, W. H. 1936. *Amer. J. Physiol.,* **116**: 309.
83. FRYERS, G. R. 1952. *Amer. J. Physiol.,* **171**: 459.
84. GELLHORN, E. 1943. *Autonomic Regulations,* p. 49. New York: Interscience Publishers.
85. GIL, J. R., and TERAN, D. G. 1948. *Blood,* **3**: 660.
86. GIRAGOSSINTZ, G., and SUNDSTROEM, E. G. 1937. *Proc. Soc. Exp. Biol. Med.,* **36**: 432.
87. GLAISTER, J., and LOGAN, D. D. 1914. *Gas Poisoning in Mining and Other Industries,* p. 209. New York: W. Wood & Co.
88. GOMEZ, G. E. 1948. *J.A.M.A.,* **137**: 1297.
89. GOODMAN, J. 1947. *Proc. Soc. Exp. Biol. Med.,* **64**: 336.
90. GORBATOW, O., and NORO, L. 1948. *Acta. Physiol. Scand.,* **15**: 77.
91. GORDON, A. S. 1959. *Physiol. Rev.,* **39**: 1.
92. GORDON, A. S.; TORNETTA, F. J.; and CHARIPPER, H. A. 1943. *Proc. Soc. Exp. Biol. Med.,* **53**: 6.
93. GRANT, W. C. 1951. *Amer. J. Physiol.,* **164**: 226.
94. ———. 1951. *Proc. Soc. Exp. Biol. Med.,* **77**: 537.
95. GRANT, W. C., and ROOT, W. S. 1953. *Amer. J. Physiol.,* **173**: 321.
96. GRAY, J. S. November 21, 1945. *USAF Sch. Aviat. Med.,* Proj. No. 386, Report No. 3.
97. GRAY, C. H.; NEUBERGER, A.; SNEATH, P. H. A. 1950. *Biochem. J.,* **47**: 87.
98. HAILMAN, H. F. 1944. *Endocrinology,* **34**: 187.
99. HALDANE, J. S., and SMITH, J. L. 1896. *J. Physiol.,* **20**: 497.
100. HALL, F. G., and BARKER, J. 1954. *Proc. Soc. Exp. Biol. Med.,* **86**: 165.
101. HARNISCHFEGER, E., and OPITZ, E. 1950. *Pflueger Arcih. Ges. Physiol.,* **252**: 627.
102. HEBER, A. R. 1921. *Lancet,* **1**: 1148.
103. HECHT, H. H., et al. 1962. *Amer. J. Med.,* **32**: 171.
104. HENDERSON, Y. 1938. *Adventures in Respiration,* p. 76. Baltimore: Williams & Wilkins Co.

105. HETHERINGTON, A. W.; LUFT, U.; and IVY, J. H. December, 1947. *Digest Ser. 4*, G. E. 61/1.
106. HIGHMAN, B., and ALTLAND, P. D. 1949. *Arch. Path.*, **48**: 503.
107. HOLLING, H. E., and ZAK, G. A. 1950. *Brit. Heart J.*, **12**: 153.
108. HOUSSAY, R. H. 1951. *Las Suprarrenales en la Hypoxia y la Intoxication por Histamina.* Buenos Aires: Liberia "El Ateneo."
109. HOUSTON, C. S. 1946. *USN Med. Bull.* **46**: 1783.
110. ———. 1947. *J. Aviat. Med.*, **18**: 237.
111. HOUSTON, C. S., and RILEY, R. L. 1947. *Amer. J. Physiol.*, **149**: 565.
112. HUERKAMP, B., and OPITZ, E. 1950. *Pflueger Arch. Ges. Physiol.*, **252**: 129.
113. HUEY, D. M., and HOLMES, J. H. 1950. *Fed. Proc.*, **9**: 64.
114. HURTADO, A. 1932. *Amer. J. Phys. Anthrop.*, **17**: 137.
115. ———. 1932. *Amer. J. Physiol.*, **100**: 487.
116. ———. Nov., 1949. "International Symposium on High Altitude Biology." Unpublished abstract, Lima.
117. HURTADO, A., and ASTE-SALAZAR, H. 1948. *J. Appl. Physiol.*, **1**: 304.
118. HURTADO, A., *et al.* 1947. *J. Aviat. Med.*, **18**: 406.
119. HURTADO, A.; ASTE-SALAZAR, H.; and REYNAFARJE, B. (See N. 116 above.)
120. HURTADO, A.; MERINO, C.; and DELGADO, E. 1945. *Arch. Intern. Med.*, **75**: 284.
121. HURTADO, A., *et al.* 1937. *Amer. J. Med. Sci.*, **194**: 708.
122. HURTADO, A., *et al.* March, 1956. *USAF Sch. Aviat. Med.*, Report No. 56–1: 1–62.
123. HUSSON, C., and OTIS, A. B. 1957. *J. Clin. Invest.*, **36**: 270.
124. IZQUIERDO, J. J. 1922. *C. R. Soc. Biol.* (Par.) , **88**: 639.
125. JENSEN, A. V., and ALT, H. L. 1945. *Proc. Soc. Exp. Biol. Med.*, **60**: 384.
126. JENSEN, A. V.; BECKER, R. F.; and WINDLE, W. F. 1948. *Arch. Neurol. Psychiat.*, **60**: 221.
127. JONES, B. F., *et al.* Jan. 1943. *C. A. M. Report No. 104.*
128. KELLOGG, R. H., *et al.* 1957. *J. Appl. Physiol.*, **11**: 65.
129. KERWIN, A. J. 1944. *Amer. Heart J.*, **28**: 69.
130. KEYS, A.; HALL, F. G.; and BARRON, E. S. G. 1936. *Amer. J. Physiol.*, **115**: 292.
131. KILLICK, E. M. 1936. *J. Physiol.*, **87**: 41.
132. ———. 1937. *Ibid.*, **91**: 229.
133. ———. 1948. *Ibid.*, **107**: 27.
134. ———. 1940. *Physiol. Rev.*, **20**: 313.
135. KINDRED, JAMES E. 1943. *Amer. J. Physiol.*, **140**: 387.
136. KOSTIAL, K.; SIMONOVIC, I.; and HAUSLER, V. 1958. *Amer. J. Physiol.*, **194**: 72.
137. KRASNO, L. R., *et al.* 1950. *J. Aviat. Med.*, **21**: 283.
138. LANGLEY, L. L., and CLARKE, R. W. 1942. *Yale J. Biol. Med.*, **14**: 529.

208 HYPOXIA

139. LANGLEY, L. L.; NIMS, L. F.; and CLARKE, R. W. 1950. *Amer. J. Physiol.*, 161: 331.
140. LANGLEY, L. L.; SCOKEL, P. W.; and WHITESIDE, J. A. 1952. *Fed. Proc.*, 11: 88.
141. LAWRENCE, J. H., *et al.* 1952. *Acta Med. Scand.*, 142: 117.
142. LEWEY, F. H., and DRABKIN, D. L. 1944. *Amer. J. Med. Sci.*, 208: 502.
143. LEWIS, R. C., *et al.* 1943. *J. Lab. Clin. Med.*, 28: 851.
144. ————. *Ibid.*, p. 860.
145. LILLEHEI, J. P.; WILKS, S. S.; and CARTER, E. T. 1954. *Fed. Proc.*, 13: 89.
146. LILIENTHAL, J. L., JR. 1950. *Pharm. Rev.*, 2: 324.
147. LIPIN, J. L., and WHITEHORN, W. V. 1950. *Fed. Proc.*, 9: 79.
148. LIPIN, J. L., and WHITEHORN, W. V. 1950. *J. Aviat. Med.*, 21: 405.
149. LOEWY, A., and MOERIKOFER, W. 1932. *Physiologie des Hohenklimas.* Berlin: J. Springer.
150. LOEWY, A., and MARTON, S. 1934. *Z. Konstitutionslehre*, 18: 148.
151. LUNDGREN, N. P. V., *et al.* July, 1954. *USAF Sch. Aviat. Med.*, Report No. 3.
152. MARSHALL, L. H.; HANNA, C. H.; and SPECHT, H. 1952. *Amer. J. Physiol.*, 171: 499.
153. MARSHALL, L., and SPECHT, H. 1950. *Amer. J. Physiol.* (Proc.), 163: 733.
154. McFARLAND, R. A., *et al.* 1939. *J. Aviat. Med.*, 10: 160.
155. MERCKER, H. 1943. *Luftfahrtmedizin*, 8: 217.
156. MERCKER, H., and OPITZ, E. 1949. *Pflueger Arch. Ges. Physiol.*, 251: 117.
157. MERCKER, H., and SCHNEIDER, M. 1949. *Pflueger Arch. Ges. Physiol.*, 251: 49.
158. MERINO, C. F. 1950. *Blood*, 5: 1.
159. ————. November, 1956. *USAF Sch. Aviat. Med.*, 56–103.
160. MERINO, C. F., and REYNAFARJE, C. 1949. *J. Lab. Clin. Med.*, 34: 637.
161. MEYER, H. H. 1912. *J. Med. Bruxelles*, 17: 409 and 424.
162. MIRANDA, A., and ROTTA, A. 1944. *An. Fac. Med. Lima*, 26: 49.
163. MONGE, C. 1942. *Science*, 95: 79.
164. ————. 1943. *Physiol. Rev.*, 23: 166.
165. ————. 1945. *An. Fac. Med. (Lima)*, 28: 307.
166. ————. 1948. *Acclimatization in the Andes.* Translated by D. F. BROWN. Baltimore: Johns Hopkins Press.
167. ————. Nov., 1949. "International Symposium on High Altitude Biology." Unpublished Abstract. Lima.
168. MONGE, C., *et al.* 1955. *Acta Physiol. Lat. Amer.*, 5: 198.
169. MONGE, C. M., *et al.* 1931. *An. Fac. Med. (Lima)*, 17: 727.
170. MOORE, C., and PRICE, D. 1948. *J. Exp. Zool.*, 108: 171.
171. MORSE, M., and CASSELS, D. E. 1953. *J. Clin. Invest.*, 32: 837.
172. MORSE, M.; CASSELS, D. E.; and HOLDER, M. 1950. *J. Clin. Invest.*, 29: 1098.

173. Mossberger, J. J. 1949. *Amer. J. Dis. Child.,* **78:** 28.
174. Nasmith, G. G., and Graham, D. A. 1906–07. *J. Physiol.,* **35:** 32.
175. Nelson, D., and Burrill, M. W. 1944. *Fed. Proc.,* **3:** 34.
176. Neuberger, A., and Niven, J. S. F. 1951. *J. Physiol.,* **112:** 292.
177. Ocaranza, F. 1926. *Rev. Mex. Biol.,* **6:** 118.
178. Oliver, T. 1916. *Diseases of Occupation* (3d ed.) , p. 68. New York: E. P. Dutton & Co.
179. Opitz, E. *In: German Aviation Medicine, World War II.* Washington, D.C.: U.S. Govt. Printing Office, 1950.
180. ———. 1951. *Exp. Med. Surg.,* **9:** 389.
181. ———. 1952. *Pflueger Arch. Ges. Physiol.,* **254:** 549.
182. Opitz, E., and Thorn, W. 1949. *Pflueger Arch. Ges. Physiol.,* **251:** 369.
183. Pace, N., *et al.* 1947. *Amer. J. Physiol.,* **148:** 152.
184. Pawel, N. E. R.; Clark, R. T., and Chinn, H. I. April, 1954. *USAF Sch. Aviat. Med.,* Report No. 4.
185. Penaloza, D., and Echevarria, M. 1957. *Amer. Heart J.,* **54:** 811.
186. Penaloza, D., *et al.* 1960. *Amer. Heart J.,* **59:** 111.
187. ———. 1961. *Ibid.,* **61:** 101.
188. Petty, T.; Bartlett, W.; and Chapin, J. L. 1955. *Proc. Soc. Exp. Biol. Med.,* **90:** 664.
189. Picon-Reategui, E. December, 1956. *USAF Sch. Aviat. Med.,* Report No. 56–105.
190. ———. November, 1956. *Ibid.,* Report No. 56–107.
191. Poel, W. E. 1949. *Amer. J. Physiol.,* **156:** 44.
192. Prystowsky, H., *et al.* 1960. *Quart. J. Exp. Physiol.,* **45:** 292.
193. Rahn, H., and Otis, A. B. 1949. *Amer. J. Physiol.,* **157:** 445.
194. Rahn, H., *et al.* 1953. *J. Appl. Physiol.,* **6:** 158.
195. Reed, D. J.; and Kellogg, R. H. 1958. *J. Appl. Physiol.,* **13:** 325.
196. Reissmann, K. R. July, 1951. *USAF Sch. Aviat. Med.,* Report No. 1.
197. ———. 1951. *Amer. J. Physiol.,* **167:** 52.
198. ———. 1952. *Blood,* **7:** 337.
199. Reissmann, K. R., *et al.* November, 1951. *USAF Sch. Aviat. Med.,* Report No. 4.
200. Rengger-Perlmann. Inaugural dissertation, Zurich, 1927; cited by A. Loewy and E. Wittkower. 1937. *The Pathology of High Altitude Climate.* London: Oxford University Press.
201. Reynafarje, C. 1959. *J. Pediatrics,* **54:** 152.
202. Reynafarje, C.; Berlin, N. I.; and Lawrence, J. H. 1954. *Proc. Soc. Exp. Biol. Med.,* **87:** 101.
203. Reynafarje, C.; Lozano, R.; and Valdivieseo, J. 1959. *Blood,* **14:** 433.
204. Reynolds, O. E. 1947. *Amer. J. Physiol.,* **150:** 65.
205. Reynolds, O. E., and Phillips, N. E. 1947. *Amer. J. Physiol.,* **151:** 147.
206. Rotta, A. 1943. *Rev. Argent. Cardiol.,* **10:** 186.

207. ——. 1947. *Amer. Heart J.*, **33:** 669.
208. ROTTA, A., *et al.* 1956. *J. Appl. Physiol.*, **9:** 328.
209. ROTTA, A., and LOPEZ, A. 1959. *Circulation,* **19:** 719.
210. ROTTA, A., MIRANDA, A., and CHAVEZ, R., cited by A. HURTADO. Nov., 1949. "International Symposium on High Altitude Biology." Unpublished abstract, Lima.
211. SAN MARTIN, M.; PRATO, Y.; and FERNANDEZ, L., August, 1956. *USAF Sch. Aviat. Med.,* Report No. 55–100.
212. SAYERS, G. 1950. *Physiol. Rev.,* **30:** 241.
213. SAYERS, R. R., *et al.* 1930. *Public Health Bull.* (U.S. Public Health Service), No. 195.
214. SCANO, A., *et al.* 1956. *Riv. Med. Aero.* (Roma), **19:** 595.
215. SCHEPERS, G. W. H. 1947. *J. Path. Bact.,* **59:** 199.
216. SCHNEIDER, E. C., and HEDBLOM, C. A. 1908. *Amer. J. Physiol.,* **23:** 90.
217. SCHNEIDER, E. C., and SISCO, D. L. 1914. *Amer. J. Physiol.,* **34:** 7 and 29.
218. SILVETTE, H. 1942. *Proc. Soc. Exp. Biol. Med.,* **51:** 199.
219. ——. 1943. *Amer. J. Physiol.,* **140:** 374.
220. SMITH, H. 1951. *The Kidney.* New York: Oxford University Press.
221. SOBEL, H., and GRABOYES, S. 1958. *Proc. Soc. Exp. Biol. Med.,* **97:** 725.
222. STEAD, E. A., JR., *et al.* 1945. *J. Clin. Invest.,* **24:** 326.
223. STICKNEY, J. C. 1946. *Proc. Soc. Exp. Biol. Med.,* **63:** 210.
224. STICKNEY, J. C.; NORTHUP, D. W.; and VAN LIERE, E. J. 1943. *Proc. Soc. Exp. Biol. Med.,* **54:** 151.
225. ——. 1951. *Amer. J. Physiol.,* **167:** 559.
226. ——. Unpublished observations.
227. STICKNEY, J. C., and VAN LIERE, E. J. 1942. *Amer. J. Physiol.,* **137:** 160.
228. ——. 1942. *J. Aviat. Med.,* **13:** 170.
229. ——. 1953. *Physiol. Rev.,* **33:** 13.
230. STROHL, J. 1910. *Zool. Jahrb.* (*Jena*), **30:** 1.
231. ——. 1912. *Actti Lab. Sci. A. Mosso* (Torino), **3:** 218.
232. SUBAUSTE, C., *et al.* September, 1958. *USAF Sch. Aviat. Med.,* 58–95.
233. SUHRIE, V., and MILLER, A. T., JR. 1944. *Proc. Soc. Exp. Biol. Med.,* **55:** 85.
234. SUNDSTROEM, E. S., and MICHAELS, G. 1942. *Mem. Univ. Calif.,* **12:** 1.
235. SWANN, H. G., and COLLINGS, W. D. 1943. *J. Aviat. Med.,* **14:** 114.
236. TALBOTT, J. H., *et al.* 1941. *Amer. Heart J.,* **22:** 754.
237. TAPPAN, D. V., and REYNAFARJE, B. 1957. *Amer. J. Physiol.,* **190:** 99.
238. TAPPAN, D. V., *et al.* 1957. *Amer. J. Physiol.,* **190:** 93.
239. TAUSSIG, H. B. 1947. *Congenital Malformations of the Heart.* New York: The Commonwealth Fund.
240. TERZIOGLU, M., *et al.* 1952. *Arch. Int. Physiol.,* **60:** 233.
241. THEILEN, E. O.; GREGG, D. E.; and ROTTA, A. 1955. *Circulation,* **12:** 383.

242. THORN, G. W., *et al.* 1946. *Bull. Johns Hopkins Hosp.,* **79:** 59.

243. THORN, G. W., *et al.* 1942. *Amer. J. Physiol.,* **137:** 606.

244. TIMIRAS, P. S., *et al.* 1956. *Fed. Proc.,* **15:** 187.

245. TIMIRAS, P. S., *et al.* 1958. *Amer. J. Physiol.,* **193:** 415.

246. TIMIRAS, P. S.; KRUM, A. A.; and PACE, N. 1957. *Amer. J. Physiol.,* **191:** 598.

247. TIMIRAS, P. S.; PACE, N.; and HWANG, C. A. 1957. *Fed. Proc.,* **16:** 340.

248. ULLRICK, W. C., *et al.* 1956. *J. Appl. Physiol.,* **9:** 49.

249. URTEAGA, O. 1942. *An. Fac. Med. (Lima)*, **25:** 89.

250. VALDIVIA, E. 1957. *Circulat. Res.,* **5:** 612.

251. ———. 1958. *Amer. J. Physiol.,* **194:** 585.

252. VAN LIERE, E. J. 1936. *Amer. J. Physiol.,* **116:** 290.

253. ———. 1942. *Anoxia, Its Effect on the Body.* Chicago: University of Chicago Press.

254. VAN LIERE, E. J.; FANG, H. S.; and NORTHUP, D. W. 1954. *Amer. J. Physiol.,* **178:** 503.

255. VAN LIERE, E. J., and FEDOR, E. J. 1955. *Proc. Soc. Exp. Biol. Med.,* **88:** 676.

256. VAN LIERE, E. J., *et al.* 1943. *Amer. J. Physiol.,* **140:** 119.

257. VAN LIERE, E. J., and STICKNEY, J. C. 1943. *J. Aviat. Med.,* **14:** 194.

258. VAN LIERE, E. J.; STICKNEY, J. C.; and NORTHUP, D. W. 1948. *Amer. J. Physiol.,* **155:** 10.

259. ———. 1951. *Proc. Soc. Exp. Biol. Med.,* **76:** 103.

260. VAUGHAN, B. E., and PACE, N. 1956. *Amer. J. Physiol.,* **185:** 549.

261. VELASQUEZ, T. November, 1956. *USAF Sch. Aviat. Med.,* 56–108.

262. VERZAR, F. 1945. *Hohenklima-Forschungen des Basler Physiologischen Institutes.* Basel: Schwabe.

263. ———. 1948. *Ibid.*

264. WANG, S. I.; WIRZ, H.; and VERZAR, F. 1951. *Schweiz. Med. Wschr.,* **81:** 82.

265. WEBER, H. 1879. *Ziemssen Handbuch des Physiologische Therapie.*

266. WETZIG, P., and D'AMOUR, F. E. 1943. *Amer. J. Physiol.,* **140:** 304.

267. WILHELM, R. E.; COMESS, M. S.; and MARBARGER, J. P., 1958. *J. Aviat. Med.,* **21:** 313.

268. WILKS, S. S.; TOMASHEFSKI, J. F.; and CLARK, R. T. November, 1953. *USAF Sch. Aviat. Med.,* Report No. 2.

269. WILL, D. H., *et al.* 1962. *Circulat. Res.,* **10:** 172.

270. WINDLE, W. F., and JENSEN, A. V. 1946. *J. Aviat. Med.,* **17:** 70.

CHAPTER XI

EFFECT OF HYPOXIA ON THE ALIMENTARY TRACT

GASTROENTERIC MOTILITY

Anoxic Hypoxia

Perhaps the earliest work reported of the effect of hypoxia on the gastrointestinal tract was that of Nolf (49, 50, 51) in 1925, who studied the motility of the gizzards of birds. Rhythmic contractions were produced by briefly stimulating the extrinsic nerves supplying the gizzard; these contractions continued for some time after the stimulus was removed. When the animals were subjected to 8–10 per cent oxygen mixture, the contractions were greatly depressed; when the hypoxia was discontinued, the gizzards continued their normal rhythm.

Swallowing movements, the esophagus, and the cardia.—No reports are available in the literature on the effect of hypoxia on swallowing movements. The swallowing mechanism is a complicated one, and there is some question as to whether the normal act of swallowing is entirely understood. The effect of hypoxia on the esophagus or on the cardia has apparently not been studied either.

Hunger contractions.—In 1930 Van Liere and Crisler (69), using the balloon method, studied the effect of hypoxia on hunger contractions in the normal, trained dog. A loss of gastric tone and a diminution in the height of hunger contractions occurred at a partial pressure of oxygen of 80 mm. Hg (18,000 feet—5,500 meters). The contractions still persisted at a partial pressure of oxygen of 40 mm. Hg (36,000 feet—11,000 meters).

In 1935 Hellebrandt *et al.* (34), using the rebreather method, studied the effect of hypoxia on man. They reported that the precoma type of hypoxia had slight effect on hunger contractions. In 1938 Krugly (40), working with dogs, found that hunger contractions were inhibited at barometric pressures from 320 to 257 mm. Hg. His findings are, for the most part, in accord with those of Van Liere and his co-workers.

Motility of stomach containing food.—It has been shown that hypoxia produces inhibition of digestive motility in barbitalized dogs

(13). The decrease in amplitude of contractions is first seen at a concentration of oxygen of about 10 per cent; at 5 per cent, contractions are greatly diminished or abolished. It was suggested that the sympathetics were sensitized by the rise in pH accompanying the initial hyperpnea and overventilation produced by hypoxia.

Hellebrandt *et al.* (34), using the rebreather, studied the effect of acute hypoxia on digestive contractions in man. They concluded that while hypoxia moderately depressed motor activity of the stomach, the precoma type of hypoxia had relatively little inhibitory effect upon digestive motility.

Gastric emptying time.—*a*) Experiments on rats: MacLachlan (43) could not demonstrate any inhibition of gastric emptying in rats which had been given corn oil by stomach tube. On the other hand, Cordier and Chanel (12) observed retarded gastric emptying of 5 per cent glucose meals in rats breathing oxygen mixtures with 12 per cent oxygen or less. The slowing was proportional to the degree of hypoxia. Since the addition of 5 per cent carbon dioxide increased the delay, the cause must be hypoxia per se and not the associated hypocapnia.

b) Experiments on dogs: It was shown by Van Liere *et al.* (70) in 1933 that dogs subjected to hypoxia showed a delay in gastric emptying. A partial pressure of 117 mm. Hg (8,000 feet—2,400 meters) was considered the threshold for the normal dog. The more severe the hypoxia, the greater the prolongation. Two dogs subjected to a partial pressure of oxygen of 73 mm. Hg (20,000 feet—6,100 meters) still had food in their stomach at the end of twenty-four hours.

Since during nitrous oxide anesthesia it is often necessary to use rather high concentrations, the subject may suffer from anoxic hypoxia. In 1938 Sleeth and Van Liere (63), working with dogs, found that administration of nitrous oxide caused a delay in gastric emptying.

c) Experiments on man: In 1936 the senior author and his co-workers (73) reported work on the effect of hypoxia on the gastric emptying of eight young adults. The threshold for man was found to be approximately that of the dog—8,000 feet (2,400 meters). At a simulated altitude of 14,000 feet (4,300 meters, partial pressure of oxygen of 94 mm. Hg), all the individuals showed a delay in gastric emptying. There were marked individual variations, with values ranging from 13.2 per cent to 166.9 per cent of the normal. Two subjects were studied at a simulated altitude of 18,000 feet (5,500 meters, partial pressure of oxygen of 80 mm. Hg). The authors concluded that in man, as in the dog, the more severe the degree of hypoxia, the greater the delay in gastric emptying time.

Confirmation of these findings was obtained by Stampfli and Endter (65) in their 1944 study of gastric emptying of an alcohol meal stained with methylene blue in eight human subjects at the moderate altitude of the Jungfraujoch (11,342 feet—3,457 meters). At this altitude, 17–20 per cent retardation was found.

The experiments of Van Liere *et al.* (71) unfortunately contained at least one uncontrolled variable—the necessity for repeated recompressions to ground level for fluoroscopic examinations. Shocket *et al.* in 1953 reported observations of gastric emptying in human subjects during experiments which did not require recompression (60). In four subjects neither exposure to a simulated altitude of 12,500 feet (3,800 meters) nor exposure to 15,000 feet (4,600 meters) was found to inhibit gastric emptying. Save for the relatively small number of subjects, these experiments are entirely admirable and reopen the question of the effect of hypoxia upon the gastric emptying mechanism.

Mechanism of the delay in gastric emptying produced by anoxic hypoxia.—Evidence (14) indicates that the delay in gastric emptying produced by moderate degrees of hypoxia is a vagospastic-pylorospastic function; that is, hypoxia stimulates the vagi, and this in turn causes contraction of the pyloric sphincter. This mechanism is an important factor up to a certain threshold, beyond which further delay is caused by the oxygen want directly affecting the gastric musculature.

Another mechanism must be mentioned. Ephedrine may delay gastric emptying in human beings (74); this is also known to occur when epinephrine is administered (64, 88). If the effects of secretion of epinephrine are capable of being augmented by hypoxia, this could cause an inhibition of gastric motility.

Pyloric sphincter.—Working with barbitalized dogs and using a pressure tonometer in the pylorus, as described by Thomas (67), Van Liere *et al.* (71) found that hypoxia produced indeterminate results. The height of the pyloric contractions was generally diminished, especially during severe grades of hypoxia. The variability of their results was attributed to the complexity of the control of the pylorus and to the general nature of the stimulus.

Using unanesthetized dogs with permanent gastric fistulae, Van Liere and Thomas (83) found that hypoxia caused a rise in the tone of the pyloric sphincter in fourteen out of seventeen trials. The threshold was found to be at a partial pressure of 108 mm. Hg (10,-000 feet—3,000 meters). The effect on pyloric contractions, however, was indeterminate. Concomitant tracings of the pyloric antrum showed a decrease in tone. Even moderately severe grades of hypoxia abolished the normal rhythmic contractions.

HEMIC HYPOXIA

Hunger contractions.—Carlson (9) in 1918 reported that gastric tone was increased and hunger contractions were intensified in dogs bled about 30 per cent of their calculated blood volume. In less than twenty-four hours this augmented effect disappeared. No satisfactory explanation was offered for this finding.

Gastric motility.—Four human beings from whom one-tenth of the calculated blood volume had been withdrawn showed an average prolongation of gastric emptying time of 41 per cent. Three of the men still showed a delay of from 15 to 20 per cent twenty-four hours after the hemorrhage. At the end of forty-eight hours, the stomach had apparently regained its normal tone (81). Two dogs from which one-tenth of their blood was withdrawn also showed a noticeable delay in gastric emptying, thus confirming the results obtained in man.

Using the balloon method, Curtis and Hamilton (16) observed an intense gastric motility in patients afflicted with pernicious anemia. This persisted during liver therapy and continued even after marked clinical improvement. The mechanism was not clear. These authors also reported continuous motility of frequent contractions of high amplitude in a case of hypoplastic anemia. Necheles *et al.* (48), using the balloon method and pentobarbital anesthesia, however, found mainly decreased motility following hemorrhage in dogs.

Carbon monoxide.—Peterson *et al.* (55), working with rats, reported that chronic carbon monoxide poisoning inhibited gastrointestinal peristalses.

STAGNANT HYPOXIA

Cardiac failure, impaired venous return, or shock may produce stagnant hypoxia. It is known clinically that certain cardiac diseases may produce nausea and vomiting as well as minor gastric disorders; in fact, any condition which impairs the circulation may produce these symptoms. No quantitative data or any carefully controlled work regarding the effect of stagnant hypoxia on gastric emptying could be found in the literature.

HISTOTOXIC HYPOXIA

In discussing histotoxic hypoxia, the cyanides should be mentioned, since they exert the greatest depression on cellular oxidation. Cyanides, however, are not widely used in medicine. No reports of the effect on the gastroenteric tract of the intact animal of cyanides or of any other agent unequivocally producing histotoxic hypoxia could be found in the literature. Some work has been done on isolated intestinal strips. In 1918 Alvarez (2) reported that the more highly active portions of the isolated strips of small intestine are inhibited more by cyanides than are less active strips.

MOVEMENTS OF THE SMALL INTESTINE AND COLON

Small intestine.—a) Anoxic hypoxia: It has been shown that severe hypoxia can markedly decrease the tone and motility of isolated loops of the small intestine (23, 87). This has also been observed in in vitro isolated intestinal strips (39).

Schnohr (58) in 1934 reported studies on the effect of hypoxia on intestinal peristalses in the unanesthetized animal. He inserted oval cellophane windows in the abdominal walls of rabbits and observed that hypoxia or an increase in carbon dioxide concentration in blood caused violent contraction of the arteries of the intestines and an immediate cessation of all intestinal movement.

Using anesthetized, intact animals, several workers (27, 28) have found that reduced oxygen tension generally decreases motility and tone of the intestine.

Van Liere and co-workers have used Macht's technique of assessing propulsive motility in unanesthetized, intact animals. A charcoal suspension in aqueous gum acacia was administered to the animal by stomach tube. The animal was kept at ground level for a few minutes so that some of the charcoal mixture would enter the duodenum before subjection to hypoxia in a decompression chamber. After a suitable time interval—thirty to forty minutes—the animal was recompressed and immediately sacrificed. The small intestine was removed, and the proportion of the length traversed by the charcoal readily determined.

Rather extensive studies (68, 79) made by the authors and their colleagues on the effect of hypoxia on the propulsive motility of the intestine in rats and mice showed inhibition. The results of their findings are shown in Table 9.

Studies were also made on pups and adult dogs. In the former, the motility was decreased at 28,000 feet (8,500 meters), but in adult dogs (79, 82) no inhibitory effect could be seen at simulated altitudes as high as 32,000 feet (9,800 meters). The epinephrine-potentiating agent, cocaine, however, when administered to adult dogs subjected to hypoxia, caused a decreased propulsive motility (78). By itself cocaine was not effective.

It is possible that adult dogs, through panting, have become tolerant to hypocapnia which accompanies the hypoxic hyperventilation. Pups would not have acquired such tolerance. Furthermore, pups have a lesser hyperglycemic response, but the significance of this is difficult to determine.

TABLE 9

EFFECT OF SIMULATED ALTITUDE ON PERISTALSIS OF SMALL INTESTINE

pO₂ (Mm. Hg)	ALTITUDE (Meters and Feet)	CONTROL		EXPERIMENTAL		P
		Number of Animals	Percentage of Gut Transversed at End of 40 Minutes	Number of Animals	Percentage of Gut Transversed at End of 40 Minutes	
		Mice*				
94...........	4,300 14,000	20	90	20	85	>0.1
80...........	5,500 18,000	25	90	25	69	<0.001
48...........	9,100 30,000	25	90	20	56	<0.001
		Rats†				
94...........	4,300 14,000	11	71	11	64	0.19
80...........	5,500 18,000	9	82	11	64	<0.01
63...........	7,300 24,000	10	76	10	50	<0.001
53...........	8,500 28,000	12	78	10	40	<0.001

* *Amer. J. Physiol.*, **140** (1943), 119.
† *Proc. Soc. Exp. Biol. Med.*, **67** (1948), 331.

Further experiments in rats (20), in which tetraethyl-ammonium chloride was used with and without hypoxia, revealed an inhibition of propulsive motility in the absence of the extrinsic nerve impulses blocked by the agent. The inhibition could have been due to epinephrine released by the direct action of hypoxia upon the adrenal medulla (92), to the direct effect upon the intestinal smooth muscle, or to both.

b) Hemic hypoxia: Peterson *et al.* (55), using a modification of Macht's technique to study the effect of carbon monoxide on gastrointestinal peristalses in rats, found that if the blood is saturated from 70 to 80 per cent with carbon monoxide gastrointestinal peristalses were inhibited 33 per cent. What they termed "the egestion time," that is, the time required for the first appearance of fecal pellets following the test meal, was prolonged 22 per cent.

In anesthetized cats, the inhibition of motility (with use of a piston recorder) in response to bleeding 30 ml. was due to adrenal secretion and not due to extrinsic innervation (38). Wakim and Mason (86) likewise found inhibition in dogs with chronic Biebl loops after bleeding 20 per cent of the blood volume and before re-infusion. The duration of hemic hypoxia, however, was brief—about nine minutes at the most. In somewhat similar experiments Hamilton and Oppenheimer (29) reported that changes occurred rarely after bleeding of about 25 per cent of the blood volume.

Van Liere et al. (77) have not been able to confirm these inhibitory effects of hemic hypoxia in unanesthetized dogs bled 3 per cent of the body weight. Indeed, the propulsive motility was significantly increased. It should be pointed out that in these experiments some time was allowed for adjustment of blood volume and presumably blood pressure. Cocaine simultaneously given with the intubated charcoal changed the excitation into inhibition (78). In pups the same relative hemorrhage produced no effect on motility (82). The results of these experiments on dogs and pups, as well as those with anoxic hypoxia, suggest that the canine species may respond uniquely to these types of stress.

Necheles et al. (48), using unanesthetized dogs with chronic fistulae and the balloon method of recording, obtained somewhat different results. They noticed increased activity usually in the lower intestinal tract but inhibition in the upper portion after hemorrhage. Since the extent of hemorrhage was not standardized, and the presence of a fistula is an unknown variable, comparison with the work of Van Liere et al. is difficult.

The colon.—Relatively little work has been done on the effect of hypoxia upon the colon. Van Liere et al. (79) in 1943 reported experiments on barbitalized dogs. Motility of both circular and longitudinal smooth muscles was recorded by means of the enterograph described by Lawson (41). The results observed in several dogs breathing low oxygen mixtures consisted generally of mild depression of motility with the threshold effect beginning between 14 and 12 per cent. In the following year Van Liere et al. (77) reported similar experiments on dogs subjected to hemic hypoxia. In general, depression was seen in the fourteen dogs used following a hemorrhage equal to about 1.5 per cent of the body weight. Occasionally, stimulation was seen just prior to the onset of depression.

Necheles et al. (48) in 1946, using the inflated balloon technique in unanesthetized chronic fistulae dogs or those under general or local anesthesia, obtained different results. Regardless of the size of the hemorrhage (within limits) , the motility generally increased, and the presence of anesthesia did not alter this action. We are at a loss to account for the discrepancy in the results between the two laboratories. Undoubtedly further work is necessary.

Summary of the effect of hypoxia on gastrointestinal motility.—It has been seen that it is necessary to subject both man and animals to a moderately severe grade of hypoxia before the movements of the alimentary tract are significantly affected. Since this is true, it may be inferred that the nausea and vomiting produced by high altitudes are not due to a direct effect on the stomach. Some people suffer from mountain sickness at altitudes as low as 7,000 feet (2,100 meters) . No pronounced change has been observed at this altitude in gastric or intestinal activity in man or in the dog.

Carlson (9) has pointed out that normal hunger contractions may produce a feeling of faintness and nausea in certain pathologic conditions. It may be that mountain sickness can cause such a condition in some people. Some aviators, before the wide use of pressure cabins, reported that moderate degrees of hypoxia were often accompanied by hunger sensations. It is not improbable that in men certain altitudes may cause stimulation of hunger contractions, although carefully controlled work on dogs gave no indication of this; in fact, the effect of hypoxia on gastrointestinal movements is generally one of depression.

It must be emphasized that the effect of hypoxia on gastric emptying shows a good deal of individual variation both in man and in animals. At an altitude of about 8,000 feet (2,435 meters) , individuals who are especially sensitive to oxygen want might show a slight retardation in gastric emptying, whereas those who are less susceptible would not be affected at all.

The effect of hypoxia on the propulsive motility of the small intestine depends somewhat upon the type of animal used. Probably more work should be done on the small intestine, since it is possible that such studies might throw light on the problems of paralytic ileus, intussusception, and other intestinal disturbances.

It must be recognized that a moderate diminution of gastric and intestinal motility is of no clinical importance. Before any significant impairment in the behavior of the stomach or intestine is noted, hypoxia probably causes cerebral manifestations and cardiac dysfunction. Compared to the central nervous system, the gastroenteric tract is relatively resistant to hypoxia.

HYPOXIA AND ABSORPTION

Gastric absorption of water.—Sleeth and Van Liere in 1937 (62) studied the effect of severe degrees of hypoxia on the permeability of gastric epithelium to water. A partial pressure of 53 mm. Hg was the most severe degree of hypoxia used. No appreciable influence on the absorption of water by the stomach was noticed even though the animals were exposed to hypoxia for an hour or more. It was concluded that hypoxia does not affect the permeability of the stomach to water.

Intestinal absorption.—In their studies on the effect of hypoxia on the alimentary tract, the senior author and his colleagues did considerable work on absorption under hypoxemic conditions.

Method of studying the problem.—In the early literature dealing with hypoxia and absorption, practically no mention is made of the degree of hypoxia used; various methods are employed to produce it, most of which are unphysiologic, such as shutting off the blood supply, producing injury to the epithelium by the application of corrosive chemical agents, and the like. These methods leave the tissues in an unphysiologic state. If the blood is completely shut off, a pronounced asphyxia is produced, which may lead to irreparable injury; corrosive agents destroy the tissues so that they become dead membranes rather than normal, semipermeable ones. It is obvious that only limited conclusions can be drawn from experiments employing these methods.

The senior author and his co-workers, in their studies on absorption, made an effort to avoid these unphysiologic methods and employed a procedure as follows: Matched pairs of dogs (or cats) which had had no food forty-eight hours previous to the experiments were used. Intravenous sodium barbital (220 mg. per kilogram) was used for an anesthetic. One animal of each pair served as a control, and the other was subjected to hypoxia. An isotonic solution of either sodium chloride or glucose, heated to body temperature, was used to wash the debris from the intestine. The entire small intestine, with the exception of the duodenum, was used for a loop. The loops of the two dogs were made of the same length by actual measurement.

The substance to be studied was brought to body temperature before it was placed in the intestine. Substances were left in long enough so that, on the average, at least 50 per cent was absorbed. Undue distention of the intestine was avoided. The contents of the loop at the end of a given time were removed, measured, and quantitatively analyzed for the substance in question. In most of the studies reported, various degrees of hypoxia were used, ranging from a partial pressure of oxygen of 117 mm. Hg (8,000 feet—2,400 meters) to one of 53 mm. Hg (28,000 feet—8,500 meters).

Absorption of water.—Recent studies on the movement of water from the lumen of the intestine suggest that osmotic forces, simultaneous transport of solute, and glucose utilization are involved, but it is too early to come to final decisions (15, 21, 42). The present concept suggests, at least, indirect dependence upon active processes for transport of water secondary to active transport of solute. Since active transport entails an oxidative supply of energy, water movement is reduced in anaerobiosis. So far, no modern studies have, to our knowledge, suggested the threshold of hypoxia for these effects. Therefore the practical effects of in vivo oxygen want in the physiologic range can be gauged only on the basis of older experiments. These will be considered below.

Absorption of sodium chloride.—Working on barbitalized dogs, Van Liere and Sleeth (80) found that absorption of isotonic sodium chloride solution was somewhat decreased even by mild degrees of hypoxia (partial pressure of oxygen of 117 mm. Hg). The absorption of fluid and the actual sodium chloride absorption ran parallel. It was concluded that oxygen aids in the absorption of physiological sodium chloride solution from the small intestine.

The senior author and his co-workers (75) found that ephedrine, administered either orally or intravenously, had no effect on the intestinal absorption of isotonic sodium chloride solution. It will be recalled that ephedrine produces a vasoconstriction of the blood vessels in the splanchnic area.

In hemic hypoxia (76), it has been observed that dogs which had been bled 3.2 per cent of their body weight absorbed more physiological salt solution from the small intestine than did the control dogs. The results obtained with hemic hypoxia were in contrast to those obtained with anoxic hypoxia. This probably may be explained on the basis that severe hemorrhage produces a depletion of chlorides throughout the tissues of the body, so that when chlorides are placed in the intestine following a hemorrhage they pass into the blood stream more rapidly because of the higher diffusion gradient.

Absorption of sodium chloride in the presence of the sulfate radical.—Although the mechanism is not understood, it is known that the chloride ion is absorbed more rapidly from the intestine in the presence of the sulfate radical (26). Van Liere and Vaughan (84) studied the effect of various degrees of anoxic hypoxia on the absorption of a solution consisting of equal parts of isotonic sodium chloride and isotonic sodium sulfate solution from the small intestine of barbitalized dogs. Although hypoxia depressed somewhat the absorption of the fluid and the sodium chloride, it did not prevent the facilitation of the absorption of the chloride ion because of the presence of the sulfate radical. This study also showed that hypoxia had no effect on the absorption of sodium sulfate.

Absorption of the sulfate radical.—The absorption of isotonic magnesium sulfate is not affected by ranges of hypoxia compatible with life in barbitalized animals (52). The absorption of sodium sulfate, as just mentioned in the preceeding paragraph, is likewise unaffected by hypoxia. These studies indicate that the permeability of the intestine to the sulfate radical is unaltered even by severe degrees of hypoxia. This is of distinct clinical importance, since magnesium sulfate especially is given, in many instances, to patients with the cardiac disorders often associated with hypoxemic states. This salt has a powerful depressant action on the central nervous system and, if absorbed in excess, may produce death.

Glucose absorption.—Gellhorn and Northup (24) have shown that while circulatory factors can affect glucose absorption the effects are so variable that in a large series they can be ignored. It has been found in anesthetized, but intact dogs, that even moderately severe degrees of anoxic hypoxia do not affect the absorption of glucose from the small intestine (54). When severe degrees of hypoxia (partial pressure of oxygen of 53 mm. Hg) are used, however, glucose absorption is increased, but the increase is not statistically significant.

Ephedrine, which is known to produce vasoconstriction of the splanchnic region, given either orally or intravenously, does not influence the absorption of glucose from the small intestine (75). It has been shown further (76) that hemic hypoxia, produced by bleeding dogs 3.2 per cent of their body weight, also has no effect on the absorption of glucose.

In modern studies of the mechanism of glucose absorption using in vitro preparations, there is unanimous evidence for the active transport of glucose (17, 90, 91). This is in part revealed by greatly reduced rates of transport in the complete absence of oxygen. The above in vivo studies, which have shown no interference with glucose absorption when degrees of hypoxia compatible with life are used, point up the ability of the organism to maintain this facet of normal physiology in the face of emergency conditions of stress.

Absorption of glucosides.—Work done on barbitalized cats shows that even a severe degree of hypoxia (partial pressure of oxygen of 53 mm. Hg) has no effect on the absorption of digitalis per se or on the fluid menstruum (72). This is of practical interest, since digitalis is often administered to cardiac patients who are markedly cyanosed and obviously suffering from considerable hypoxia.

Absorption of amino acids.—The absorption of glycine (54) is unaffected by moderately severe degrees of hypoxia (partial pressure of oxygen of 80–63 mm. Hg), but at more severe degrees of hypoxia it is significantly decreased. It has been shown with modern in vitro methods that complete hypoxia or cyanide poisoning (histotoxic hypoxia) severely restrict the transport of l-methionine (91), l-alanine (22), and of l-histidine and l-phenylalanine (1). Whether degrees of hypoxia compatible with life are capable of influencing the uptake of these amino acids remains to be proved.

Summary of the effect of hypoxia on absorption.—Evaluation of the studies made on absorption suggests that any conclusion about whether hypoxia interferes with intestinal absorption so as to prevent the proper nourishment of the body must await further work.

Probably the main value of the studies of hypoxia and absorption is the light they throw on the fundamental mechanisms of absorption processes and especially of the role of physiologic oxidations. These studies, however, are not solely of academic interest; some clinical importance may be attached to some of them. It is of interest, for example, that digitalis absorption is not influenced by hypoxia. It is also important that the absorption of the sulfate radical is not increased by hypoxia, since it is so widely used in conditions which are associated with hypoxia. Negative findings are at times as important as are positive findings. Much more work is needed on the effect of hypoxia on absorption; thus far only a few simple substances have been studied.

SECRETION

Anoxic hypoxia and salivary secretion.—Three studies have come to our notice in which the effect of hypoxia upon pilocarpine-stimulated secretion in anesthetized dogs has been followed. Eddy in 1929 (19) reported a threshold decrease in secretion with the respiration of an oxygen-nitrogen mixture with 18 per cent oxygen. Greater decreases in oxygen percentage caused greater inhibition. Similar findings were later reported by Brody and Shilling in 1930 (8) and Brass-field in 1936 (7). Brody and Shilling recounted the puzzling finding that whereas pilocarpine-induced secretion was inhibited by hypoxia, that due to chorda tympani stimulation was not.

Anoxic hypoxia and gastric secretion.—*a*) Experiments on dogs: In 1911 Bayeux (6), working with dogs at an altitude of 14,000 feet (4,300 meters), found that while the total acid was not affected the volume of gastric juice was diminished. Delrue in 1934 (18) reported that when his dogs were transported from his laboratory to an altitude of 8,000 feet (2,400 meters), the gastric juice showed an increase in pH and a decrease in total acid. In 1935 Hellebrandt *et al.* (34), using a rebreather apparatus, subjected human beings to short periods of hypoxia. They reported that anoxic hypoxia of the precoma type caused no appreciable decrease in gastric acidity.

In 1936 Sleeth and Van Liere (61) subjected barbitalized dogs which had had water placed in their stomachs to various degrees of hypoxia. Only after a partial pressure of oxygen of 52 mm. Hg (28,-000 feet—8,500 meters) was reached did there occur definite diminution in the acidity and chlorides in the gastric contents.

Pickett and Van Liere in 1939 (56) studied the effect of various degrees of hypoxia on gastric secretion after a standard meal in a series of dogs with Pavlov pouches and in a series with Heidenhain pouches. In this connection, it must be remembered that a stomach pouch made according to the method of Pavlov has a normal blood supply and a relatively normal nerve supply; the Heidenhain pouch, however, is an isolated pouch, and while it has an adequate blood supply, it presumably has no vagal nerve supply. In these experiments no significant decrease in gastric secretion was obtained until a partial pressure of 80 mm. Hg (18,500 feet—5,500 meters) was used. Greater decreases were seen at 63 mm. Hg (24,000 feet—7,300 meters). Since acclimatization may have inadvertently affected these results, it is entirely possible that the true inhibition due to hypoxia was underestimated. The work should be repeated, and the effects of acclimatization on gastric secretion should also be studied. These results have been confirmed by more recent reports in the literature of the hypoxic inhibition of gastric secretion in pouch dogs exposed to reduced ambient pressure (45, 46, 59).

b) Experiments on man: Experiments by Selmanova in 1940 (59), on a man and a woman at 4,000 meters (13,000 feet) with a test meal, in which inhibition of gastric secretion was reported have been cited. Later studies have confirmed this report. With human subjects the method of study is necessarily restricted to the use of gastric intubation for collection of samples. The volume of secretion cannot be accurately determined, because gastric emptying may affect the amounts recovered in unpredictable ways. Stampfli and Endtner in 1944 (65) reported their studies on eight young subjects during a three-day sojourn on the Jungfraujoch at 3,457 meters (11,342 feet). An alcohol test meal was used to stimulate secretion. The concentration of free and total acid usually did not change at altitude. However, the volume of secretion was low on the second day. Hartiala and Karvonen (33) and Karvinen and Karvonen (36), in each of two later studies on three young students, reported essentially the same sort of findings at a simulated altitude of 5,000 meters (16,000 feet). The most that can be said for the experiments on human subjects is that the investigators have the impression that secretion is inhibited by hypoxia, but this has not been proved in a rigorous manner.

Basal gastric secretion.—It has been shown (85) that anoxic hypoxia, within ranges compatible with consciousness in unacclimatized dogs, has no effect on the chlorides, acids, or pH of the basal secretion of Pavlov pouch dogs. Moderate ranges of hypoxia do not affect the volume of basal secretion as much as the secretion provoked by food; severe hypoxia, however, depresses the basal secretion as it does the secretion called forth by food.

Hemic hypoxia and gastric secretion.—A number of interesting observations have been made on the relation between the hemoglobin content of the blood and gastric acidity. Alvarez and Vanzant (3) in 1936 reported a study of this relationship in a large number of human beings. It was found that the incidence of achlorhydria rose rapidly and that the mean gastric acidity fell off sharply when the hemoglobin fell below 12 g/100 ml. They concluded from their work that loss of blood in both animals and man can temporarily lower gastric acidity.

Hartfall and Witts (31), studying cases of idiopathic microcytic anemia, found in a series of one hundred and thirty-seven cases that 80 per cent gave evidence of achlorhydria; they did not feel, however, that the low acidity was secondary to the anemia. In subjects afflicted with pernicious anemia, Goldhamer (25) found a direct relation between the red cell count and the amount of gastric juice secreted within a given time.

In 1936 Apperly and Cary (4) showed experimentally that when the red cell count of the blood fell below a certain critical level, free acid disappeared from the stomach.

When the effects of hemic hypoxia and anoxic hypoxia are compared, it appears that hemic hypoxia has more profound effect on depressing gastric juice than has the anoxic type. The loss of chlorides during hemorrhage may be one reason for this.

Pancreatic secretion.—In secretin-stimulated secretion of the pancreas in anesthetized dogs, Chardon and Gross in 1946 (10) found a decreased volume but no change in amylase activity due to breathing 2–5 per cent oxygen mixtures. In thirteen barbitalized dogs under 8 per cent oxygen with secretion stimulated with a secretin-pancreozymin mixture, Hartiala (32) in 1951 found decreases in volume, bicarbonate content, and amylase concentration.

In the same paper, Hartiala also described studies on fourteen medical students in the decompression chamber at three different simulated altitudes: 3,500, 4,000 and 5,500 meters (11,000, 13,000, and 18,000 feet). A double tube technique was used to collect pancreatic secretion uncontaminated with gastric juice from the duodenum. Pancreatic secretion was stimulated with intravenous secretin. During hypoxic exposure there was a significant decrease in volume of pancreatic juice as well as in the amounts of bicarbonate, amylase, and trypsin. Volume and bicarbonate were decreased most at the highest altitude; the decrease in the other components was not significantly increased in going from 3,500–4,000 meters to 5,500 meters.

Bile flow.—The effect of hypoxia upon the flow of bile has been studied almost entirely with anesthetized animals. Archdeacon *et al.* (5), using oxygen-nitrogen mixtures for ten to twenty minute periods in three rabbits, found 11.8 per cent oxygen of no effect; 9.1 per cent, depressing; and 6.1 per cent, drastically effective in decreasing bile flow.

Hanson (30) similarly in rats found 6 per cent oxygen capable of decreasing the flow to one-half to one-quarter of the control rate. On the other hand, MacLachlan *et al.* (44), using unanesthetized chronic bile fistulae rats, found no change in the secretion of bile salts during four-hour exposures to the simulated altitudes of 24,000 and 28,000 feet (7,300 and 8,500 meters) in the decompression chamber. As seen by the fact that two rats died at the latter altitude, the degree of hypoxia was quite severe. Although bile salt output is measured here, and not bile flow, the failure to confirm the inhibition on liver secretion in anesthetized rats raises the question of the complication introduced by the use of anesthesia.

In the dog under sodium pentobarbital breathing 10 and 7.5 per cent oxygen in nitrogen, Tanturi and Ivy in 1938 (66) failed to find a general decrease in bile flow during brief exposures. In 1941 Schnedorf and Orr (57) found decreased flow in the dog, similarly anesthetized, during periods of thirty to forty-five minutes of 15 per cent oxygen in nitrogen. Reduction of the percentage of oxygen to as low as 5 per cent caused greater decreases, with acholia appearing in two dogs. Decreased biliary secretion has also been reported by Chardon *et al.* (11) in the dog inhaling a 3 per cent oxygen in nitrogen mixture.

Some experiments by Kaufman *et al.* (37) on sulfobromophthalein sodium retention in fourteen normal human subjects breathing 10 per cent oxygen in nitrogen are interesting. The subjects were, of course, not anesthetized, and no depression of liver function was observed. However, in seven subjects who had impaired liver function due to liver disease, the hypoxia caused further retention of the drug, indicating inhibition of function by hypoxia.

Hemic hypoxia and liver function.—In 1944 Ireneus and Puestow (35) reported their studies during ten days of liver function in eleven dogs surviving a hemorrhage of about 3 per cent of their body weight. In several tests given (BSP, galactose tolerance, prothrombin time, serum phosphate), the dogs seemed abnormal only in the case of the galactose test in which eight of the eleven dogs were deficient.

The work of Wilhelmi *et al.* (89) in 1945 on rats bled 2.8 to 3.0 per cent of the body weight suggested that the hemic hypoxia interfered with the function of the liver in handling amino acids and in urea synthesis.

Effect of intestinal secretion.—In 1939 Northup and Van Liere (53) studied the effect of various degrees of hypoxia on intestinal secretion in barbitalized dogs. In order to secure sufficient secretion, the small intestine was made to secrete by injecting intravenously a peptone extract prepared according to the method described by Nasset and Pierce (47). It was only when a partial pressure of oxygen of 53 mm. Hg (28,000 feet—8,500 meters) was reached that a slight depression of secretion occurred; this decrease, moreover, was not statistically significant even though fifteen animals were used. The authors concluded that the intestine had a low energy requirement.

Summary of the effect of hypoxia on secretion.—While experimental work shows that anoxic hypoxia is capable of diminishing gastric secretion, it can be seen that, for the most part, the gastric glands are relatively resistant to oxygen want. Only during severe degrees of hypoxia is the secretion appreciably decreased. Hemic hypoxia apparently affects gastric secretion more than does the anoxic type. Since pernicious anemia is associated with achlorhydria, more research could be done profitably in this particular field. From the limited studies of the effect of hypoxia on pancreatic secretion, it is apparent that function is affected only with severe degrees of stress.

The animal studies of the effect on bile flow are complicated by the unknown side effects which the use of anesthesia presumably introduces. In the single human study, liver function did not seem to be affected by a rather severe degree of hypoxia in normal subjects, but it was impaired in those already suffering from liver deficiency. The secretion of the intestine seems to be so resistant to oxygen want that, for practical purposes, the effect of hypoxia on its secretion is largely of academic interest.

REFERENCES

1. AGAR, W. T.; HIRD, F. J. R.; and SIDHU, C. S. 1953. *J. Physiol.*, **121:** 255.
2. ALVAREZ, W. C. 1918. *J. Phrmacol. Exp. Ther.* (Proc.), **11:** 171.
3. ALVAREZ, W. C., and VANZANT, F. R. 1936. *Proc. Mayo Clin.*, **11:** 385.
4. APPERLY, F. L., and CARY, M. K. 1936. *Amer. J. Dig. Dis.*, **3:** 466.
5. ARCHDEACON, J. W.; DANFORTH, J. T.; and DUMMIT, G. D. 1954. *Amer. J. Physiol.*, **178:** 499.
6. BAYEUX, M. R. 1911. *C. R. Acad. Sci.* (Par.), **152:** 396.
7. BRASSFIELD, C. R. 1936. *Amer. J. Physiol.*, **116:** 174.
8. BRODY, H., and SHILLING, M. S. 1930. *Amer. J. Physiol.*, **91:** 399.
9. CARLSON, A. J. 1916. *The Control of Hunger in Health and Disease.* Chicago: University of Chicago Press.
10. CHARDON, G., and GROSS, A. 1946. *C. R. Soc. Biol.* (Par.), **140:** 1004.
11. CHARDON, G.; NEVERRE, G.; and JEANNOEL, G. 1949. *C. R. Soc. Biol.* (Par.), **143:** 697.
12. CORDIER, D., and CHANEL, J. 1950. *C. R. Soc. Biol.* (Par.), **144:** 535.
13. CRISLER, G.; VAN LIERE, E. J.; and BOOHER, W. T. 1932. *Amer. J. Physiol.*, **102:** 629.
14. CRISLER, G.; VAN LIERE, E. J.; and WILES, I. A. 1935. *Amer. J. Dig. Dis.*, **2:** 221.
15. CURRAN, P. S., and SOLOMON, A. K. 1957. *J. Gen. Physiol.*, **41:** 143.
16. CURTIS, G. M., and HAMILTON, F. E. 1938. *Trans. West. Surg. Ass.*, pp. 447–73.
17. DARLINGTON, W. A., and QUASTEL, J. H. 1953. *Arch. Biochem.*, **43:** 194.
18. DELRUE, G. 1934. *Arch. Int. Physiol.*, **38:** 126.
19. EDDY, N. B. 1929. *Amer. J. Physiol.*, **88:** 534.
20. FANG, H. S.; NORTHUP, D. W.; and VAN LIERE, E. J. 1953. *Amer. J. Physiol.*, **173:** 459.
21. FISHER, R. B. 1955. *J. Physiol.*, **130:** 655.
22. FRIDHANDLER, L., and QUASTEL, J. H. 1955. *Arch. Biochem.*, **56:** 424.

23. FURCHGOTT, R. F., and SHORR, E. 1950. *Amer. J. Physiol.*, **162**: 88.
24. GELLHORN, E., and NORTHUP, D. 1934. *Amer. J. Physiol.*, **108**: 469.
25. GOLDHAMER, S. M. 1936. *Amer. J. Med. Sci.*, **191**: 405.
26. GOLDSCHMIDT, S., and DAYTON, A. B. 1919. *Amer. J. Physiol.*, **48**: 459.
27. GRANDPIERRE, R., and FRANCK, C. 1944. *Contribution à l'étude des anoxemies, action physiologique des anoxemies sur l'appareil digestif.* Cannes: Imprimerie Devaye.
28. ———. 1944. *C. R. Acad. Sci. (Par.)* , **218**: 808.
29. HAMILTON, A. S., and OPPENHEIMER, M. J. 1944. *Fed. Proc.*, **3**: 17.
30. HANSON, V. 1952. *Acta Physiol. Scand.*, 28 (Suppl.) : 101.
31. HARTFALL, S. J., and WITTS, L. J. 1933. *Guy Hosp. Rep.*, **83**: 3.
32. HARTIALA, K. J. V. 1951. *Ann. Acad. Sci. Fenn.*, No. 25: 66.
33. HARTIALA, K., and KARVONEN, M. 1946. *Acta Physiol. Scand.*, **11**: 85.
34. HELLEBRANDT, F. A.; BROGDON, E.; and HOOPES, S. L. 1935. *Amer. J. Physiol.*, **112**: 451.
35. IRENEUS, C., and PUESTOW, C. B. 1944. *A. M. A. Arch Surg.*, **49**: 100.
36. KARVINEN, E., and KARVONEN, M. J. 1949. *Ann. Med. Exp. Biol. Fenn.*, **27**: 59.
37. KAUFMAN, P. J., *et al.* 1950. *New Engl. J. Med.*, **242**: 90.
38. KOCK, N. G. 1959. *Acta Physiol. Scand.*, **47** (Suppl.) : 164.
39. KROEGER, D. C., and EDWARDS, L. D. 1953. *J. Amer. Pharm. Ass. (Sci.)* , **42**: 564.
40. KRUGLY, A. N., cited by J. P. QUIGLEY. 1940. *Ann. Rev. Physiol.*, **2**: 50.
41. LAWSON, H. 1935. *J. Lab. Clin. Med.*, **20**: 496.
42. LIFSON, N., and PARSONS, D. S. 1957. *Proc. Soc. Exp. Biol. Med.*, **95**: 532.
43. MACLACHLAN, P. L. 1946. *Proc. Soc. Exp. Biol. Med.*, **63**: 147.
44. MACLACHLAN, P. L.; SLEETH, C. K.; and GOVER, J. 1947. *Proc. Soc. Exp. Biol. Med.*, **66**: 275.
45. MALKIMAN, I. V., cited by GRANDPIERRE and FRANCK. (See reference 27 above.)
46. MALLISON, R., cited by GRANDPIERRE and FRANCK. (See reference 27 above.)
47. NASSET, E. S., and PIERCE, H. B. 1935. *Amer. J. Physiol.*, **113**: 568.
48. NECHELES, H.; WALKER, L.; and OLSON, W. H. 1946. *Amer. J. Physiol.*, **146**: 449.
49. NOLF, P. 1925. *C. R. Soc. Biol. (Par.)* , **93**: 455.
50. ———. *Ibid.*, p. 480.
51. ———. 1925. *Ibid.*, **93**: 1049.
52. NORTHUP, D. W., and VAN LIERE, E. J. 1939. *Arch. Int. Pharmacodyn.*, **62**: 175.
53. ———. 1939. *Proc. Soc. Exp. Biol. Med.*, 42: 162.
54. ———. 1941. *Amer. J. Physiol.*, **134**: 288.
55. PETERSON, C. A.; SMITH, E.; and HALE, H. B. 1938. *Proc. Soc. Exp. Biol. Med.*, **39**: 509.

56. PICKETT, A. D., and VAN LIERE, E. J. 1939. *Amer. J. Physiol.*, **127:** 637.
57. SCHNEDORF, J. G., and ORR, T. G. 1941. *Amer. J. Dig. Dis.*, **8:** 356.
58. SCHNOHR, E. 1934. *Hospitalstidende,* **77:** 29.
59. SELMANOVA, E. S., cited by GRANEPIERRE and FRANCK. (See reference 27 above.)
60. SHOCKET, E.; JACKSON, M. M.; and DYME, H. C. 1953. *J. Aviat. Med.*, **24:** 113.
61. SLEETH, C. K., and VAN LIERE, E. J. 1936. *Proc. Soc. Exp. Biol. Med.*, **36:** 208.
62. ———. 1937. *Proc. Soc. Exp. Biol. Med.*, **36:** 571.
63. ———. 1938. *J. Pharmacol. Exp. Ther.*, **63:** 65.
64. SMITH, M. I. 1918. *Amer. J. Physiol.*, **46:** 232.
65. STAMPFLI, R., and ENDTNER, B. 1944. *Helv. Physiol. Pharmacol. Acta,* **12** (Suppl. III) : 189.
66. TANTURI, C. A., and IVY, A. C. 1938. *Amer. J. Physiol.*, **121:** 61.
67. THOMAS, J. E. 1927. *Amer. J. Physiol.*, **82:** 727.
68. VAN LIERE, E. J., *et al.* 1948. *Proc. Soc. Exp. Biol. Med.*, **67:** 331.
69. VAN LIERE, E. J., and CRISLER, G. R. 1930. *Amer. J. Physiol.*, **93:** 267.
70. VAN LIERE, E. J.; CRISLER, G.; and ROBINSON, D. H. 1933. *A. M. A. Arch. Intern. Med.*, **51:** 796.
71. VAN LIERE, E. J.; CRISLER, G.; and WILES, I. A. 1935. *Amer. J. Physiol.*, **111:** 330.
72. VAN LIERE, E. J., and EMERSON, G. A. 1937. *Arch. Int. Pharmacodyn.*, **57:** 45.
73. VAN LIERE, E. J.; LOUGH, D.; and SLEETH, C. K. 1936. *A. M. A. Arch. Intern. Med.*, **58:** 130.
74. ———. 1936. *J.A.M.A.*, **106:** 535.
75. VAN LIERE, E. J.; NORTHUP, D. W.; and SLEETH, C. K. 1937. *J. Pharmacol. Exp. Ther.*, **60:** 434.
76. ———. 1938. *Amer. J. Physiol.*, **124:** 102.
77. VAN LIERE, E. J.; NORTHUP, D. W.; and STICKNEY, J. C. 1944. *Amer. J. Physiol.*, **142:** 260.
78. ———. *Ibid.*, p. 615.
79. VAN LIERE, E. J., *et al.* 1943. *Amer. J. Physiol.*, **140:** 119.
80. VAN LIERE, E. J., and SLEETH, C. K. 1936. *Amer. J. Physiol.*, **117:** 309.
81. VAN LIERE, E. J.; SLEETH, C. K.; and NORTHUP, D. W. 1936. *Amer. J. Physiol.*, **117:** 226.
82. VAN LIERE, E. J.; STICKNEY, J. C.; NORTHUP, D. W. 1951. *Amer. J. Physiol.*, **167:** 103.
83. VAN LIERE, E. J., and THOMAS, J. E. 1936. *Amer. J. Dig. Dis.*, **3:** 94.
84. VAN LIERE, E. J., and VAUGHAN, P. E. 1940. *Amer. J. Physiol.*, **129:** 618.
85. ———. 1941. *Amer. J. Dig. Dis.*, **8:** 155.
86. WAKIM, K. G., and MASON, J. W. 1945. *Gastroenterology,* **4:** 92.

87. WEST, T. C.; HADDEN, G.; and FARAH, A. 1951. *Amer. J. Physiol.*, 164: 565.
88. WILDER, R. L., and SCHULTZ, S. W. 1931. *Amer. J. Physiol.*, **96**: 54.
89. WILHELMI, A. E., *et al.* 1945. *Amer. J. Physiol.*, **144**: 674.
90. WILSON, T. H., and VINCENT, T. N. 1955. *J. Biol. Chem.*, **216**: 851.
91. WILSON, T. H., and WISEMAN, G. 1954. *J. Physiol.*, **123**: 116.
92. ZWEMER, R. L., and NEWTON, H. F. 1928. *Amer. J. Physiol.*, **85**: 507.

CHAPTER XII

HYPOXIA AND THE SECRETION OF URINE

URINE VOLUME

A fairly large number of experiments have been done on the rat, the dog, and man concerning the effect of anoxic hypoxia upon the volume flow of urine.

Animals.—Silvette in 1942 (29) reported that rats maintained for three hours at the simulated altitude of 15,000 feet (4,600 meters) have a marked polyuria. Contrary results were later found by Swann and Collings (35). On the basis of their studies in 1943 on rats at 18,-000 feet (5,500 meters) simulated altitude for various periods of time from six to twenty-three hours, they concluded that the rat does not show a diuresis at altitude. Other work by Stickney (32) and Van Middlesworth *et al.* (40), like that of Silvette, failed to confirm this conclusion. As a matter of fact, all these workers found increases in urine flow three- to sevenfold greater during hypoxia than in the control periods. However, Van Middlesworth *et al.* found that the diuresis gradually disappeared over a five-hour period of exposure to 27,000 feet (8,200 meters) simulated altitude interrupted hourly for measurements. This decline in urine flow was not altered by replacement of fluid volume by intraperitoneal saline injections.

Hoy and Adolph in 1956 (16) reported that the newborn rat, during hypoxia produced by low-oxygen mixtures, responds with oliguria and develops the diuretic response only with age. An uncontrolled variable here was that the rats were under close restraint.

Most of the experiments using dogs have been complicated by the use of anesthesia (9, 20, 33, 36, 39). The usual response to exposure to hypoxia in these has been reduced urine flow or oliguria. Stickney *et al.* (33) found, however, that oliguria was usually associated with severe hypoxia (7 per cent or less oxygen in nitrogen) and polyuria, with mild hypoxia. Toth (36) also studied unanesthetized dogs with bladder fistulae. In these, hypoxia almost invariably produced polyuria even though the severity of the hypoxia was as great as that with 6.5 per cent oxygen mixtures. Similarly, Alexander in 1953 (2) reported only polyuria in his saline-infused dogs breathing 8 per cent oxygen in nitrogen.

On the other hand, even in the unanesthetized dog, oliguria may be the rule if the hypoxic exposure is severe enough. Thus, Ferguson and Smith (15) in 1953 reported mostly decreased urine flows in repeated decompressions to 30,000 feet (9,100 meters) simulated altitude in six dogs. Axelrod and Pitts (4) found both increased and decreased flows at times in their two unanesthetized dogs breathing 9.4 and 6.3 per cent oxygen in nitrogen mixtures. They suggested that mild hypoxia might enhance urine flow by inhibiting the release of antidiuretic hormone from the posterior pituitary. They pointed out that the oliguria of severe hypoxia is associated with circulatory, central nervous system, and other derangements. Further, it is not clear whether the reduction in urine flow arises from pituitary stimulation or from a decreased glomerular filtration rate.

Man.—In three human subjects decompressed to 450 mm. Hg ambient pressure (about 14,000 feet or 4,300 meters), Asmussen and Nielsen in 1945 (3) found marked polyuria in two and a moderate oliguria in one. Kleinschmidt in 1948 (17) studied twelve human subjects in the decompression chamber at ground level and at 9,800, 13,000, 16,000, and 20,000 feet (3,000, 4,000, 5,000, and 6,000 meters) simulated altitudes. After the subjects had drunk a liter of tepid water, their urine volume was determined at half-hour intervals. Hypoxia had no effect on the resulting water diuresis until the altitude of 13,000 feet, where it was increased during the two and a half hours of exposure. At 16,000 feet the diuresis was decreased below that found during the control period, and at 20,000 feet the decrease was even greater. On the other hand, Burrill *et al.* (10), in six human subjects exposed one hour to a simulated altitude of 18,000 feet (5,500 meters), found increases in urine volume.

In 1961 Ullmann (38), in an interesting study of human subjects, found polyuria as a rule; but whenever there was distress during the experimental procedure, oliguria and even temporary anuria became manifest. The role of respiratory alkalosis was evaluated in this study by having subjects hyperventilate in normal room air to produce hypocapnia, by having them breathe 11 per cent oxygen, or by giving carbon dioxide along with 10 per cent oxygen to produce a hypoxia without hypocapnia. Polyuria of about the same degree was produced by each procedure, in spite of differences in total solute excretion.

A second paper by Currie with Ullmann as co-worker in 1961 (13) reported a further study of the common denominator in the above work, that is, respiratory modifications, which particularly increased changes in intrathoracic pressure variation. The hypothesis suggested was that the increased filling of the central vascular bed produced by the "respiratory pump" reflexly decreased the secretion of antidiuretic hormone from the posterior pituitary.

The final conclusion in regard to the renal effects of hypoxia was that they are produced by extra-renal events and not by the direct effect of hypoxia upon renal structures. The oliguria following upon the occasion of distress during hypoxia was suggested as due to the increased secretion of antidiuretic hormone. Other workers studying human subjects during mild hypoxia have failed to find significant changes on the average (7, 14).

In summary, the above findings indicate on the whole that mild degrees of hypoxia, if effecting a change, produce polyuria while severe degrees may produce oliguria. The exact mechanism for these changes remains yet to be determined.

RENAL BLOOD FLOW

The alterations in urine volume during hypoxia may be secondary to changes in renal blood flow. However, the relationship may be complicated by local vascular changes within the kidney such as preferential vasoconstriction adjacent to the glomerulus, the possible presence of shunting mechanisms, or other presently obscure reactions.

Local vascular mechanisms.—An example of local vascular changes is the response to the secretion of the adrenal medulla which was suggested as a possible explanation for the urine flow changes during hypoxia (39). That the adrenal medullary secretion can affect the kidney in such ways has been known for a long time. Richards and Plant in 1922 proved that the diuretic response to epinephrine was due to local vasoconstriction of the efferent arteriole of the glomerulus (25). In 1937 Toth (37) found that the diuretic response could be produced regularly in anesthetized dogs by slow rates of intravenous infusion of epinephrine but that fast rates of infusion produced oliguria. These results seem to mimic those seen with moderate and severe degrees of hypoxia, respectively. However, it still remains to be seen whether the actual changes during hypoxia are functions of the epinephrine mechanism.

Unanesthetized dog.—The only experiments assessing the effect of hypoxia upon renal blood flow in unanesthetized dogs that have come to our notice are those of McDonald and Kelley in 1948 (21). Actually, the effective renal plasma flow was determined indirectly with the use of creatinine for glomerular filtration and para-aminohippuric acid for tubular secretion. Exposures to both 18,000 feet (5,500 meters) and 24,000 feet (7,200 meters) simulated altitudes were made in an altitude chamber. Urine collection periods of ten to fifteen minutes each, beginning at least seventy-five minutes after reaching the desired altitude, were used.

All three dogs had increases in effective renal plasma flow at 18,000 feet, while at 24,000 feet one had a further increase, and the other two had decreases. Rate of glomerular filtration did not appear to change regularly with altitude except in the case of one dog where it was strikingly increased at 18,000 feet. The filtration fractions determined in these experiments at simulated altitudes could be interpreted as reflecting local changes in the circulation adjacent to the glomerulus. In some there were decreases with altitude which could be due to efferent arteriolar dilatation, while in others there were increases suggesting vasoconstriction in that locus. It is not possible to make sweeping generalizations on the basis of such scant data, but the variations in blood flow and the changes secondary to such variations are not incompatible with the effects that could be produced by varying amounts of circulating adrenal medullary hormones.

Anesthetized dog.—As might have been anticipated from the urine volume studies of anesthetized dogs under hypoxia, values of the renal blood flow determined under such conditions are remarkably different from those in the unanesthetized animal. Kreienberg *et al.* in 1949 (18) reported the results in seventeen anesthetized dogs given 6.5 to 7.5 per cent oxygen mixtures to breathe. The renal blood flow, measured with the quantitatively inaccurate Rein thermostromuhr, was invariably reduced drastically by the hypoxia. This occurred whether the systemic blood pressure rose or fell during the episode. In 1960 Balint *et al.* (5) reported their comparison of directly measured blood flows with those determined indirectly from inulin-para-aminohippuric acid clearance values. Chloralosed dogs breathing 10 per cent oxygen had no changes of consequence. On 8 per cent oxygen, renal blood flow was decreased markedly. However, the decrease determined indirectly was vastly greater than that directly measured from the renal vein. Such discrepancy between the two types of measurement have been noted before (28, 34). It follows that renal blood flow cannot be determined accurately with the indirect method when urine flow is greatly decreased. Presumably under other circumstances the method is reliable.

Man.—Determination by clearance methods of renal blood flow in the human subject during hypoxia were reported in 1949 by

Berger *et al.* (7) with 14 per cent oxygen mixtures and by Caldwell *et al.* (11) with 9.3 per cent mixtures. No changes were found by either group. However, 14 per cent oxygen is very mild hypoxia, and in the work of Caldwell *et al.*, the periods of exposure were rather short. Aas and Blegen, also in 1949 (1), found by similar methods increases of renal blood flow during twenty minutes of breathing 9.5 per cent oxygen mixtures in two normal human subjects. Obviously, more subjects should be studied before one can say what the effect of hypoxia is.

ELECTROLYTES

Urinary excretion of solutes during anoxic hypoxia reflects largely the homeostatic function of the kidney in meeting the concomitant respiratory alkalosis. Accordingly, one finds increased secretion of sodium, potassium, and bicarbonate. Since the demands for ammonia production by the kidney, which serves to spare plasma alkaline reserve, are lessened, the ammonia excretion is usually reduced. The rise in urine pH is part of this picture.

Dogs.—In the studies of Ferguson and Smith (15), six unanesthetized dogs were exposed for thirty-minute periods to the simulated altitude of 30,000 feet (9,100 meters). The urinary excretion of sodium approximately doubled, while that of potassium was increased about one-third. In the seven unanesthetized dogs of Alexander (2), which were breathing 8 per cent oxygen and were given continuous saline infusion, both electrolytes had about a 25 per cent increased excretion.

Man.—The nine human subjects of Berger *et al.* (7), breathing 14 per cent oxygen, had over 58 per cent increase in sodium excretion and 20 per cent in potassium excretion. Most of these electrolytes must have been excreted as chlorides, since the excretion of those anions increased by a little over 50 per cent. Similar changes were observed in the two subjects of Asmussen and Nielsen (3) who had polyuria but not in the subject having oliguria. In the study of Ochwadt (22), there is evidence that bicarbonate excretion is also increased; for in five healthy young men for two or three hours in the decompression chamber at 20,000 feet (6,000 meters) the urinary bicarbonate output increased from control values of 0.1–1.6 millimols to 5–6 during hypoxia.

In the studies of Currie and Ullman (13, 38) referred to above, data on electrolyte excretion was obtained in human subjects under combinations of hypoxia with and without hypocapnia and with pure hypocapnia. It is questionable whether equal degrees of hypoxia occurred in the hypoxia experiments with and without hypocapnia. Also, in the voluntary overbreathing experiments, the hypocapnia was more extreme than that in the hypoxic hypocapnia instances. It is impossible, therefore, to come to final conclusions. However, the results seemed to indicate that electrolyte excretion was dominated largely by the homeostatic response to the respiratory alkalosis when hypocapnia was present. In the absence of hypocapnia, there was no increased excretion of sodium and potassium in spite of the polyuria.

Ammonia.—Brassfield and Behrmann (9) observed ammonia excretion decreased in five of their six anesthetized dogs while breathing 6–10 per cent oxygen for ten to thirty-five minutes. Transient decreases were also seen by Schonholzer and Gross (27) in eight human subjects, mainly during the first day on the Jungfraujoch (about 11,300 feet, 3,450 meters).

pH.—In the work of Alexander (2) cited above, urinary pH rose from the control value of 7.00 to 8.05. Lesser rises were seen by Brassfield and Behrmann (9). Berger *et al.* (7), also cited above, found pH values in their human subjects rising from the control reading of 6.1 to 6.7 during hypoxia.

HEMIC HYPOXIA AND RENAL FUNCTION

Urine volume.—The only study to come to our attention concerning the effect of toxic hypoxia (carbon monoxide poisoning) on the flow of urine has been that of Silvette (30). During three hours following one hour's exposure to 0.4 per cent carbon monoxide, urine output in rats was decreased about 19 per cent as compared to the control rate. The excretion of intraperitoneally injected phenolsulphonphthalein in the same experiments was decreased about 12 per cent by the hypoxia. Since the severity of hypoxia was not quantified, the contrast with the polyuria of rats exposed to anoxic hypoxia cannot be readily evaluated.

Renal blood flow.—Several adequate studies have been made over the last twenty years on renal blood flow during hemic hypoxia. In every instance the reduction in oxygen capacity has been attended by decreases in the flow of blood through the kidneys.

Animals.—Sapirstein (26) studied the effect of hemorrhage on the fractional distribution of the cardiac output in rats with the use of $K^{42}Cl$. Whereas coronary and bronchial fractions were increased and hepatic and skin fractions unchanged, the renal fraction fell from 19.4

to 10.1 per cent of the cardiac output. He also found that this distribution could be precisely mimicked by epinephrine (5 gammas/rat).

In 1951 Paterson (23) produced a chronic anemia in two dogs over a period of five months. Renal studies employing creatinine, glucose, and para-aminohippurate were made at intevrals as hemoglobin concentration declined to as low as 2.45 and 3.75 g/100 ml. in the two dogs. Renal blood flow decreased proportionately with the anemia. Renal plasma flow and glomerular filtration rate were not particularly affected until hemoglobin concentration fell to around 5 g/100 ml and below. Both filtration fraction and the tubular maxima for glucose and para-aminohippurate were unchanged.

Corcoran and Page (12) concluded from their experiments in 1943 on the bled, anesthetized dog that diodrast does not measure accurately the renal blood flow in severe hypotension but exaggerates the decrease in blood flow. Selkurt in 1946 (28) found in eight similarly anesthetized dogs that reducing the mean blood pressure to 60 mm. Hg by bleeding decreased the directly measured renal blood flow to 41.5 per cent of the control value. Since complete anuria was usually present under these conditions, the renal blood flow calculated from clearance (creatinine and para-aminohippurate) was obviously nil. Actually, however, 66.5 ml. of blood per minute was passing through the kidney early in the period. An interesting observation in this study was that after reinfusion of blood there was immediate, though not complete, restoration of blood pressure and renal blood flow, which suggested a neural rather than a humoral basis of the derangement. Similar observations were made by Phillips *et al.* (24) and reported the same year. Balint *et al.* in 1961 (6) described their studies of twenty-six chloralosed dogs subjected to bleeding in order to reduce the blood pressure to 50 to 60 mm. Hg. Comparisons of renal blood flow directly determined, with that indirectly measured with inulin and para-aminohippurate clearances, demonstrated the previous exaggeration of the reduction of renal blood flow by the indirect methods.

Man.—Three reports have come to our attention concerning the renal blood flow in human cases of hemic hypoxia. In general the findings are similar to those reported for animals. That this should prevail in the absence of anesthesia in the human studies suggests that in hemic hypoxia anesthesia does not produce a qualitative change in the adaptation to this stress. Lauson *et al.* in 1944 (19) described their studies of nine patients with post-hemorrhagic shock. They found rate of glomerular filtration and renal plasma flow decreased and roughly proportionate to the degree of shock. Since the decrease was more than could be accounted for by the arterial hypotension, the kidney was visualized as having its vascular resistance increased, thereby shunting blood away during shock.

The study of fifteen cases of chronic anemia in human subjects was described by the Bradleys in 1947 (8). In these subjects, hematocrits varied between 13 and 28 per cent, while arterial blood pressure was essentially in the normal range. Hemic hypoxia was thus relatively pure and not accompanied by the fluid loss and hypotension that have been complications in most of the studies described above. The various parameters of kidney function were compared to the standards of Smith *et al.* (31). Most noteworthy was the reduction in renal blood flow by 32 per cent in females and 46 per cent in males. Glomerular filtration and filtration fraction were moderately decreased on the average. Of particular interest was the observation that the handling of diodrast by the tubule was depressed in a majority of the cases, while that of glucose was normal in six out of seven.

In two cases of anemia reported by Aas and Blegen in 1949 (1), the reduced renal blood flow indirectly determined with inulin and paraaminohippurate was reversed upon recovery of oxygen capacity to normal.

The ubiquitous reduction in renal blood flow during hemic hypoxia indicates increased vascular resistance within the kidney. Although the condition may be mimicked by epinephrine injection, there is good evidence that it is mediated physiologically through the renal efferent nerves. The benefits to the organism appear to be the shunting of blood to more vital organs during hypotension and reduced effective oxygen carrying capacity of the blood. Since there is no dominant respiratory change, one sees neither polyuria secondary to increased venous return nor the electrolyte changes related to alkalosis that characterize moderate anoxic hypoxia.

REFERENCES

1. Aas, K., and Blegen, E. 1949. *Scand. J. Clin. Lab. Invest.,* 1: 22.
2. Alexander, J. D. September, 1953. *USAF Sch. Aviat. Med.,* Project No. 21–1201–0001, Report No. 1.
3. Asmussen, E., and Neilsen, M. 1945. *Acta Physiol. Scand.,* 9: 75.
4. Axelrod, D. R., and Pitts, R. F. 1952. *J. Appl. Physiol.,* 4: 593.
5. Balint, P., *et al.* 1960. *Pflueger Arch. Ges. Physiol.,* 271: 705.
6. Balint, P.; Kiss, E.; and Sturcz, J. 1961. *Pflueger Arch. Ges. Physiol.,* 272: 307.
7. Berger, E. Y., *et al.* 1949. *J. Clin. Invest.,* 28: 648.

8. Bradley, S. E., and Bradley, G. P. 1947. *Blood,* 2: 192.
9. Brassfield, C. R., and Behrmann, V. G. 1941. *Amer. J. Physiol.,* 132: 272.
10. Burrill, W. M.; Freeman, S.; and Ivy, A. C. 1945. *J. Biol. Chem.,* 157: 297.
11. Caldwell, F. T.; Rolf, D.; and White, H. L. 1949. *J. Appl. Physiol.,* 1: 597.
12. Corcoran, A. C., and Page, I. H. 1943. *J. Exp. Med.,* 78: 205.
13. Currie, J. C. M., and Ullmann, E. 1961. *J. Physiol.,* 155: 438.
14. D'Angelo, S. A. 1946. *Proc. Soc. Exp. Biol. Med.,* 62: 13.
15. Ferguson, F. P., and Smith, D. C. 1953. *Amer. J. Physiol.,* 173: 503.
16. Hoy, P. A., and Adolph, E. F. 1956. *Amer. J. Physiol.,* 187: 32.
17. Kleinschmidt, K. 1948. *Pflueger Arch. Ges. Physiol.,* 250: 79.
18. Kreienberg, W.; Prokop, L.; and Schiffer, T. 1949. *Pflueger Arch. Ges. Physiol.,* 251: 675.
19. Lauson, H. D.; Bradley, S. E.; and Cournand, A. 1944. *J. Clin. Invest.,* 23: 381.
20. Malmejac, J. 1944. *J. Aviat. Med.,* 15: 167.
21. McDonald, R. K., and Kelley, V. C. 1948. *Amer. J. Physiol.,* 154: 193.
22. Ochwadt, B. 1947. *Pflueger Arch. Ges. Physiol.,* 249: 452.
23. Paterson, J. C. S. 1951. *Amer. J. Physiol.,* 164: 682.
24. Phillips, R. A., et al. 1946. *Amer. J. Physiol.,* 145: 314.
25. Richards, A. N., and Plant, O. H. 1922. *Amer. J. Physiol.,* 59: 191.
26. Sapirstein, L. A. 1957. *Fed. Proc.,* 16: 111.
27. Schonholzer, G. and Gross, F. 1948. *Helv. Physiol. Pharmacol. Acta,* 6: 699.
28. Selkurt, E. E. 1946. *Amer. J. Physiol.,* 145: 699.
29. Silvette, H. 1942. *Proc. Soc. Exp. Biol. Med.,* 51: 199.
30. ———. 1943. *Amer. J. Physiol.,* 140: 374.
31. Smith, H. W., et al. 1943. *J. Mount Sinai Hosp. (N.Y.),* 10: 59.
32. Stickney, J. C. 1946. *Proc. Soc. Exp. Biol. Med.,* 63: 210.
33. Stickney, J. C.; Northup, D. W., and Van Liere, E. J. 1946. *Amer. J. Physiol.,* 147: 616.
34. Study, R. S., and Shipley, R. E. 1950. *Amer. J. Physiol.,* 163: 442.
35. Swann, H. G., and Collings, W. D. 1943. *J. Aviat. Med.,* 14: 114.
36. Toth, L. A. 1937. *Amer. J. Physiol.,* 119: 127.
37. ———. *Ibid.,* p. 140.
38. Ullman, E. 1961. *J. Physiol.,* 155: 417.
39. Van Liere, E. J., et al. 1935. *Proc. Soc. Exp. Biol. Med.,* 33: 479.
40. Van Middlesworth, L., et al. 1948. *Proc. Soc. Exp. Biol. Med.,* 69: 288.

CHAPTER XIII

EFFECT OF HYPOXIA ON THE ENDOCRINE GLANDS

ADRENAL CORTEX

Exhaustion of the adrenal cortex by hypoxia.—In 1937 Giragossintz and Sundstroem (28), working with rats under atmospheric pressures which either were very low or extended for lengthy periods of time, believed that the functional alterations observed were identical with those seen in adrenal cortical insufficiency in adrenalectomized animals. When cortical hormone was administered to these animals, the effects were ameliorated. These workers further observed that histologic sections of the adrenals showed that prolonged hypoxia produced cellular necrosis and hemorrhage. It was felt that structural damage was due to the overwhelming demand made by hypoxia on the glands and that this eventually resulted in exhaustion.

A year later Armstrong and Heim (3), working with rabbits and subjecting them daily for four hours to a simulated altitude of 18,000 feet (5,500 meters), made findings similar to those reported by the workers previously mentioned. They first noted a hypertrophy of the whole adrenal gland and later observed degenerative changes in the cortex. In one group of animals exposed daily for a period of five weeks, the average weight of the adrenal glands as compared to the control showed a gain of 28 per cent, based on the adrenal weight–body weight ratio. Armstrong suggested the possibility that the fatigue seen in both acute and chronic altitude sickness might be related to adrenal insufficiency or exhaustion.

Activation of the adrenal cortex by hypoxia.—*a*) Increased adrenal weight: In 1942 Thorn *et al.* (70) reported the results of their experiments on rats and rabbits exposed intermittently (four hours per day) to 18,000 feet (5,500 meters) simulated altitude in decompression chambers. They confirmed the finding of Armstrong and Heim, that adrenal weight is increased as a result of hypoxic stress, in both

241

species. At 25,000 feet (7,600 meters) in the rabbit, the increase was even more striking. In the rat, they concluded that the greater part of the enlargement of the adrenal involved the adrenal cortex. Dohan, and Langley and Clarke in the same year reported similar increase in adrenal weight in decompressed rats (18, 39). Confirmation in rats was also reported by Dalton *et al.* in 1944 (16) and by Edelmann in 1945 (19). Negative results were found by Darrow and Sarason (17) and by Levin (44), which would suggest that the enlargement is not invariable but may be related to the specific schedule of exposures or to severity of the hypoxic stress.

In 1958 Holland (35) reported the rather paradoxical finding that newborn rats whose mothers were decompressed to a simulated altitude of 18,000 feet (5,500 meters) for the last three days of gestation have a significant atrophy of the adrenal glands. The interpretation was that excess maternal adrenal corticoids induced by the hypoxia crossed the placenta to inhibit the output of fetal corticotrophin.

b) Secondary evidences of activation: Both Aschan (4) and Tepperman *et al.* (68) have found depletion of ascorbic acid content in the adrenal cortex of rats exposed to anoxic hypoxia. Biddulph *et al.* (6) failed to confirm this in anesthetized dogs breathing 5 per cent oxygen in nitrogen for thirty minutes.

Decreases of about 50 per cent in eosinophils in the peripheral blood of unanesthetized dogs submitted to a simulated altitude of 30,000 feet (9,100 meters) in a decompression chamber were found by Ferguson and Smith (22). Similarly, decreases of 18 and 40 per cent have been reported by Hale and Keator (32) in human subjects decompressed to an "altitude" of 15,000 feet (4,600 meters) without oxygen or to 40,000 feet (12,200 meters) with oxygen, respectively. Thorn *et al.* in 1953 (69) reported an average fall of 32 per cent in ten human subjects rebreathing a carbon dioxide–free mixture with decreasing inspired oxygen tension until the conditions equivalent to an altitude of about 27,000 feet (8,200 meters) were attained. The latter authors determined that this fall would have been accompanied by an insignificant increase in the output of corticoids. Eosinopenia, therefore, may not necessarily indicate adrenal cortical activation.

Several studies have been made of the depletion of adrenal cortical cholesterol and lipids as a result of anoxic hypoxia. Cullumbine (15) in 1952 reported decreases in adrenal cholesterol content in mice during twenty-four to forty-eight hours of decompression to

460 mm. Hg (13,000 to 14,000 feet, or about 4,000 meters). Levin (44), Nichols (54), and Tepperman *et al.* (68) had earlier found depletion in adrenal cholesterol in rats after one to fifteen hours at simulated altitudes between 23,000 and 33,000 feet (7,000–10,000 meters). Both Dalton *et al.* (16) and Darrow and Sarason (17), also in rats, found disappearance of lipid in stained sections of the adrenal cortex as a result of anoxic hypoxia. The latter authors found that at 25,000 feet (7,600 meters) the depletion was complete by the second day but that by the seventh day of continuous exposure the lipids had been restored in spite of the hypoxia.

c) Adrenal cortical secretion: Fowler *et al.* (23) found no increase in adrenal 17-hydroxycorticosteroid output in anesthetized dogs breathing 7.1 per cent oxygen in nitrogen.

In 1943 Pincus and Hoagland (57) reported results obtained on three human subjects by simulating both pilot fatigue on a pursuit meter and altitude with the use of oxygen-nitrogen mixtures. As the concentration of oxygen was lowered to 18, 16, and 14 per cent in different experiments, there was a sharp increase in the urinary excretion of 17-ketosteroids. However, the physiologic significance of 17-ketosteroid output by the adrenal is still not known (62).

Attempts to find evidence for increased output of 17-hydroxycorticoids during anoxic hypoxia in man have been unsuccessful. Hale *et al.* (33) used oxygen mixtures equivalent to about 14,000 feet (4,300 meters). No increased concentration of plasma 17-hydroxycorticoids was evident within forty-five minutes. As mentioned above, Thorn *et al.* (69) concluded that rebreathing of oxygen mixtures even to the point of unconsciousness within some twenty-five to thirty minutes failed to produce convincing evidence of adrenal cortical activation.

Evidence for increased adrenal cortical secretion during anoxic hypoxia has been convincing in the mouse, the rat, and the rabbit. The lack of such evidence in the dog and in man may be due to failure to continue the exposure sufficiently long. There is some indication that the adrenal cortical involvement is more the result of the hypocapnia and alkalosis than of the hypoxia per se (31, 41, 42).

d) Anemic hypoxia: Carpenter *et al.* in 1961 (14) reported the effects of 250 ml. hemorrhage in two 15–20 kg. dogs. The left adrenal had been transplanted to the neck where effluent adrenal venous blood could be collected without inducing stress, and so control values for aldosterone, corticosterone, and Porter-Silber chromogens were low. Within 60 to 120 minutes following hemorrhage, there were marked increases in all the adrenal corticoids in the venous effluent. It is not possible to say whether these are the results of hypotension, of hypoxia, or of both.

e) Histotoxic hypoxia: In 1949 Nichols and Miller (55) reported that repeated sublethal doses of sodium cyanide administered over a period of twenty to twenty-eight hours caused moderate increases in adrenal weight and marked depletion of adrenal cortical lipids. These findings, of course, are similar to those seen in anoxic hypoxia.

ADRENAL MEDULLA

Asphyxia.—Although a number of workers (10, 11, 12, 13, 24, 36) have reported that asphyxia stimulates the adrenal medulla, leading to an increased liberation of adrenal medullary hormones, there has been considerable controversy, with Stewart and Rogoff and their associates presenting conflicting evidence (66). Since space does not permit our giving details of the evidence, the reader is referred to the original work of these investigators. It is questionable whether asphyxia should be considered further here because it is hypoxia complicated by hypercapnia. However, early work by Kellaway suggested that hypoxia was more important than hypercapnia in stimulating the adrenals (38). Recent evidence (67) proves that rather severe hypercapnia, with percentages of carbon dioxide elevated to 12–20 in the alveolar air, of anesthetized cats is capable of causing a discharge of epinephrine as indicated by contraction of the denervated nictitating membrane. Furthermore, Gellhorn and Packer (27) have found that carbon dioxide potentiates the effect of hypoxia upon the sympathetico-adrenal system. The exact role of hypoxia per se in stimulating the adrenal medulla cannot, therefore, be gauged in experiments with asphyxia.

Anoxic hypoxia.—The English worker Kellaway (38) in 1919 presented some evidence that hypoxia can stimulate the adrenals of unanesthetized as well as of anesthetized cats to increase their output of epinephrine. In 1926 Houssay and Molinelli (36), using blood-pressure rise and heart rate in cross-transfused anesthetized dogs, found evidence of increased adrenal medullary secretion with three dogs breathing oxygen-nitrogen mixture with 5.7–6.3 per cent oxygen. This was confirmed later by Malmejac *et al.* using similar methods (45). Lehmann and Michaelis (43) are reported to have found in 1942 increased epinephrine in the blood of human subjects breathing 16 per cent or less oxygen mixtures. Also, in rats at 31,000 feet

(9,500 meters) simulated altitude, the plasma epinephrine content rose 21.3 per cent. Fowler *et al.* (23) in a recent study found three-fold increases in norepinephrine-like substances in the adrenal venous blood of eleven anesthetized dogs breathing 7.1 per cent oxygen mixtures. The rabbit aortic strip was used for assay.

A few studies have been made on the epinephrine content of the adrenal glands before and after exposure to hypoxia. It is agreed that decreases of contents in such work does not permit distinguishing between a decreased rate of formation of epinephrine and an exhaustion of adrenal stores. In 1936 Binet and Lanxade (7) reported marked increases in adrenal concentration of epinephrine in anesthetized dogs exposed approximately twenty to forty minutes to 33,000–36,000 feet (10,000–11,000 meters) simulated altitude by decompression. On the other hand, Emerson and Van Liere in 1938, (20) in unanesthetized cats subjected for three hours to a simulated altitude of 28,000 feet (8,500 meters), found a 40 per cent depletion of epinephrine content. In 1943 Raab (59) reported similar results in rats similarly treated. However, when the duration of exposure was increased to sixty-two hours, no decrease occurred. These reports do not add great clarity to the picture of adrenal medullary activity during hypoxia. However, with the modern techniques of estimation of the catechol amines and the use of isotopic tracers, it should be possible to advance our knowledge in this area.

Hypoxia stimulates the adrenal medulla largely through the sympathetics. Section of the sympathetic branches to the adrenal glands, at least, greatly reduces the output of adrenal medullary hormones (38, 50). According to some workers, the adrenal medulla may be excited directly (8, 38, 53); but Malmejac *et al.* (46) have denied this. Manger *et al.* (47) have noted hypoxic elevation of epinephrine-like substances in the venous blood of the dog after section of the spinal cord. This result may be due to the direct effect of hypoxia upon the adrenal glands, upon sympathetic centers in the spinal cord, or both. It points up secretion in the absence of chemoreceptor impulses from carotid and aortic bodies impinging upon higher centers, such as those in the hypothalamus or medulla of the brain. For a detailed review of the role of the central nervous system in the control of the adrenal medulla, the reader is referred to the monographs of Gellhorn (25, 26).

Hemic hypoxia: anemic type.—No studies have come to our notice in which the effect of pure anemic hypoxia upon the adrenal medulla has been assessed. A large number of studies have been made of the effect of hemorrhage upon adrenal medullary secretion, but these have invariably involved hypotension (23, 74, 76, 77). Fowler *et al.* (23) in 1961 rapidly infused saline or Kreb's solution into six anesthetized dogs so that hematocrit was reduced, from an average of 48 per cent to 25 per cent. In spite of the production of this anemic hypoxia, the output of norepinephrine-like substances in adrenal venous blood fell during the infusion from a rather high control value of 13.9 microg/kg/min $\times$ 10^{-2} to 4.1 microg/kg/min $\times$ 10^{-2}. Ten minutes later the original control value had been attained. The authors felt that their results supported the hypothesis of Walker *et al.* (74) that blood volume (rather than anemia) may be an important factor in the control of adrenal medullary secretion. In 1959 Walker *et al.* (74), in experiments on dogs, had found a similar suppression of catechol-amine secretion in the adrenal vein outflow as saline or dextrin infusion restored blood volume after hemorrhage. Justus *et al.* (37), in dogs subjected to chronic anemia after six daily bleedings, found evidence in the blood stream, after the original hypotension had passed, of a humoral factor that increased cardiac output and heart rate in a recipient assay dog.

Hemic hypoxia: toxic type.—In 1912 Starkenstein (65) studied the effect of very severe, acute carbon monoxide poisoning in dogs and rabbits. The presence of hyperglycemia and glycosuria, the loss of hypertensive factor in adrenal extract, and the loss of intensity of stain in chromaffin tissue in the adrenal medulla were considered proof of adrenal medullary involvement. Mikami (50) in 1927 found hyperglycemia and glycosuria after several hours exposure in rabbits. Later, in 1936, Schulze (64) reported that carbon monoxide poisoning in mice leads to blood sugar rise and glycogen fall, which were interpreted to be the results of adrenal medullary secretion.

Histotoxic hypoxia.—Houssay and Molinelli (36) reported the results of one experiment in which repeated potassium cyanide injections produced evidence of adrenal medullary secretion in the anesthetized dog.

Summary of Adrenal Function in Hypoxia

If the stress of hypoxia is of critical severity or of effective duration, the nervous discharge over the sympathetics causes an emergency release of adrenal medullary hormones. These hormones enable the organism to cope with the stress by increasing cardiac output, by mobilizing glucose from liver glycogen producing hyperglycemia, and by furthering glycolysis and energy production in the muscles. Continued exposure to the stress of hypoxia and/or associated hypocapnia causes, through the hypothalamo-pituitary axis, secretion of corticotrophin which leads to discharge of adreno-cortical hormones. Of these, the glucocorticoids promote gluconeogenesis from protein and carbohydrate metabolism in general. The action of cortical steroids upon lymphocytes, eosinophils, and the thymus is difficult at present to relate to the organism's coping with the stress of hypoxia. It is likewise not easy to see the value of the increased mineralocorticoids, particularly in combating the respiratory alkalosis of anoxic hypoxia.

THE HYPOPHYSIS

Corticotrophin (adrenocorticotrophic hormone) .—The present concept of one of the effects of stress upon the mammalian organism is that stress causes the median eminence of the hypothalamus to release a hormonal factor: corticotrophin-releasing-factor. This factor is thought to be transported by way of the pituitary portal venous system to the anterior hypophysis where it acts to accelerate the release of corticotrophin (adrenocorticotrophin) (60) . In 1952 Porter (58) , using cats and monkeys under cyclopropane anesthesia, which is considered to cause minimal stress, found that hypoxia, among other types of stress, caused a marked increase of electrical activity limited to the posterior hypothalamus. It is possible that the increased electrical activity is involved in the above-mentioned mediation with the pituitary. In the absence of the hypophysis, one would not expect adreno-cortical activation and the consequent secondary changes. This expectation has been supported by the finding of Malmejac and Gross (46) , that hypophysectomy in rats prevented the lymphopenia ordinarily induced by decompressing rats to a simulated altitude of 28,000 feet (8,500 meters) . Hale *et al.* (33) found no change in the titer of adrenocorticotrophic hormone in the peripheral blood of human subjects exposed for forty-five minutes to 12 per cent oxygen mixtures. Perhaps longer exposures would have been significantly stressful.

A preliminary finding of increased adrenocorticotrophic hormone outputs following hemorrhage has been made in dogs, but this may not necessarily be due to the anemic hypoxia (52) .

Gonadotrophin: toxic hypoxia.—Patterson *et al.* (56) in 1938 subjected a group of male rats to carbon monoxide poisoning (a gas-air mixture was used which contained 0.34 per cent carbon monoxide) for an hour a day for periods from 50 to 131 days. The hypophysis upon histologic section showed vacuolated and enlarged basophils;

the histologic picture resembled that produced by castration as described by Addison (1) in 1917. The gonadotropic potency of the hypophyses was measured by noting the response of the ovaries and uteri of immature female rats. It was observed that the gonadotropic hormone was increased. It appears, therefore, that the effect of carbon monoxide poisoning on the hypophysis is secondary to a deleterious effect on the gonads. (For further evidence, see p. 249 below.)

Gonadotrophin: anoxic hypoxia.—In 1943 Gordon *et al.* (29, 30) reported their study of rats exposed six hours per day for two to three weeks to altitudes of 25,000–28,000 feet (7,600–8,500 meters) simulated by decompression. In neither males nor females were there changes in the pituitary weight–body weight ratio. Histologically, the pituitary of the decompressed males was similar to that found by Patterson *et al.* (56), cited above, in carbon monoxide poisoned rats. Similarly, the gonadotrophin content of the pituitaries was greatly increased.

Thyrotrophin.—In the study of Gordon *et al.* (30), just cited, thyrotropic hormone of the sera and pituitaries of rats exposed to anoxic hypoxia was assayed in tadpoles. The serum concentration of the hormone was greatly decreased in the experimental animals, but there was no difference from the control rats in the concentration in the pituitary glands.

Other pituitary functions.—Since the hyperglycemic response to epinephrine secreted during exposure of rats to 280 mm. Hg barometric pressure is present for several days after hypophysectomy, Safford and Gellhorn (61) concluded that the hypophysis plays no direct role in sympathetico-adrenal reactions.

Langley and Gunthorpe (40) in 1957 found that the ability of hypophysectomized-adrenalectomized rats to deposit liver glycogen was impaired when they were exposed to a simulated altitude of 20,-000 feet (6,100 meters). This occurred in spite of the fact that the rats were on minimal hypophyseal, but adequate adrenocortical, hormone therapy. This led to the suggestion by the same authors that in altitude stress the hypophysis has a role in carbohydrate metabolism.

THE GONADS

Anoxic hypoxia.—It has been known for several hundred years that inhabitants at high altitudes, both man and animals, lose their fertility and may not be able to bear young. Monge (51) has studied the early records of the Spaniards, relative to their experiences in the Andes. It was related by Father Cobo that, while the natives were quite prolific, the Spaniards showed a greatly reduced birth rate and that miscarriages and stillbirths were common. There are records stating that so many animals died at birth that the capital of Peru was transferred from the altitude of 10,000 feet (3,000 meters) to sea level.

In 1943 Gordon *et al.* (29) reported that male rats exposed six hours per day by decompression to the simulated altitudes of 25,000–28,000 feet (7,600–8,500 meters) for two or three weeks showed marked degeneration of spermatogenic cells. Since the germinal damage could not be prevented by administration of gonadotropic hormone, it was concluded that hypoxia acted directly upon the testis. Only slight atrophy was seen in the interstitial tissue of the testis and in the epithelium of the seminal vesicles and prostate gland. In another report (30) of a study of female rats similarly stressed, the degenerative changes in the ovaries were not very great, and there were no changes in the uterus. In the males there was a marked loss of weight of the testis and lesser losses in seminal vesicles and ventral prostate. In the females there were moderate losses of weight in the ovaries and in the uterus.

Altland and Allen in 1952 (2) exposed rats from birth to forty-eight days of age to the simulated altitude of 25,000 feet (7,600 meters) for four hours per day. No mode of degeneration of primordial sex cells not seen in the control was induced by the hypoxia, but spermatogenesis was prevented in the experimental series. Increased incidence of degeneration in leptotene cells was seen in the hypoxic series, which was independent of degeneration by exfoliation. Support for the direct action of hypoxia is thus seen.

Toxic hypoxia.—Not only does anoxic hypoxia produce a loss of fertility, but the hypoxia produced by carbon monoxide poisoning may likewise do so. Campbell (9) in 1935 exposed white mice to increasing concentrations of pure carbon monoxide (24 parts per 10,-000 were reached on the forty-sixth day) and found that after prolonged exposures the mice lost their fertility, although there was little disturbance in their growth.

In the same year Williams and Smith (78) exposed rats to 1.43 per cent illuminating gas daily for a certain length of time. Fertility was decidedly reduced, and the testes weighed only one-third to one-half of those of the control group. After sixty days of treatment, no living spermatozoa were found by the hanging-drop method. The females which were mated with normal males were less fertile than the control animals. On histologic examination the ovaries were not found to be abnormal, although they were smaller.

Patterson *et al.* (56) in 1938, working with rats, reported that the combined testis and epididymis weight in rats was reduced about one-half after fifty or more one-hour exposures to illuminating gas, that the number of spermatozoa was greatly decreased, and that the motility of the few viable sperm was impaired.

THE UTERUS

It has been shown that the uterus of the dog is extremely resistant to both anoxic and hemic hypoxia. In 1952 Van Liere *et al.* (71), using lightly barbitalized pregnant or estrogenized dogs, found that an oxygen concentration as low as 5 per cent had no effect on uterine contractions. When the animals were subjected to a brisk hemorrhage (hemic hypoxia), uterine contractions were greater in amplitude. The authors suggested that hemorrhage produced a stimulation of the sympathetic fibers supplying uterine musculature. In a subsequent study (72), it was found that mixtures of 85, 90, or 95 per cent nitrous oxide and oxygen administered intratracheally had no effect on the amplitude or on the frequency of contractions of the uterus.

Hilton and Woodbury (34) in 1951 studied the influence of low oxygen tension on the activity of isolated uterine strips of rabbits which had been estrogenized. A reduction in response to oxytocic agents was observed during hypoxia.

THE THYROID

It was pointed out by Asher and Streuli (5) in 1918 that thyroidectomized animals are considerably less susceptible to oxygen want than are normal animals. While statistical data probably are needed to establish this point indisputably, it is reasonable to suppose that these observations are correct; inasmuch as metabolism is lowered after thyroidectomy, the animal requires less oxygen. In this connection, it is of interest to recall that Haldane pointed out long ago that small animals, which are known to have a high metabolic rate, are more sensitive to carbon monoxide than are large animals.

Schulze (63) in 1936 subjected white mice ten minutes daily to carbon monoxide, 5 parts in 10,000, a concentration which was capable of causing symptoms and even death in some animals. After twelve to sixteen days of treatment, certain changes in the staining of the thyroid occurred, consisting of a heavy basophilic staining of the colloid material. These animals also showed an increase in basal metabolism, measured on days when the mice were not exposed to carbon monoxide.

On the other hand, Walters in 1927 (75) had found that metabolism was depressed during the exposure to the carbon monoxide atmosphere. The extent of the depression was correlated with the carbon monoxide concentration of inspired air and the duration of exposure. There was also a concomitant fall in body temperature. In these experiments the oxygen consumption following exposure to carbon monoxide was not determined.

In 1951 Van Middlesworth and Berry reported the effect of anoxic hypoxia on iodine metabolism of male rats (73) that had been kept on a low-iodine diet. The uptake of I^{131} by the thyroid was measured during the last twenty-four hours of a thirty-six-hour exposure to 260 mm. Hg ambient pressure at 15° C. The uptake was found greatly depressed and the level of protein-bound I^{131} in the plasma was only one-tenth that in the controls. Since the disappearance rate of protein-bound I^{131} from the plasma was normal in the hypoxic rats, it is concluded that the function of the thyroid was severely inhibited by the hypoxia. The inhibition is not at all unexpected since Gordon *et al.* (30) had found decreased levels of serum thyrotrophin under similar circumstances.

THE ISLETS OF LANGERHANS

McQuarrie *et al.* (49) in 1939 reported that in adrenalectomized dogs the breathing of 5 per cent oxygen in nitrogen produced a fall in blood sugar instead of the usual rise seen in intact animals. This was confirmed in 1940 by Feldman *et al.* (21) in rabbits with bilaterally denervated adrenal glands and in adrenalectomized rats, both breathing a mixture with 7 per cent oxygen. The hypoglycemia in the latter group was due to impulses over the abdominal vagus nerve, since sub-diaphramatic vagotomy abolished it in other adrenalectomized rats subjected to hypoxia. Furthermore, since the insulin content of the blood of the adrenalectomized rats was increased by the hypoxic exposure, and this increase was lacking in the adrenalectomized-vagotomized, it was concluded that the above hypoglycemia was due to the increased secretion of insulin. This interpretation was confirmed later by McQuarrie *et al.* (48) in adrenalectomized-depancreatized dogs exposed to hypoxia, which produced neither the rise in blood sugar characteristic of the intact dog nor the fall seen in the adrenalectomized animal.

In 1957 Langley and Gunthorpe (40) suggested that insulin may be involved in the glycogen deposition in the liver induced by hypoxia, since this deposition is impaired in rats made diabetic with alloxan.

In summary, regarding carbohydrate metabolism, it is well known that hypoxia induces the outputs of adrenal medullary hormones, first pointed out by Cannon (13). This response is mediated through the sympathetics. The adrenal cortex also is activated by way of the hypothalmo-pituitary release of corticotrophin. Finally, there is simultaneous parasympathetic activity with a discharge over the vagal branches to the Islets of Langerhans, resulting in the release of insulin.

REFERENCES

1. Addison, W. H. F. 1917. *J. Comp. Neurol.,* 28: 441.
2. Altland, P. D., and Allen, E. 1952. *J. Morph.,* 91: 541.
3. Armstrong, H. G., and Heim, J. W. 1938. *J. Aviat. Med.,* 9: 92.
4. Aschan, G. 1953. *Acta Soc. Med. Upsal.,* 58: 265.
5. Asher, L., and Streuli, H. 1918. *Biochem. Z.,* 87: 359.
6. Biddulph, C.; Finerty, J. C.; and Ellis, J. P., Jr. 1959. *Amer. J. Physiol.,* 197: 126.
7. Binet, L., and Lanxade, J. 1936. *C. R. Soc. Biol. (Par.),* 122: 1011.
8. Bulbring, E.; Burn, J. H.; and De Elio, F. J. 1948. *J. Physiol.,* 107: 222.
9. Campbell, J. A. 1935. *Quart. J. Exp. Physiol.,* 24: 271.
10. Cannon, W. B. 1924. *Endocrinology and Metabolism,* II, 174. New York: D. Appleton & Co.
11. ———. 1929. *Bodily Changes in Pain, Hunger, Fear and Rage.* 2d ed. New York and London: Appleton.
12. ———. 1932. *The Wisdom of the Body.* New York: Norton.
13. Cannon, W. B., and Hoskins, R. G. 1911–12. *Amer. J. Physiol.,* 29: 274.
14. Carpenter, C. C. J., *et al.* 1961. *J. Clin. Invest.,* 40: 196.
15. Cullumbine, H. 1952. *Amer. J. Physiol.,* 169: 515.
16. Dalton, A. J., *et al.* 1944. *J. Nat. Cancer Inst.,* 4: 527.
17. Darrow, D. C., and Sarason, E. L. 1944. *J. Clin. Invest.,* 23: 11.
18. Dohan, F. C. 1942. *Proc. Soc. Exp. Biol. Med.,* 49: 404.

19. EDELMANN, A. 1945. *Proc. Soc. Exp. Biol. Med.,* **58:** 271.
20. EMERSON, G. A., and VAN LIERE, E. J. 1938. *Proc. Soc. Exp. Biol. Med.,* **38:** 500.
21. FELDMAN, J.; CORTELL, R.; and GELLHORN, E. 1940. *Amer. J. Physiol.,* **131:** 281.
22. FERGUSON, F. P., and SMITH, D. C. 1953. *Amer. J. Physiol.,* **173:** 503.
23. FOWLER, N. O.; SHABETAI, R.; and HOLMES, J. C. 1961. *Circulat. Res.,* **9:** 427.
24. GASSER, H. S., and MEEK, W. J. 1914. *Amer. J. Physiol.,* **34:** 48.
25. GELLHORN, E. 1943. *Autonomic Regulations,* p. 131. New York: Interscience Publishers.
26. ———. 1957. *Autonomic Imbalance and the Hypothalamus.* Minneapolis: University of Minnesota Press.
27. GELLHORN, E., and PACKER, A. 1939. *Proc. Soc. Exp. Biol. Med.,* **42:** 475.
28. GIRAGOSSINTZ, G., and SUNDSTROEM, E. 1937. *Proc. Soc. Exp. Biol. Med.,* **36:** 432.
29. GORDON, A. S.; TORNETTA, F. J.; and CHARIPPER, H. A. 1943. *Proc. Soc. Exp. Biol. Med.,* **53:** 6.
30. GORDON, A. S., *et al.* 1943. *Endocrinology,* **33:** 366.
31. HAILMAN, H. F. 1944. *Endocrinology,* **34:** 187.
32. HALE, H. B., and KEATOR, J. E. 1952. *Fed. Proc.,* **11:** 63.
33. HALE, H. B., *et al.* 1957. *J. Clin. Invest.,* **36:** 1642.
34. HILTON, J. G., and WOODBURY, R. A. 1951. *Fed. Proc.,* **10:** 309.
35. HOLLAND, R. C. 1958. *Anat. Rec.,* **130:** 177.
36. HOUSSAY, B. A., and MOLINELLI, E. A. 1926. *Amer. J. Physiol.,* **76:** 538.
37. JUSTUS, D. W.; CORNETT, R. W.; and HATCHER, J. D. 1957. *Circulat. Res.,* **5:** 207.
38. KELLAWAY, C. H. 1919–20. *J. Physiol.,* **53:** 211.
39. LANGLEY, L. L., and CLARKE, R. W. 1942. *Yale J. Biol. Med.,* **14:** 529.
40. LANGLEY, L. L., and GUNTHORPE, C. H. 1957. *Amer. J. Physiol.,* **191:** 342.
41. LANGLEY, L. L.; NIMS, L. G.; and CLARKE, R. W. 1950. *Amer. J. Physiol.,* **161:** 331.
42. LANGLEY, L. L.; SCOKEL, P. W.; and WHITESIDE, J. A. 1952. *Fed. Proc.,* **11:** 88.
43. LEHMANN, G., and MICHAELIS, H. F. 1942. *Luftfahrtmedizin,* **7:** 292.
44. LEVIN, L. 1945. *Endocrinology,* **37:** 34.
45. MALMEJAC, J.; CHARDON, G.; and NEVERRE, G. 1949. *C. R. Soc. Biol.* (*Par.*), **143:** 1526.
46. MALMEJAC, J., and GROSS, A. 1950. *C. R. Soc. Biol.* (*Par.*), **144:** 528.
47. MANGER, W. M.; WAKIM, K. A.; and BOLLMANN, I. L. 1959. *Chemical Quantitation of Epinephrine and Norepinephrine in Plasma,* p. 169. Springfield, Ill.: Thomas.

48. McQuarrie, I.; Ziegler, M. R.; and Hay, L. J. 1942. *Endocrinology*, **30:** 898.
49. McQuarrie, I., *et al.* 1939. *Proc. Soc. Exp. Biol. Med.*, **42:** 513.
50. Mikami, S. 1927. *Tohoku J. Exp. Med.*, **8:** 113.
51. Monge, C. M. 1935. *An. Fac. Med. (Lima)*, **17:** 233.
52. Mulrow, P. J., and Ganong, W. F. 1960. *Fed. Proc.*, **19:** 152.
53. Nahas, G. G., *et al.* 1954. *Amer. J. Physiol.*, **177:** 13.
54. Nichols, J. 1948. *J. Aviat. Med.*, **19:** 171.
55. Nichols, J., and Miller, A. T., Jr. 1949. *Proc. Soc. Exp. Biol. Med.*, **70:** 300.
56. Patterson, C. A.; Smith, E.; and Pickett, A. D. 1938. *Proc. Soc. Exp. Biol. Med.*, **38:** 455.
57. Pincus, G., and Hoagland, H. 1943. *J. Aviat. Med.*, **14:** 173.
58. Porter, R. W. 1952. *Amer. J. Physiol.*, **169:** 629.
59. Raab, W. 1943. *J. Aviat. Med.*, **14:** 284.
60. Royce, P. C., and Sayers, G. 1960. *Proc. Soc. Exp. Biol. Med.*, **103:** 447.
61. Safford, H.; Wells, L.; and Gellhorn, E. 1946. *Amer. J. Physiol.*, **146:** 386.
62. Sayers, G.; Redgate, E. S.; and Royce, P. C. 1958. *Ann. Rev. Physiol.*, **20:** 243.
63. Schulze, E. 1936. *Naunyn Schmiedeberg Arch. Exp. Path.*, **180:** 639.
64. ————. *Ibid.*, p. 649.
65. Starkenstein, E. 1912. *Z. Exp. Path. Ther.*, **10:** 78.
66. Stewart, G. N. 1924. *Endocrinology and Metabolism*, II, 127. New York: D. Appleton & Co.
67. Tenney, S. M. 1956. *Amer. J. Physiol.*, **187:** 341.
68. Tepperman, J., *et al.* 1947. *Endocrinology*, **41:** 356.
69. Thorn, G. W.; Jenkins, D.; and Laidlaw, J. C. 1953. *Recent Progress in Hormone Research*, p. 171. New York: Academic Press.
70. Thorn, G. W., *et al.* 1942. *Amer. J. Physiol.*, **137:** 606.
71. Van Liere, E. J.; McCarty, G. B.; and Matthews, J. G. 1952. *Amer. J. Physiol.*, **171:** 245.
72. Van Liere, E. J., and Northup, D. W. 1958. *Fed. Proc.*, **17:** 167.
73. Van Middlesworth, L., and Berry, M. M. 1951. *Amer. J. Physiol.*, **167:** 576.
74. Walker, W. F., *et al.* 1959. *Amer. J. Physiol.*, **197:** 773.
75. Walters, F. M. 1927. *Amer. J. Physiol.*, **80:** 140.
76. Watts, D. R. 1956. *Amer. J. Physiol.*, **184:** 271.
77. Watts, D. T., and Bragg, A. D. 1957. *Proc. Soc. Exp. Biol. Med.*, **96:** 609.
78. Williams, I. R., and Smith, E. 1935. *Amer. J. Physiol.*, **110:** 611.

CHAPTER XIV

METABOLISM AND HYPOXIA

OXIDATIVE METABOLISM

Man: acute exposures to anoxic hypoxia.—Loewy et al. (43), as early as 1897, using a low-pressure chamber and working at a barometric pressure of 448 mm. Hg (14,000 feet or 4,300 meters), found that the exchange of carbon dioxide and oxygen remained normal both at rest and during muscular exercise.

A number of observations on metabolism have been made on Monte Rosa. One of the early reports was that of Durig and Zuntz (15) in 1904. Working at an altitude of 15,000 feet (430 mm. Hg and 4,600 meters) during a sojourn of two and a half weeks, they found that the resting metabolism increased as much as 15 per cent above that of sea level. It was not due to cold, since the readings were taken while the subject was in a warm bed. At an altitude of 10,500 feet (2,200 meters), negative results were reported. Durig (14) in 1909, working with six subjects on Monte Rosa, found increases in the amount of oxygen absorbed ranging between 9.9 and 45.5 per cent. In the same year Fuchs and Deimler (20), also working on Monte Rosa, found an increase in carbon dioxide production and oxygen absorption above that of sea level, and it was proportionately greater during standing than while reclining at rest.

Studies in metabolism were also reported by members of the Anglo-American Expedition to Pike's Peak in 1911 (12). The respiratory exchange of Douglas was only slightly greater on Pike's Peak than at sea level. The gaseous metabolism during muscular exercise was found unchanged with altitude.

In 1915 Hasselbalch and Lindhard (28) found no change in the exchange of carbon dioxide and oxygen in a low-pressure chamber at atmospheric pressures ranging from 589 mm. Hg (7,000 feet or 2,100 meters) to 448 mm. Hg (14,000 feet or 4,300 meters). Each man spent a number of days in the chamber.

Viale (59) in 1919 reported work with two subjects at the Mosso

Scientific Institute on Monte Rosa. One showed an increase in metabolism the first five days and a return to normal during the succeeding five days. The other subject showed no initial rise, as did the first, but showed and maintained an increment of about 11 per cent oxygen. The respiratory quotient was increased at high altitude.

In 1923 Schneider (49) reported some studies on respiratory exchange, during a sojourn on Pike's Peak, in men sitting at rest and during a moderate amount of exercise. At rest, two of the three men showed no change in the gaseous metabolism above the normal established at sea level; the third man showed a slight rise for the first forty-eight hours and then returned to normal. During moderate exercise, there was some increase in the rate of metabolism for the first few days; but within one to three days, six of the seven men showed no exchange above that of sea level.

In 1927 Kestner and Schadow (36), reporting work done on the Jungfraujoch, concluded that the slight increase found in the basal metabolic rate was attributable to the increased activity of the respiratory muscles.

In 1946, in connection with another study, Lilienthal et al. (41) noted a trend of about 10 per cent toward a reduction in oxygen consumption on the average in six men breathing oxygen-nitrogen mixtures simulating approximate pressure-altitudes of 16,500 feet (5,000 meters).

Frank and Wezler reported in 1948 their studies of three young men (unclothed) under carefully controlled conditions (19). Room temperature was maintained at 30° C.; relative humidity, at 50 per cent; and air velocity, at 10 cm/sec. Hypoxia was produced during one to three hours with the use of oxygen-nitrogen mixtures having 12, 10, and 8 per cent oxygen. In two of the subjects, oxygen uptake was increased in proportion to the degree of hypoxia. The increases with 8 per cent oxygen were 33 and 67 per cent above the control for the two subjects. This occurred in spite of the fact that rectal temperature declined with the percentage of oxygen used, particularly with the lower two percentages. The third subject, on the other hand, suffered decreases in oxygen uptake of 10 and 35 per cent when breathing 12 and 10 per cent oxygen, respectively, the only mixtures studied with him.

Huckabee in 1958 (32) found no change in thirteen human subjects breathing 10 per cent oxygen for fifteen to thirty minutes.

In the same year, Cross et al. (10) reported that in fourteen newborn infants oxygen consumption decreased 17 per cent on a 15 per cent oxygen mixture. Presumably rectal temperature was not changed, in spite of the fact that crude direct calorimetry under similar conditions suggested lesser heat production in the hypoxic infants (6). The immediate environmental temperature of the infants in the latter related study was 26° C.

In summary, the work on human subjects as a whole would seem to indicate that gaseous metabolism is independent of variations in inspired oxygen tensions. However, there have been distinct exceptions noted in past research. In the following review of the work done on other, and particularly, smaller, mammals it will be seen that environmental temperature is a very important variable. Perhaps not enough attention has been paid to this aspect in the work on human subjects in the past. Finally, one may well question the inclusion of the newborn infant with the human adult series, because the results will be seen to resemble more those on the small mammal at non-neutral environmental temperatures.

Animals: acute exposure to anoxic hypoxia.—Since 1923 when Ogata (45) reported that rabbits showed a decrease in oxygen consumption breathing 16.5 per cent oxygen or less, much work has been done on the rabbit as well as on other species of animals.

Chevillard and Mayer reported findings in mice in 1935 similar to those of Ogata (8).

In 1931, Lintzel (42) studied oxygen consumption and rectal temperature in rats decompressed for four hours to barometric pressures between 274 and 290 mm. Hg (approximately 24,000–26,000 feet or 7,300–7,900 meters) at different ambient temperatures from 18° to 34.5° C. Below the neutral temperature, 29°–32° C., the oxygen uptake decreased in proportion to the external temperature with a 60 per cent reduction at 18° C. Rectal temperatures fell proportionately. At 34.5° C., oxygen consumption increased 11–12 per cent. When external temperature was held at 24.5° C., oxygen consumption declined with the barometric pressure, decreasing from −23 to −39 per cent of the control from 460 mm. Hg to 280 mm. Hg. As the author pointed out, the rats under hypoxia resembled poikilothermal, or hibernating, animals.

The findings of Blood *et al.* (5) in 1949 were rather similar even though the rats used were acclimated to 5,280 feet (1,610 meters) and lightly anesthetized. The authors pointed out that although there is a close parallelism between oxygen consumption and body temperature in hypoxia, there are several indications that they may vary independently.

Fluckiger in 1956 (18), using rats under rather close restraint at an ambient temperature of 21°–22° C., found decreased oxygen uptake and fall of body temperature on 10 per cent oxygen. An interesting finding was that no oxygen debt was found on the average following the hypoxic period in a group of eight rats.

Two reports on infant rats appeared in 1960. One was by Taylor (54) and the other by Adolph and Hoy (2). Both found oxygen consumption decreased under hypoxia in spite of maintenance of animals at neutral temperature. Like Fluckiger, the latter authors found no repayment of an oxygen debt in the recovery periods.

Guinea pigs were studied by Rothschuh in 1947 (47). Oxygen uptake was found unchanged at 25° C. as the barometric pressure was lowered to 404 mm. Hg (16,000 feet, or 5,000 meters). Below that pressure, uptake of oxygen fell as did body temperature. A peculiar finding was that, during recovery, not only was the hypoxic oxygen debt paid but oxygen in excess of the deficit was consumed amounting to some 15–48 per cent of the control metabolic rate. It would seem that this unique result needs confirmation, if, indeed, this is possible.

The adult guinea pig was chosen by Hill (31) in 1959 for comparison with the kitten in order to discover whether size or maturity is responsible for the hypoxic reduction of oxygen consumption. Both animals were restrained for study. Since 10–15 per cent oxygen in the inspired air reduced the oxygen uptake in both, it was concluded that immaturity is not a factor. Ambient temperature, however, was found to be important. At the neutral ambient temperature peculiar to each species, oxygen consumption was not affected from 21 per cent down to 10 per cent inspired oxygen, and rectal temperature did not fall. The author suggested that when the metabolic rate is elevated for maintenance of body temperature at lower than neutral ambient temperatures, hypoxia depresses the extra oxygen consumption and body temperature is not maintained. It was further pointed out that the body temperature quickly returns to normal in recovery and there is an extra oxygen consumption to provide for this. There is no evidence of the repayment of any other possibly existent oxygen debt.

The above findings of Hill were quite completely confirmed by Moore (44) on the kitten in the same year. Since no restraint was used by Moore, this factor can be dismissed in the results of Hill. Moore's results also showed rather clearly that the state of oxygen consumption determines the fall of rectal temperature during hypoxia as well as the rise during recovery.

The original finding by Ogata (45) in rabbits was confirmed by Hamon *et al.* in 1935 (26) and by Ivanov in 1959 (33).

In anesthetized, newborn lambs both Acheson *et al.* (1) and Cross *et al.* (9) have found depression of oxygen consumption by hypoxia. The latter authors found that this occurred in spite of maintenance of a neutral ambient temperature. They also found that in the anesthetized adult sheep oxygen consumption was well maintained on 6 per cent oxygen in the inspired air. The report of Hemingway and Birzis suggests that the anesthetized adult cat is apparently quite resistant to the hypoxic reduction of oxygen uptake (29).

In 1952, Hemingway and Nahas (30) reported the results of their study of four unanesthetized dogs breathing oxygen mixtures by mask from 20.9 down to 6 per cent for a period of one hour with ambient temperature maintained at 23° C., presumably the neutral temperature. Whereas rectal temperatures fell uniformly with the three lowest oxygen mixtures, the oxygen consumption, after a fall during the early part of the hypoxic exposure, regained control or higher levels subsequently. There appeared to be an excess oxygen consumption in the after-period on air during which time rectal temperatures regained their control values.

The experiments of Gorlin and Lewis (22) on anesthetized dogs and those of Alpert *et al.* (3) on the spinal cord–transected dog showed decreases of oxygen consumption during short-term experiments in which severe degrees of hypoxia were imposed. Under the circumstances, these results are not necessarily incompatible with those of Hemingway and Nahas.

In summary, the experiments on animals have brought out the necessity of maintenance of a neutral ambient temperature if the oxygen consumption during hypoxia is to be properly evaluated. Under such circumstances, the consumption does not fall until severe degrees of hypoxia are encountered. Otherwise the fall begins almost immediately after the inspired oxygen tension is lowered below normal. In the recovery from hypoxia, the impression is strong that extra oxygen may be involved in returning the rectal temperature to normal but that no other excess oxygen consumption is involved. No true hypoxic oxygen debt is thus seen. In comparing the various species of animals, the larger animals, such as the cat, dog, and sheep, seem less susceptible to a hypoxic reduction in oxygen consumption than the smaller mouse, rat, guinea pig and rabbit. It would seem that man behaves like the larger animals. Most of the experiments with newborn animals, including man, strongly indicate a particular susceptibility to hypoxic reductions of oxygen consumption in spite of maintenance of a neutral ambient temperature. It is possible, however, that more attention must be paid, not only to species, but to individual neutral ambient temperature.

Toxic hypoxia and metabolism.—Conflicting results have been reported in the literature on the effect of carbon monoxide on metabolism. Some workers (24, 60) have reported that carbon monoxide produces a decrease in metabolic rate in animals, while others (46, 50) have reported the opposite results. Killick (37) has pointed out that when the experimental findings are summed up it seems that if the animals are exposed to low concentrations of carbon monoxide and if hypoxia develops slowly, the metabolic rate is slowed; but, on the other hand, if the hypoxia is severe and rapid, the metabolic rate may actually rise as a result of increased activity of the respiratory muscles (23). She further points out that it must be recognized in experiments (46, 50) in which the animals were subjected to repeated severe poisonings that the ductless glands were affected; hence the metabolism was increased.

Only a few observations have been reported on the effect of carbon monoxide on the metabolism in the human being. Beck (4) in 1936 found that the metabolic rate was significantly reduced in just over half of his patients who had been exposed repeatedly to carbon monoxide. Drinker (13) in 1938 made the observation that acute carbon monoxide poisoning was frequently accompanied by a marked fall in body temperature presumably because of depressed metabolism.

In 1946 Tepperman *et al.* (55) studied the effects of methemoglobinemia produced with p-amino-propiophenone in both trained and untrained human subjects in short bouts (three minutes) of moderately heavy work loads on the bicycle ergometer. Increased production of blood lactate in the recovery period occurred in those cases in which the methemoglobinemia was relatively high: between 17.0 and 27.1 per cent of methemoglobin in total hemoglobin.

Anemic hypoxia and metabolism.—Human subjects with anemia (5.2–9.3 g/100 ml hemoglobin) were compared, by Sproule *et al.* (51), with normals exercising two and a half minutes on the treadmill. Grade and speed were standardized by adjustment to a maximum amount of oxygen extracted from air inspired by the exercising subject. Whereas resting oxygen consumptions were nearly identical in the two groups, that of the anemic group during exercise was increased only 5.75-fold compared to 9.76-fold for the normal group. If, indeed, the exercise were truly standardized, it is difficult to account for the difference, for venous pH was not unusually depressed in the anemic group, nor was their symptomatic distress greater than in the normal group.

CARBOHYDRATE METABOLISM

Liver glycogen in anoxic hypoxia.—In 1934 and 1936 Evans (16, 17) observed that there is an increase of glycogen, mostly in the liver, of fasted rats exposed for twenty-four hours to one-half atmosphere of pressure. The adrenal cortex and the pituitary but not the adrenal medulla were found necessary for the phenomenon to occur. Since there was an increase of total urinary nonprotein nitrogen under these conditions, it was concluded that protein was the source of the carbohydrate. These findings were confirmed in part in 1942 by Lewis *et al.* (40), not only in the rat, but also in the rabbit and the monkey. Since the addition of carbon dioxide to the inspired air under decompression reduced the glycogen deposition, Langley *et al.* (38) suggested that the increased glycogen deposition might be a response to the associated hypocapnia rather than to the hypoxia per se. Since carbon dioxide stimulates respiration, however, there is a reduction in the severity of the hypoxia under these circumstances, and the results could also be explained on this basis.

Different results in respect to liver glycogen were found by Van Middlesworth in 1946 (58). Rats were given glucose by stomach tube or by intraperitoneal injection and exposed for four hours to the simulated altitude of 27,000 feet (8,200 meters). In both cases, glycogen concentration in the liver ninety minutes after the glucose administration was only about half as great as in the controls similarly treated at ground level.

More recently (1958) Timiras *et al.* (56) have found both decreases and increases in liver-glycogen concentration of rats at 12,470 feet (3,800 meters), depending upon the experimental conditions.

Glucose tolerance: animals.—Several investigations have been made of glucose tolerance at altitude. Kelley and co-worker (34) and Keyes and Kelley (35), with the intravenous glucose-tolerance test in unanesthetized dogs at both 18,000 and 24,000 feet (5,500 and 7,300 meters) simulated altitude, finally concluded that glucose tolerance was increased. Similar glucose-tolerance curves were found by Stickney *et al.* (52) in unanesthetized dogs decompressed to a simulated of 28,000 feet (8,500 meters). Since the curves have an early maximum which is lower than that obtained at ground level but have a later portion characterized by elevations above the control curves, they are difficult to interpret. Technically one could conclude that since the total area under the curves is greater at "altitude" than at ground level, tolerance is decreased. If one assumes with Keyes and Kelley (35) that the initial depression of the experimental curve indicates greater conversion of glucose to glycogen, then tolerance must be increased. The delayed return of the curve beyond this point must indicate either decreased tolerance or continued mobilization of blood glucose by the experimental animal.

In Van Middlesworth's experiments on rats (58) mentioned above, tolerance to fed glucose was distinctly reduced, and the animals had a striking glycosuria.

Glucose tolerance: man.—In 1942 Leipert and Kellersmann (39) ran glucose-tolerance tests on six young men in the decompression chamber at 18,000–20,000 feet (5,500–6,200 meters) for three hours. The tolerance curves at simulated altitude were markedly different than the ground-level ones in three of the men. In these, as in those of the dogs of Kelley and Keyes (34, 35) and of Stickney *et al.* (52), the terminal portions were elevated. As a whole, the early hyperglycemic maxima were no greater at altitude than at ground level. The later hypoglycemic phase seen regularly in the control curves was missing in all but one of the subjects at "altitude."

In five young men on the Jungfraujoch (about 11,000 feet or 3,457 meters) for eight days, Schaffeler and Flury (48) found glucose tolerance slightly increased.

Summary.—Carbohydrate metabolism is definitely altered by hypoxia. The hyperglycemic response is well known (see chapter iv, p. 65). The changes in glycogen deposition in the liver depend largely upon the experimental conditions. In some cases, the glycogen concentration is increased; in others, decreased. There is some question whether hypoxia per se, the associated hypocapnia, or both are the important variables inducing the alterations. Glucose tolerance is not greatly changed except in very severe hypoxia. The tolerance curves usually show a terminal elevated blood sugar which may be interpreted as either reduced tolerance or as persistence of the hypoxic hyperglycemia.

NITROGEN METABOLISM

It has been shown by a number of workers (11, 25, 27, 28, 53) that anoxic hypoxia produces a decrease in the excretion of ammonia.

It is thought that this decrease is a response, as previously mentioned (p. 236), to the alkalosis of hyperpnea. Brunquist *et al.* (7) in 1924 found an increase in severe hypoxia in the rate of total nitrogen excretion, as well as of urea, ammonia, and creatine excretion in little pigs. This increase in total nitrogen excretion is like that in urinary, nonprotein nitrogen more recently seen in fasting rats under hypoxia (16, 17, 38, 40). The explanation is that during hypoxia there may be increased gluconeogenesis from protein.

Toxic hypoxia and nitrogen metabolism.—An increase in urinary excretion of total nitrogen and of ammonia in carbon monoxide poisoning has been reported by several workers (21, 57). In 1928 Tscherkess and Melnikova (57) reported that urinary nitrogen increased during and after periods of severe carbon monoxide hypoxia in various animals. These workers claimed that this indicated increased destruction of protein, a conclusion which is compatible with the present viewpoint.

REFERENCES

1. ACHESON, G. H.; DAWES, G. S.; and MOTT, J. C. 1957. *J. Physiol.,* **135:** 623.
2. ADOLPH, E. F., and HOY, P. A. 1960. *J. Appl. Physiol.,* **15:** 1075.
3. ALPERT, N. R.; KAYNE, H.; and HASLETT, W. 1958. *Amer. J. Physiol.,* **192:** 585.
4. BECK, H. G. 1936. *J.A.M.A.,* **107:** 1025.
5. BLOOD, F. R., *et al.* 1949. *Amer. J. Physiol.,* **156:** 62.
6. BRODIE, H. R.; CROSS, K. W.; and LOMER, T. R. 1957. *J. Physiol.,* **138:** 156.
7. BRUNQUIST, E. H.; SCHNELLER, E. J.; and LOEVENHART, A. S. 1924. *J. Biol. Chem.,* **62:** 93.
8. CHEVILLARD, L., and MAYER, A. 1935. *Ann. Physiol.,* **11:** 225.
9. CROSS, K. W.; DAWES, G. S.; and MOTT, J. C. 1959. *J. Physiol.,* **146:** 316.
10. CROSS, K. W.; TIZARD, J. P. M.; and TRYTHALL, D. A. H. 1958. *Acta Paediat. (Upps.),* **47:** 217.
11. DAVIES, H. W., *et al.* 1920. *J. Physiol.,* **54:** 32.
12. DOUGLAS, C. G., *et al.* 1913. *Phil. Trans. Roy. Soc., London,* B, **203:** 185.
13. DRINKER, C. K. 1938. *Carbon Monoxide Asphyxia,* p. 30. New York: Oxford University Press.
14. DURIG, A. 1909. *Physiologische Ergebnisse der im Jahr 1906 durchgeführten, Monte Rosa Expedition,* p. 160. Vienna.

15. Durig, A., and Zuntz, N. 1904. *Pflueger Arch. Ges. Physiol.,* Suppl.: p. 147.
16. Evans, G. 1934. *Amer. J. Physiol.,* 110: 273.
17. ————. 1936. *Ibid.,* 114: 297.
18. Fluckiger, E. 1956. *Helv. Physiol. Pharmacol. Acta,* 14: 369.
19. Frank, E., and Wezler, K. 1948. *Pflueger Arch. Ges. Physiol.,* 250: 320.
20. Fuchs, R. F., and Deimler, T. 1909. *Sitzungsb. d. phys.-Med. Soz. zu Erlangen,* 41: 125.
21. Glaubitz, G. 1921. *Z. Ges. Exp. Med.,* 25: 230.
22. Gorlin, R., and Lewis, B. M. 1954. *J. Appl. Physiol.,* 7: 180.
23. Haggard, H. W., and Henderson, Y. 1921. *J. Biol. Chem.,* 47: 421.
24. Haldane, J. S. 1895. *J. Physiol.,* 18: 201.
25. Haldane, J. S.; Kellas, A. M.; and Kennaway, E. L. 1919–20. *J. Physiol.,* 53: 181.
26. Hamon, F.; Kolodny, S.; and Mayer, A. 1935. *Ann. Physiol.,* 11: 211.
27. Hasselbalch, K. A. 1916. *Biochem. Z.,* 74: 48.
28. Hasselbalch, K. A., and Lindhard, J. 1915; 1916. *Biochem. Z.,* 68: 265, 295; 74: 1.
29. Hemingway, A., and Birzis, L. 1956. *J. Appl. Physiol.,* 8: 577.
30. Hemingway, A., and Nahas, G. G. 1952. *Amer. J. Physiol.,* 170: 426.
31. Hill, J. R. 1959. *J. Physiol.,* 149: 346.
32. Huckabee, W. E. 1958. *J. Clin. Invest.,* 37: 264.
33. Ivanov, K. P. 1959. *Sechenov Physiol. J. (U.S.S.R.),* 45: 81.
34. Kelley, V. C., and McDonald, R. K. 1948. *Amer. J. Physiol.,* 152: 250.
35. Keyes, G. H., and Kelley, V. C. 1949. *Amer. J. Physiol.,* 158: 358.
36. Kestner, O., and Schadow, H. 1927. *Pflueger Arch. Ges. Physiol.,* 217: 492.
37. Killick, E. M. 1940. *Physiol. Rev.,* 20: 313.
38. Langley, L. L.; Nims, L. F.; and Clarke, R. W. 1950. *Amer. J. Physiol.,* 161: 331.
39. Leipert, T., and Kellersmann, E. 1942. *Hoppe Seyler Z. Physiol. Chem.,* 276: 214.
40. Lewis, R. A., *et al.* 1942. *J. Clin. Invest.,* 21: 33.
41. Lilienthal, J. L., Jr. *et al.* 1946. *Amer. J. Physiol.,* 147: 199.
42. Lintzel, W. 1931. *Pflueger Arch. Ges. Physiol.,* 227: 693.
43. Loewy, A.; Loewy, J.; and Zuntz, L. 1897. *Pflueger Arch. Ges. Physiol.,* 66: 477.
44. Moore, R. E. 1959. *J. Physiol.,* 149: 500.
45. Ogata, H. 1923. *J. Biophysics (Japan),* 1: 1.
46. Reploh, H. 1932. *Arch. Hyg.,* 107: 283.
47. Rothschuh, K. E. 1947. *Pflueger Arch. Ges. Physiol.,* 249: 175.
48. Schaffeler, K., and Flury, M. 1948. *Helv. Physiol. Pharmacol. Acta,* 6: 596.

49. SCHNEIDER, E. C. 1923. *Amer. J. Physiol.,* **65:** 107.
50. SCHULZE, E. 1936. *Naunyn Schmiedeberg Arch. Exp. Path.,* **180:** 639.
51. SPROULE, B. J.; MITCHELL, J. H.; and MILLER, W. F. 1960. *J. Clin. Invest.,* **39:** 378.
52. STICKNEY, J. C.; NORTHUP, D. W.; and VAN LIERE, E. J. 1948. *Amer. J. Physiol.,* **154:** 423.
53. SUNDSTROEM, E. S. 1919. *Univ. Calif. Publ. Physiol.,* **5:** 121.
54. TAYLOR, P. M. 1960. *J. Physiol.,* **154:** 153.
55. TEPPERMAN, J.; BODANSKY, O.; and JANDORF, B. J. 1946. *Amer. J. Physiol.,* **146:** 702.
56. TIMIRAS, P. S., *et al.* 1958. *Amer. J. Physiol.,* **193:** 415.
57. TSCHERKESS, A., and MELNIKOVA, W. 1928. *Arb. Materielen d. Ukrainischen Staatsinst f. Arbeitspath. u. Arbeitshyg. Charkow.*
58. VAN MIDDLESWORTH, L. 1946. *Amer. J. Physiol.,* **146:** 491.
59. VIALE, G. 1919. *G. Accad. Med. Torino,* **67:** 9.
60. WALTERS, F. M. 1927. *Amer. J. Physiol.,* **80:** 140.

CHAPTER XV

HYPOXIA AND HEAT REGULATION

ANOXIC HYPOXIA

Rabbits.—Bayeux reported in 1909 (1) that rabbits which had been transported to a height of 14,272 feet (4,350 meters) showed a decrease in body temperature. Several years previously he had made observations on himself and his wife on the summit of Mount Blanc and found a reduction in the axillary temperature. Bayeux regarded the hypothermia observed at high altitudes as resulting not from fatigue or cold but from an actual decrease of the physiologic oxidations of the body.

Behague *et al.* (2) in 1927 placed rabbits at 14°–16° C. in a chamber from which air could be withdrawn and reported that reduction in the air pressure was paralleled by fall of temperature in the animals. They concluded that the hypothermia was produced by the reduced oxidation resulting from the oxygen deficiency.

Rats and mice.—In 1931 Lintzel (11) exposed rats to reduced barometric pressures at different environmental temperatures. He noted that between 24,000 and 26,000 feet (7,300 and 7,900 meters) simulated altitude, at the neutral temperature between 29° and 32° C., body temperature was maintained constant but that at lower external temperatures body temperatures fell proportionately and at a higher temperature they rose. He pointed out the similarity to poikilothermal or hibernating animals. Lintzel's findings on the rat were confirmed by Blood *et al.* in 1949 (3). Lintzel's study and particularly the later one by Hill (8) emphasize the importance of taking into account neutral ambient temperature as well as other external temperatures if one is to appreciate the exact effect of hypoxia upon temperature regulation. In many studies this has not been done.

Gellhorn in 1937 (5) found that mice at room temperature have striking falls in rectal temperature when decompressed to 295 mm. Hg (about 24,000 feet, or 7,300 meters). Under these conditions, the rectal temperature fell 2.5° C. in five minutes, 3.0° C. in ten minutes, and 4–6° C. in fifteen or twenty minutes. Elevation of the ambient temperature at this simulated altitude prevented the fall in body temperature, but mortality was 90 per cent compared to 8.4 per cent at the lower room temperature. A more severe degree of hypoxia and a longer exposure were required in order to depress the rectal temperature in rats at room temperature as much as in mice. Gellhorn also found that the addition of carbon dioxide to the inspired low-oxygen mixture intensified the fall in rectal temperature. Since the carbon dioxide should have offset the effects of oxygen deficiency to a certain extent, the result seems to indicate that reduced oxygenation in the tissues is not the only factor producing the decline in body temperature. Increased blood flow through the skin was suggested as an important factor. Since the mouse has relatively a greater surface area than the rat, it should lose heat more rapidly under these circumstances.

Man and dog.—Kottke *et al.* in 1948 (10), in experiments on mice, dogs, and men exposed to hypoxia at low environmental temperatures, saw shivering stop under the effect of hypoxia and recorded an increase in skin temperature in man under these conditions. These experiments suggest that hypoxia inhibits increased heat production against cold and at the same time increases the heat loss through the skin.

In the same year Wezler and Frank (13) reported that hypoxia decreases rectal temperature in man even under conditions of neutral ambient temperature (30° C.). Increased heat loss was concluded to be the mechanism.

In the unanesthetized dog, Hemingway and Nahas (7) found that, in the cold, hypoxia reduces but does not eliminate the elevated oxygen consumption caused by shivering.

Kittens and guinea pigs.—In 1959 Hill (8) compared the responses to hypoxia of kittens and adult guinea pigs at various environmental temperatures. She found rectal temperature under moderate hypoxia (down to 10 per cent oxygen) well maintained in both species if a neutral ambient temperature were maintained. If the animal were placed at a lower temperature, however, even moderate hypoxia would induce a fall in rectal temperature and decrease the rate of oxygen consumption. It is the author's hypothesis that hypoxia eliminates the extra oxygen consumption required to maintain body temperature and in so doing prevents the maintenance of body temperature. The author presumably dismisses any effect of hypoxia upon mechanisms of heat loss and the decreased oxygen consumption and heat production secondary to fall in body temperature, as suggested by Gellhorn (6). Moore, also in 1959 (12), studied the kitten's responses to hypoxia. He suggested that the initial decline in oxygen consumption seems to precede the fall in body temperature. The later and slower decline of oxygen consumption may be secondary to reduced body temperature.

Effect of various agents.—In the experiments of Blood *et al.* (3), thyroid agents were used to demonstrate an independence of oxygen consumption and rectal temperature. More recently, Jarai and Lendvay (9) have also shown that the hypothermic response to hypoxia is not diminished by dinitrophenol in spite of increased heat production. However, these experiments are difficult to interpret.

Summary.—One may go along with Hill's suggestion (8) that the changes in body temperature and oxygen consumption in hypoxia are not the consequences of a specific effect of the hypoxia but of the general limitation of the organism to absorb oxygen from the atmosphere. The changes could also be seen as stemming from a specific impairment of the heat-regulating function of the hypothalamus. It has long been known that the brain is particularly vulnerable to hypoxia. The temperature-regulating mechanism in the hypothalamus is known to respond to reductions in skin and core temperature by reducing heat loss through the skin (vasoconstriction) and by increasing heat production through initiating shivering and perhaps increasing skeletal muscle tone. The effect of hypoxia may be on either a part or on all of these responses depending upon the species, the ambient temperature, or the degree of hypoxia. It is possible that the hypothalamus of the immature animal may respond in different ways than the adult.

TOXIC HYPOXIA

Drinker (4), as noted previously (p. 260), has frequently observed marked falls in body temperature in acute carbon monoxide poisoning.

REFERENCES

1. BAYEUX, M. R. 1909. *C. R. Acad. Sci. (Par.)*, **148**: 1691.
2. BEHAGUE, P.; RICHET, G.; and RICHET, C. 1927. *C. R. Soc. Biol. (Par.)*, **96**: 766.
3. BLOOD, F. R., *et al.* 1949. *Amer. J. Physiol.*, **156**: 62.

4. DRINKER, C. K. 1938. *Carbon Monoxide Asphyxia,* p. 30. New York: Oxford University Press.
5. GELLHORN, E. 1937. *Amer. J. Physiol.,* 120: 190.
6. ———. 1943. *Autonomic Regulations,* p. 49. New York: Interscience Publishers.
7. HEMINGWAY, A., and NAHAS, G. G. 1952. *J. Appl. Physiol.,* 5: 267.
8. HILL, J. R. 1959. *J. Physiol.,* 149: 346.
9. JARAI, I., and LENDVAY, B. 1958. *Acta Physiol. Acad. Sci. Hung.,* 13: 147.
10. KOTTKE, F. J., *et al.* 1948. *Amer. J. Physiol.,* 153: 10.
11. LINTZEL, W. 1931. *Pflueger Arch. Ges. Physiol.,* 227: 693.
12. MOORE, R. E. 1959. *J. Physiol.,* 149: 500.
13. WEZLER, K., and FRANK, E. 1948. *Pflueger Arch. Ges. Physiol.,* 250: 439.

CHAPTER XVI

EFFECT OF ANOXIC HYPOXIA ON WATER DISTRIBUTION IN THE BODY

In 1947 Lawless and Van Liere (1) made a study of the effect of various degrees of hypoxia on the water content of several different tissues in the white rat. The tissues studied were the cerebrum, kidney, liver, striated muscles, skin, and adrenals. The animals were exposed to hypoxia for three and a half hours. Barometric pressures of 564, 379, and 247 mm. Hg, corresponding to altitudes of 8,000, 18,000, and 28,000 feet (2,400, 5,500, and 8,500 meters), were used.

At each level of hypoxia a significant reduction in body weight occurred. At a barometric pressure of 564 mm. Hg, there was no significant change in the water content of any of the tissues examined; but at 379 mm. Hg, there was a significant reduction in percentage of water in striated muscle and in the skin. At a barometric pressure of 247 mm. Hg, no significant changes in the water content of any tissue was found except in the adrenals of one of the three groups studied. In that case there was an increase in the water content. It was concluded that the water content of the tissues does not change following hypoxia. That of the muscles and skin in particular is indeterminate; in some instances the amount of water was increased and in others decreased.

It had been known for some time that rats subjected to anoxic hypoxia lose weight. Swann et al. had shown this in 1942 (5) and 1943 (4); and Stickney, in 1946 (3). In the study of Swann et al. in which the losses due to feces, urine, and insensible water loss were analyzed after exposure to the simulated altitude of 18,000 feet (5,500 meters), only the insensible loss was found significantly increased. At the various durations of exposure varying from six to twenty-three hours, total water loss increased from about 50 to 100 per cent over the control values.

Stickney also found significant increases in fecal excretion, urine secretion, and insensible water loss during three and a half hours at all simulated altitudes above 8,000 feet (2,400 meters) in rats. Total water loss increased over the control values from about 75 per cent at 8,000 feet to about 180 per cent at 28,000 feet (8,500 meters). Part of the difference between the results of Swann *et al.* and those of Stickney is explained by the fact that no water was provided during hypoxia in the experiments of the latter.

More recently Picon-Reátegui *et al.* (2) have analyzed the body weight and water loss of rats during continuous exposure to 15,000 feet (4,600 meters) simulated altitude. They found water and weight loss maximal during the first week of exposure. At this time 20 per cent of the body water content had been lost and this loss accounted for 94 per cent of the reduction in body weight.

In the experiments of Lawless and Van Liere (above), since there was a loss of body weight but no organs were found to have lost water, the authors postulated that hemoconcentration must have taken place. Such hemoconcentration during hypoxia has been noted elsewhere (see p. 37). Presumably under longer durations of hypoxia, the tissue cells would also suffer a loss of water. Picon-Reátegui *et al.* (2) suggest that in addition there may be outright loss of tissue in order to account for the marked water loss.

REFERENCES

1. LAWLESS, J. J., and VAN LIERE, E. J. 1947. *Amer. J. Physiol.,* **149:** 103.
2. PICON-REÁTEGUI, E., *et al.* 1953. *Amer. J. Physiol.,* **172:** 33.
3. STICKNEY, J. C. 1946. *Proc. Soc. Exp. Biol. Med.,* **63:** 210.
4. SWANN, H. J., and COLLINGS, W. D. 1943. *J. Aviat. Med.,* **14:** 114.
5. SWANN, H. J., *et al.* 1942. *Science,* **96:** 588.

CHAPTER XVII

HYPOXIA AND NUTRITION

Reference has already been made to the fact that beyond a certain critical altitude animals will not eat (5) (see chap. x, p. 187). While working on production of cardiac hypertrophy by anoxic hypoxia, the senior author (18) in 1926 noticed that his animals, although receiving the choicest of foods, did not eat well and that all of them lost weight. In 1931 Lintzel (15) reported that rats which had been kept at a barometric pressure of 280 mm. Hg (about 28,000 feet—8,535 meters) lost 20 per cent of their weight within three weeks.

Observations made on men at high altitudes parallel the findings made on experimental animals. The newcomer to high altitude, of course, often suffers from mountain sickness, does not eat substantial meals, and consequently loses weight. In this section we will not consider the food habits of airplane passengers or those who are at altitude for a relatively short time but will limit our discussion to those people who make relatively long sojourns to high regions.

Barcroft (1), the leader of the expedition to the Peruvian Andes in 1921–22, called attention to the fact that the appetite of the members was often capricious and irregular. He emphasized that one of the most notable physiologic features was the loss of weight which the men suffered; all members of the party were affected. The individual who sustained the greatest loss declined in weight from 155 to 131 pounds in twenty-seven days.

Hingston (12), medical officer for the 1924 Mount Everest Expedition, observed that at great altitudes (beyond 21,000 feet—6,400 meters) the appetite became impaired and most of the men lost their taste for solid foods but still enjoyed sweets, fruits, and soups. The consensus was that at extreme altitudes sweets were the most, and meats the least, palatable. These men were, of course, well acclimated. The Mount Everest climbers who lived from six to seven weeks above 20,000 feet (6,095 meters) lost from thirty to fifty pounds (11). Bauer (2) also reported that subjects who had remained for six weeks at 20,000 feet or higher lost a great deal of weight.

In nine members of the International High Altitude Expedition to Chile, there was a mean loss of weight of eighteen pounds (16). Keys (14) has emphasized that the appetite may be capricious at high altitudes but that sweet foods, such as chocolate and jams, are often relished. Although it would be expected, it is interesting that those who had the greatest difficulty in becoming acclimated showed the greatest loss of weight.

Gray (8) reported studies of appetite and acclimatization to altitude on eight companies of troops. During the winter of 1943 a survey was made of the nutritional status of troops at Camp Hale, Colorado, situated at an approximate altitude of 9,000 feet (2,745 meters). The troops maneuvered at heights between 10,000 feet (3,050 meters) and 13,000 feet (3,960 meters). At the end of one month the daily average caloric intake was about 3,750; at the end of two months, 3,870; and at the end of three and a half months, about 5,000. There was an increase in carbohydrate consumption; initially carbohydrates constituted 39.8 per cent of the diet; after acclimatization this rose to 44.1 per cent. On the other hand, fat consumption decreased; initially it amounted to 46.9 per cent; it was decreased to 43.4 per cent.

The relatively recent observations of Pugh and Ward (17) on members of the expedition to Mount Everest agree in general with those of earlier workers, namely, the appetite may be capricious, and weight loss is common. The members of one group at a camp situated at 17,000 feet (5,180 meters) complained of poor appetites, and there was an average weight loss of eleven pounds in twenty-six days. A few of the men developed a craving for particular foods, in this instance tinned salmon and pineapple cubes. These articles were not available, but rather than eat foods which did not appeal to them, some refused to eat anything. On the whole, however, appetite for sweets increased.

At another camp, situated at 18,000 feet (5,485 meters), there was initially a depression of the appetite, but this symptom passed off in about two weeks. This probably was associated with acclimatization. It was observed that going without food too long at altitudes over 20,000 feet (5,095 meters) caused considerable fatigue. This could promptly be relieved by eating sugar. At approximately 21,000 feet (6,400 meters) the average intake of food was about 3,900 calories. The European type "Compo" rations were used but were supplemented with fresh meat, eggs, and potatoes. The four weeks spent at this altitude caused an average weight loss of about four pounds.

Work has been reported on vitamin needs of animals which have been subjected to oxygen want. Bronshtein (4) reported in 1944, after working with guinea pigs, that hypoxia lowers the level of ascorbic acid in the blood and hastens the development of scurvy on a normal diet. This work was confirmed five years later by Borsuk (3).

Grieg and Govier (9) demonstrated in 1943 that extensive dephosphorylation of the tissues occurred in animals which had been subjected to either hemic or anoxic hypoxia. Govier (7) feels that this may be extended to dephosphorylation of cocarboxylase and subsequently may lead to a rise of blood thiamine.

In 1945 Gusman *et al.* (10) noted a rise in the pyruvic acid content in the blood of aviators; this would fit in with the findings of Govier. Furthermore, Friedemann and Ivy and their collaborators (6) in 1949, using men as subjects, found that exposure to hypoxia at simulated altitudes above 15,000 feet (4,570 meters) produced a rise in concentration of lactic and pyruvic acids in the blood. There was also a rise in the lactate-pyruvic ratio.

As far as the authors of this monograph are aware, the requirements of man for ascorbic acid, thiamine, or nicotinic acid have not been found to be higher at altitude.

Dwellers at high altitudes.—A number of investigators have observed that people who make their home at high altitudes are not, as a rule, obese. Hurtado (13) reported that the Andean native children are significantly underweight in comparison with similar racial stock at sea level. Barcroft (1) has stated that he was informed that newcomers to the high plateau region of Peru all lost weight. If the subjects remained at high altitude, they subsequently regained some of it, although the former sea-level weight was seldom reached.

The fact that people who live at high altitudes are not obese cannot be accounted for by the effect of oxygen want on the gastrointestinal tract alone. It has been shown (see chapter xi, p. 219) that the gastroenteric tract is relatively resistant to hypoxia; this is true not only for motility but for secretion and absorption as well. There are several likely reasons to account for the initial loss of weight of the newcomer to high altitudes, as well as for the subnormal weight of the native dweller of high plateau regions. As has been mentioned, the appetite is not normal, and there are often minor gastrointestinal disturbances, such as diarrhea. In many instances it is difficult for these men to procure sound, refreshing sleep; this would tend to prevent them from gaining weight. Exertion at high altitudes, even in the well-acclimated individual, leads to dyspnea, although it is known that metabolism during moderate exercise is unchanged at high altitudes; so presumably the wear and tear of the body machinery is no greater.

There may be more subtle reasons which, as yet, are not understood thoroughly. It may be that the reduction in cellular oxidation brought about by the oxygen want is partially responsible for the inability of these people to maintain their normal weight. At any rate, it is known that the entire body often shows an impairment of function at high altitudes, and it may be this general impairment which is responsible for the subnormal weight of people at high altitude.

REFERENCES

1. BARCROFT, J. 1925. *The Respiratory Function of the Blood,* Part I, "Lessons from High Altitudes." Cambridge: Cambridge University Press.
2. BAUER, P. 1931. *Im Kampf um den Hamalaya,* p. 161. Munich: Knorr & Hirth.
3. BORSUK, V. N. 1949. *Chem. Abst.,* 42: 4740.
4. BRONSHTEIN, Y. E. 1944. *Amer. Rev. Soviet. Med.,* 1: 314.
5. CAMPBELL, J. A. 1935. *Brit. J. Exp. Path.,* 16: 39.
6. FRIEDEMANN, T. E., et al. 1949. *Quart. Bull. Northw. Univ. Med. Sch.,* 23: 438.
7. GOVIER, W. M. 1944. *J.A.M.A.,* 126: 749.
8. GRAY, E. L. 1955. *Milit. Med.,* 117: 427.
9. GREIG, M. E. and GOVIER, W. M. 1943. *J. Pharmacol. Exp. Ther.,* 79: 169.
10. GUSMAN, S. M.; SHTEINGART, D. M.; and KHARADZE, K. M. 1946. *Chem. Abst.,* 40: 2213.
11. HARTMAN, A. H. 1935. *Verh. Deutsch. Ges. Inn. Med.,* 47: 48.
12. HINGSTON, R. W. G., cited by J. BARCROFT. 1925. *The Respiratory Function of the Blood,* Part I, "Lessons from High Altitudes," p. 185. Cambridge: Cambridge University Press.
13. HURTADO, A. 1932. *Amer. J. Phys. Anthrop.,* 17: 137.
14. KEYS, A. 1936. *Sci. Monthly,* 43: 289.
15. LINTZEL, W. 1931. *Pflueger Arch. Ges. Physiol.,* 227: 685.
16. McFARLAND, R. A. 1937. *J. Comp. Psychol.,* 24: 189.
17. PUGH, L. G. C., and WARD, M. P. 1956. *Lancet,* 271: 1115.
18. VAN LIERE, E. J. 1936. *Amer. J. Physiol.,* 116: 290.

CHAPTER XVIII

EFFECT OF HYPOXIA ON THE NERVOUS SYSTEM

Of all the tissues in the body, nervous tissue is the least capable of withstanding oxygen want. Whereas cartilage tissue, for example, may withstand total deprivation of oxygen for several hours without suffering any apparent deleterious effects, nervous tissue can withstand deprivation of oxygen for only a few minutes. Since nervous tissue is so sensitive to oxygen want, it is obvious that the effect of hypoxia on the central nervous system of the intact organism is of paramount importance.

BLOOD SUPPLY TO THE BRAIN

The literature on cerebral circulation was reviewed by Wolff (109) in 1936. In 1943 Schmidt (86) published a monograph on cerebral circulation. The effect of hypoxia on cerebral circulation was reviewed by Opitz (76) in 1950, by Kety (62) in 1958, and by Lassen (65) in 1959. The reader is referred to these reviews for details of this important subject.

Schmidt (85) and Schmidt and Pierson (87) showed that oxygen deficiency produces vasodilatation and an increased volume of blood flow to the medulla oblongata and hypothalamus. A number of investigators in the early 1930's (20, 67, 110) also demonstrated that hypoxia produces dilatation of the pial vessels. These findings have been confirmed by later workers (65).

Wolff (109) stated that inhalation of carbon dioxide produces a more marked vasodilatation of the vessels which supply the brain than does oxygen want. If this were true, there would be a greater dilatation of the cerebral vessels during asphyxia than during anoxic hypoxia. On the other hand, Dumke and Schmidt (31) in 1943 observed that both hypoxia and hypercapnia increased cerebral blood flow but that the effect of hypoxia was more striking than that produced by carbon dioxide.

The consensus is that slight variations of oxygen tensions do not affect cerebral blood flow; however, a moderate decrease in oxygen tension may produce a significant increase. Courtice (23) in 1941, working with chloralosed cats, found that there was no increase in cerebral circulation until the inspired air contains less than 15 per cent oxygen. Kety and Schmidt (63) in 1948 reported that in subjects breathing 10–13 per cent oxygen the cerebral blood flow increased about 35 per cent. Lassen (65) reported similar findings. The latter worker has emphasized that the pronounced vasodilatory response to oxygen lack means that a greater degree of arterial oxygen unsaturation can be tolerated than would be the case if this response did not occur.

Opitz and Schneider (76) reported in 1950 that cerebral blood flow increased by anemia and that vasodilatation commences when the pO_2 of the cerebral venous blood falls to about 28 mm. Hg.

Although there is sound evidence that anoxic hypoxia and probably hemic hypoxia cause an increased blood supply to the brain, it is likely that in spite of this the diminished oxygen tension during hypoxia produces a deficient oxygen supply to the brain. It is generally conceded that during anoxic hypoxia the brain is one of the first organs to be affected.

SURVIVAL TIME OF DIFFERENT NERVE TISSUES DEPRIVED OF BLOOD

It has been known for a long time that different parts of the nervous system are more sensitive to deprivation of blood supply, that is, stagnant and hemic hypoxia, than are others. According to Heymans[1] (49), Stenon (93) in 1667 and Legallois (66) more than a century and a half later, were the first to investigate this important problem.

Many workers have experimentally produced anemia of the brain by occluding the arterial supply; among the early investigators were: Cooper (22) in 1836; Hill (51) in 1896 and in 1900 (52); Crile and Dolley (25) in 1908; and Pike, Guthrie, and Stewart (78) also in 1908. Others have reported studies on the effect of acute anemia on nervous centers (4, 16, 17, 25, 28, 39, 43, 50, 60, 61, 72, 77, 94, 95, 103).

Cannon and Burkett (19) in 1913 reviewed the literature of the

[1] C. Heymans in 1950 reviewed the literature concerning survival and revival of nervous tissues after arrest of circulation. The reader is referred to this extensive review which lists 246 references. (C. Heymans, *Physiol. Rev.*, 30 [1950], 395.)

effect of anemia on nerve cells of different classes. Table 10, which was compiled by Drinker (30) from the literature cited by Cannon and Burkett, shows the survival time of different nerve tissues when completely deprived of blood.

TABLE 10

SURVIVAL TIME OF DIFFERENT NERVE TISSUES
COMPLETELY DEPRIVED OF BLOOD*

Tissue	Survival Time (Minutes)
Cerebrum, small pyramidal cells	8
Cerebellum, Purkinje's cells	13
Medullary centers	20–30
Spinal cord	45–60
Sympathetic ganglia	60
Myenteric plexus	180

* From W. P. Drinker, *Carbon Monoxide Asphyxia* (New York: Oxford University Press, 1938), p. 133.

Drinker, interestingly enough, has pointed out that Table 10 indicates that individuals who have suffered from severe hypoxia, such as may be produced by carbon monoxide poisoning, may be practically decerebrated.

Heymans *et al.* (50) in 1937 studied the effect of acute anemia on the nerve centers by perfusion of the isolated head of the dog. The circulation was interrupted for varying periods of time, and the ability of the centers to revive after the circulation had been completely interrupted was noted.

Table 11 shows that the cortical regions are the most sensitive to oxygen want. It is of interest that Davies and Bronk (26a), in studies

TABLE 11

ABILITY OF CENTERS AT VARIOUS LEVELS OF THE NERVOUS SYSTEM
TO WITHSTAND COMPLETE INTERRUPTION OF BLOOD SUPPLY*

Interruption of Central Circulation up to	Cortical	Palpebral Pupillary	Cardio-regulatory	Vaso-motor	Respiratory
1–5 min	+	+	+	+	+
5–10	−	+	+	+	+
10–15	−	−	+	+	+
15–30	−	−	+	+	+
30	−	−	−	−	−

* From W. P. Drinker, *Carbon Monoxide Asphyxia* (New York: Oxford University Press, 1938), p. 134.

on oxygen tension in the mammalian brain, reported that the cortex (at least locally) is on the verge of oxygen insufficiency even in its normal state. Actually the cortex has but a small reserve of dissolved oxygen should the circulation fail completely. Their experiments suggest, however, that the cortex ought to function normally as long as its oxygen tension is well above 5 mm. Hg.

It is of especial interest (Table 11) that the respiratory center, which is generally regarded as being extremely sensitive to oxygen want, may be revived after it has been deprived of its circulation for a considerable time. Heymans *et al.* (50) pointed out that their experiments demonstrated that the respiratory and circulatory centers possessed great resistance to hypoxia and could be revived after the circulation had been arrested for as long as thirty minutes. They stated, however, that certain centers, which probably were situated in the cerebrum, were more sensitive to anemia and were irreparably damaged if the circulation were arrested for more than five minutes.

Arrest of circulation in spinal cord.—As early as 1667 Stenon (93) reported that anemia of the spinal cord produces paralysis at the end of one minute and suppression of sensitivity and motor functions after three minutes. Legallois (see 66) in 1830 reported that ligation of the abdominal aorta produced paralysis of motor spinal functions but that the spinal centers may recover their function if the circulation has not been obstructed too long.

Since this early work a number of investigators (12, 13, 14, 15, 21, 36, 69, 84, 92, 97, 100) have reported the effects of interruption of the circulation of the spinal cord. Many of these studies were made following obstruction of the abdominal aorta.

HISTOLOGIC STUDIES OF STRUCTURAL CHANGES

*Anoxic hypoxia.*Thorner and Lewy (96) in 1940 reported experiments performed on guinea pigs and cats which had been subjected to complete hypoxia by being placed in an environment of pure nitrogen for various periods of time. These workers found that exposures to sublethal periods of pure hypoxia produced vascular and degenerative changes in the central nervous system. It was emphasized that some of these changes were irreversible and became summated in animals repeatedly subjected to hypoxia.

Following fatal cases of nitrous oxide-oxygen anesthesia, lesions of the brain, especially in the cortex and basal ganglia, have been observed (41, 70). These changes have been attributed to anoxic hypoxia.

It has been suggested by van der Molen (98) that cortical cell changes occur at partial pressures of oxygen equivalent to an altitude of 28,000 feet (8,535 meters) and, moreover, that some of these changes might be irreversible. It will be remembered, however, that the average unacclimatized individual cannot live much beyond an altitude of 25,000 feet (7,620 meters). Only individuals thoroughly acclimated could withstand an altitude of 28,000 feet; it is known, of course, that several members of the various Mount Everest expeditions were reasonably well acclimated to this great height.

Windle and his co-workers (105, 106, 107, 108), during the early 1940's, carried out extensive researches on the central nervous system of full-term guinea pig fetuses which had been subjected to severe grades of hypoxia (and of asphyxia). (Some of these animals were resuscitated and later subjected to learning tests.) Controlled histopathologic studies were made. Neuropathologic changes of various degrees of severity were observed, which were not necessarily related to the duration of the hypoxia. Among the changes noted were capillary hemorrhages, clouding of Nissl substances, shrinkage of the neuron, and loss of stainability. In some instances, there was a generalized necrosis of the brain and spinal cord with chromatolysis and edema. Glial proliferation and loss of nerve cells, especially in the pyramidal layers of the cerebral cortex, were also found.

Morrison (74) in 1946 made comprehensive histologic observations on twenty-five dogs and ten monkeys which had been subjected to various degrees of hypoxia. He observed that a single exposure to a simulated altitude of 32,000 feet (9,755 meters) for twenty-five minutes produced extensive lamina necrosis in the cortex of the monkey.

Repeated exposures of moderate hypoxia (12–13 volumes per cent of oxygen in the blood) showed that the first histologic changes occurred in the cell bodies of the cortical gray matter. When 10 volumes per cent oxygen were used, and the animals subjected to repeated exposures, the white matter became involved, demyelinization appearing in the corpus callosum and centrum semiovale.

It was observed further that during severe hypoxia the frontal lobe was most often, and the temporal lobe least often, involved. The cerebellum was more often affected than the basal ganglion. The spinal cord and medulla were not affected by hypoxia compatible with life.

In 1945 Hoff, Grenell, and Fulton (57), working with guinea pigs, reported that hypoxia caused marked changes in the cell, which involved the cytoplasm, nuclei, and Nissl substance. Damaged cells were found in various locations of the brain, but those in the medulla and cerebellar cortex were especially involved.

Metz (73) in 1949, after subjecting several different species of vertebrates (goldfish, frogs, turtles, pigeons, and rats) to severe grades of hypoxia, commented on the fact that he did not see much histologic nerve damage. He emphasized the possibility that the changes which may have occurred were not morphologic in nature but rather were biochemical phenomena at a submicroscopic level. This is an interesting observation and suggests further researches along this line.

Recently Hager *et al.* (46) studied electron-microscopic changes in brain tissue of hamsters following acute hypoxia. The studies suggested that there is a rise of intracellular osmotic pressure and disintegration in both the perikaryon and the mitochondria.

Gerard (38), from his studies on hypoxia and neural metabolism, has concluded that one of the functions of oxygen is to keep the cell membrane polarized and, further, that proteolytic processes are initiated by complete hypoxia. It is thought that the accumulation of lactic acid in severe degrees of hypoxia may be partially responsible for this reaction.

Gellhorn *et al.* (37) have suggested that hypoxia and hypoglycemia have a similar physiologic action on the central nervous system and that they act synergistically in the production of convulsive seizures. Sugar and Gerard (95) have also suggested that hypoglycemia acts much like hypoxia on the function of the brain, since it leads to interference with oxidation in that organ.

Hemic and stagnant hypoxia.—Histologic studies of nervous tissue have been made on the differential effects of hypoxia following anemia. Gomez and Pike (41) in 1909, working with cats, reported histologic changes in nerve cells brought about by total anemia of the central nervous system. The order of susceptibility of the cells of the central nervous system to oxygen want, as shown by histological studies, was as follows: small pyramidal cells, Purkinje cells, cells of the medulla oblongata, cells of retina, cells of cervical cord, cells in lumbar cord, and sympathetic ganglionic cells.

Gildea and Cobb (39) in 1930, studying pathologic effects of cerebral anemia, observed nonspecific cortical lesions, such as focal areas of necrosis and swollen and shrunken ganglion cells. The most pronounced effect was noted in the cells of lamina III and IV of the cortex.

In 1938 Greenfield (42) reviewed previous work on neuronal damage from stagnant and anoxic hypoxia. He emphasized that there are considerable differences in the responses of different nerve cells.

Weinberger *et al.* (101) in 1940, working with cats, produced temporary anemia by occluding the pulmonary artery. At the end of three minutes and ten seconds, permanent and severe pathologic changes were found in the cerebral cortex. Longer periods of hemic hypoxia produced lesions in the Purkinje cells of the cerebellum and in nerve cells in the basal ganglion.

Effect of anemia on cells of spinal cord: A number of investigators (34, 47, 81, 92, 99) have made histologic studies of certain nerve cells after the circulation of the spinal cord had been partially or totally arrested. For the most part, severe anemia (ischemia) produced grave damage to the cells, and in some instances necrosis and destruction occurred. The amount of damage, of course, depended upon the severity and duration of the anemia. Some cells—for example, those of the spinal ganglia—withstood anemia much better than others.

These studies on the cells of the spinal cord have important clinical significance. They are especially pertinent in surgical operations involving important blood vessels, particularly the aorta. Recently, however, the use of extracorporeal circulation has removed many dangers in this area.

As might be expected, arrest of circulation produces grave organic changes in the cells of the central nervous system within a relatively short time. It has been emphasized by Sugar and Gerard (95), however, that while the damages which follow sudden anemia are primarily due to hypoxia, there are other important contributing factors. Those which they mention are hypoglycemia, hypercapnia, and the increased extracellular potassium.

Carbon monoxide poisoning.—The effect of carbon monoxide on the nervous system has engaged the attention of numerous workers (53, 54, 58, 75, 91, 96, 111). Not only has necrosis of nerve fibers in the brain been observed, but necrosis in the peripheral nerves, as well (58, 91).

In 1934 Yant *et al.* (111) made extensive investigations of histologic changes produced in the central nervous system of dogs following administration of carbon monoxide; various pronounced lesions were found.

In 1946 Lhermitte and De Ajuriaguerra (68) reported that if death rapidly followed carbon monoxide poisoning, hemorrhages, necrosis, and edema occurred. These changes primarily involved the lenticular nuclei; but the subcortical white matter, the hippocampus, the substantia nigra, and the cerebellum also were affected. If carbon monoxide poisoning is continued for long, changes appear in the vascular network with infiltration of the walls by neutral lipids and other substances, such as ferric salts and calcium.

These authors suggest that a toxic factor in addition to the anoxic factor in carbon monoxide poisoning affects the neuroglia and the vascular network with specific involvement of the basilar region and the white fibers of the centrum ovale. In this connection, Thorner and Lewy (96) in 1940 raised the interesting question whether the cerebral changes in carbon monoxide poisoning are actually typical of hypoxia or are caused by other factors.

Dutra (32) in 1952, studying the brain of man, reported that cerebral lesions which occur as residua of carbon monoxide poisoning consist essentially of dilatation of blood vessels, edema, perivascular hemorrhages, degeneration and death of ganglionic cells, focal demyelinization, and foci of necrosis. He felt that these lesions were either directly or indirectly caused by diminution of the supply of oxygen.

Obviously, carbon monoxide poisoning is capable of producing severe damage to nervous tissue. Some of the histologic changes following severe poisoning are irreversible, so that permanent damage has been done, and as Drinker has pointed out, individuals may be practically decerebrated.

CHEMISTRY OF THE BRAIN

During the past two decades or so, considerable research has been done on the chemistry of the brain during hypoxia. Several investigators (6, 7, 44, 45) have found an increase in lactic acid during anoxic hypoxia. Gurdjian *et al.* (44, 45) in 1944 reported that cerebral lactic acid rose when the oxygen content of inspired air fell to 10–13 per cent. Criscuolo and Biddulph (26) in 1958, working with rats, found that adrenalectomy prevented an increase in lactic acid of the brain during hypoxia. If, however, epinephrine were administered, the usual rise of lactic acid during hypoxia was observed. The authors felt that this finding suggested that blood sugar is the substrate for lactic acid.

There is evidence that hypoxia causes a decrease in phosphocreatine. Gurdjian *et al.* (44) reported a decrease of phosohocreatine when animals breathed 7 per cent oxygen. No change, however, was noted in cerebral adenosine triphosphate. In 1953 Albaum *et al.* (2), working with rabbits, subjected them to progressive stages of hypoxia and correlated the chemical changes in the brain with electrical measurement of function. Moderate decreases of adenosine triphosphate, creatine phosphate, and glycogen were observed. These decreases, however, were not noted until the stage of inexcitability had been reached.

Welsh (102) subjected rats to anoxic hypoxia (200–100 mm. Hg barometric pressure) for one to two hours and observed that the acetylcholine in the brain was decreased by approximately one-third to one-half. Insulin hypoglycemia was found to cause a greater decrease in acetylcholine than anoxic hypoxia. It was suggested that the decline in free acetylcholine might account for the decrease in excitability of the cortex under conditions of hypoxia and of hypoglycemia.

Dixon (29) in 1949 studied changes in the concentration of potassium in slices of rabbit cerebral cortex, which were bathed in a bicarbonate-Ringer's solution. In the absence of glucose a loss of potassium from the tissues was noted. With active utilization of glucose, however, there was an increase in the uptake of potassium. In this respect brain tissue resembles other tissues of the body.

The chemistry of the brain during hypoxic states obviously needs further investigation. Studies which correlate the chemical changes with electrical activity of the brain are especially needed.

ABILITY OF YOUNG ANIMALS TO WITHSTAND ASPHYXIA AND HYPOXIA

It has been known for well over two centuries that young animals are considerably less susceptible to asphyxia than adults. As early as 1725 Robert Boyle (10) commented on the resistance of kittens to asphyxia, and Paul Bert (5) in 1870 called attention to the fact that newborn animals were capable of withstanding prolonged asphyxia. Since that time many observers have reported studies on asphyxia and also on hypoxia in young animals and have confirmed and extended the earlier work.

Studies have been made on rats (1, 8, 9, 11, 18, 27, 35, 48, 55, 83, 88, 89, 90, 104), on dogs (33, 35, 40, 55, 61, 64, 88, 90, 104), on guinea pigs (18, 35, 40, 104), on rabbits (35, 40, 88, 90, 104), on cats (35, 64, 90, 104), and on mice (3, 59, 79, 80). A few observations have also been made on chicks and ducklings (82) and on the opossum (64). Newborn human infants, too, are capable of withstanding considerable periods of hypoxia; several workers have emphasized this (24, 71, 104).

Space does not permit giving details concerning all these experiments. Suffice it to say that the problem has been approached in numerous ways, and various grades and different types of hypoxia were used; the length of exposure was also varied. A few typical experiments may be cited.

Kabat (60) in 1940, studying resistance of very young puppies to arrest of brain circulation, found they were much more resistant to acute hypoxia than adult animals. The respiratory center in the newborn animal continued to function seventeen times as long as in the adult. The newborn also achieved complete functional recovery much more quickly than did the adult animal. At the age of four months, the resistance was diminished to the adult level.

Fazekas, Alexander, and Himwich (35) in 1941 studied the tolerance of the adult and infant of various species (rat, dog, cat, rabbit, and guinea pig) to hypoxia. The newborn exhibited a much greater tolerance to hypoxia than adults. Tolerance varied in the different species; for example, tolerance was longest in the physiologically immature newborn rats and shortest in the comparatively mature guinea pig. The authors suggested that in the newborn puppy and rat the factor permitting survival was poikilothermia, the fall of temperature diminishing the metabolic demands. It has also been demonstrated that in these two animals there is a lower cerebral metabolic rate.

Glass, Snyder, and Webster (40) in 1944, working with dogs, rabbits, and guinea pigs, subjected to pure nitrogen, concluded that tolerance to hypoxia is related to the stage of development rather than to environment. Interesting results were obtained with suckling rabbits breathing pure nitrogen. The survival period at one week was ten minutes; at two weeks, four minutes; and at three weeks, one and a half minutes, the last value being the same as that of the matured animal. These authors emphasized that the defense of the fetus against asphyxia is important because of the increased hazard of respiratory failure during the terminal phase of intrauterine life and the early neonatal period.

Selle (89) has pointed out that the increased tolerance of young animals to hypoxia is apparently due to several factors: (*a*) a low metabolic rate of the central nervous system, (*b*) poikilothermia, and (*c*) an anaerobic source of energy. Kabat (60) and Jelinek (59) also feel that the newborn can obtain anaerobic energy from glycolysis to a greater extent than adults. It has been shown by Himwich and his associates (55) that insulin reduces, and glucose increases, the survival of young animals placed in pure nitrogen. He and his coworkers (56), studying the survival of young animals which had been given sodium cyanide (which inhibits the cytochrome system), demonstrated clearly that anaerobic energy is available to young animals.

De Haan and Field (27) in 1959, working with rats, felt that young animals can withstand hypoxia better than adults because of high glycogen levels and the infant's ability to metabolize lactic and pyruvic acids to lipids.

REFERENCES

1. ADOLPH, E. F. 1948. *Amer. J. Physiol.,* **155:** 366.
2. ALBAUM, H. G.; NOELL, W. K.; and CHINN, H. I. 1953. *Amer. J. Physiol.,* **174:** 408.
3. AVERY, R. C., and JOHLIN, J. M. 1932. *Proc. Soc. Exp. Biol. Med.,* **29:** 1184.
4. BATTELLI, F. 1900. *J. Physiol. Path. Gen.,* **2:** 443.
5. BERT, P. 1870. *Physiologie de la respiration.* Paris.
6. BIDDULPH, C., *et al.* 1958. *Amer. J. Physiol.,* **193:** 345.
7. ———. 1959. *J. Appl. Physiol.,* **13:** 486.
8. BOLLMAN, J. H.; FAZIO, A. N.; and FAULCONER, A. 1951. *Anesthesiology,* **12:** 420.
9. BORGARD, W., and HOFFMAN, F. 1939. *Arch. Gynaek.,* **168:** 873.
10. BOYLE, R. 1725. *The Philosophical Works of Boyle.* London: W. and J. Innys.
11. BRITTON, S. W., and KLINE, R. F. 1945. *Amer. J. Physiol.,* **145:** 190.
12. BROWN-SEQUARD, E. 1851. *C. R. Soc. Biol. (Par.)* , **32:** 855.
13. ———. 1855. *Ibid.,* **41:** 628.
14. ———. 1855. *Ibid.,* **45:** 562.
15. ———. 1858. *J. Physiol. Homme,* **1:** 95, 117, 353.
16. BRUKHONENKO, S., and TCHETCHULINE, S. 1929. *J. Physiol. Path. Gen.,* **27:** 64.
17. BUNCE, D. F. M. 1961. *Fed. Proc.,* **20:** 100.
18. CAMERON, J. A. 1941. *J. Cell. Comp. Physiol.,* **18:** 379.
19. CANNON, W. B., and BURKETT, I. R. 1913. *Amer. J. Physiol.,* **32:** 347.
20. COBB, S., and FREEMONT-SMITH, F. 1931. *Arch. Neurol. Psychiat.,* **26:** 731.
21. COLSON, C. 1890. *Arch. Biol. (Par.)* , **10:** 431.
22. COOPER, A. 1836. *Guy Hosp. Rep.,* **7:** 457.
23. COURTICE, F. C. 1941. *J. Physiol.,* **100:** 198.
24. CREHAN, E. L.; KENNEDY, R. L. J.; and WOOD, E. H. 1950. *Proc. Mayo Clinic,* **25:** 392.
25. CRILE, G., and DOLLEY. 1908. *J. Exp. Med.,* **10:** 782.
26. CRISCUOLO, D., and BIDDULPH, C. 1958. *Proc. Soc. Exp. Biol. Med.,* **98:** 118.
26a. DAVIES, P. W., and BRONK, D. W. 1957. *Fed. Proc.,* **16:** 689.
27. DE HAAN, R. L., and FIELD, J. 1959. *Amer. J. Physiol.,* **197:** 445.
28. D'HALLIUM, M. 1904. *Presse Med.,* **12:** 345.
29. DIXON, K. C. 1949. *Biochem. J.,* **44:** 187.

30. DRINKER, C. K. 1938. *Carbon Monoxide Asphyxia,* p. 133. New York: Oxford University Press.
31. DUMKE, P. R., and SCHMIDT, C. F. 1943. *Amer. J. Physiol.,* **138:** 421.
32. DUTRA, F. R. 1952. *Amer. J. Clin. Path.* **22:** 925.
33. EDERSTROM, H. E. 1959. *Proc. Soc. Exp. Med. Biol.,* **100:** 741.
34. EHRLICH, P., and BRIEGER, L. 1884. *Z. Klin. Med.,* **8** (Suppl.) : 155.
35. FAZEKAS, J. F.; ALEXANDER, F. A. D.; and HIMWICH, H. E. 1941. *Amer. J. Physiol.,* **134:** 281.
36. GELFAN, S., and TARLOV, I. M. 1953. *Fed. Proc.,* **12:** 50.
37. GELLHORN, E.; INGRAHAM, R. C.; and MOLDAVSKY, L. 1938. *J. Neurophysiol.,* **1:** 301.
38. GERARD, R. W. 1938. *Arch. Neurol. Psychiat.,* **40:** 985.
39. GILDEA, E. F., and COBB, S. 1930. *Arch. Neurol. Psychiat.,* **23:** 876.
40. GLASS, H. G.; SNYDER, F. F.; and WEBSTER, E. 1944. *Amer. J. Physiol.,* **140:** 609.
41. GOMEZ, L., and PIKE, F. H. 1909. *J. Exp. Med.,* **11:** 257.
42. GREENFIELD, J. G. 1938. *J. Neurol. Psychiat.,* **1:** 306.
43. GRENELL, R. G. 1946. *J. Neuropath. Exp. Neurol.,* **5:** 131.
44. GURDJIAN, E. S.; STONE, W. E.; and WEBSTER, J. E. 1944. *Arch. Neurol. Psychiat.,* **51:** 472.
45. GURDJIAN, E. S.; WEBSTER, J. E.; and STONE, W. E. 1949. *Amer. J. Physiol.,* **156:** 149.
46. HAGER, H.; HIRSCHBERGER, W.; and SCHOLZ, W. 1960. *Aerospace Med.,* **31:** 379.
47. HAGGQUIVST, G. 1940. *Acta Med. Scand.,* **104:** 8.
48. HERRLICH, H. C.; FAZEKAS, J. F.; and HIMWICH, H. E. 1941. *Proc. Soc. Exp. Biol. Med.,* **48:** 466.
49. HEYMANS, C. 1950. *Physiol. Rev.,* **30:** 395.
50. HEYMANS, C., et al. 1937. *Arch. Neurol. Psychiat.,* **38:** 304.
51. HILL, L. 1896. *The Cerebral Circulation.* London: Churchill.
52. ―――. 1900. *Trans. Roy. Soc., London,* B, **193:** 69.
53. HILL, L., and SEMERAK, C. B. 1918. *J.A.M.A.,* **71:** 649.
54. HILLER, F. 1924. *Z. Ges. Neurol. Psychiat.,* **93:** 594.
55. HIMWICH, H. E.; ALEXANDER, F. A. D.; and FAZEKAS, J. F. 1941. *Amer. J. Physiol.* (*Proc.*) , **53:** 193.
56. HIMWICH, H. E., et al. 1942. *Amer. J. Physiol.,* **135:** 387.
57. HOFF, E. C.; GRENELL, R. G.; FULTON, J. F. 1945. *Medicine,* **24:** 161.
58. HSU, Y. K., and CHENG, Y. L. 1938. *Brain,* **61:** 384.
59. JELINEK, V. 1950. *Biol. Listy* (Prague) , **31:** 76.
60. KABAT, H. 1940. *Amer. J. Physiol.,* **130:** 588.
61. KABAT, H.; DENNIS, C.; and BAKER, A. B. 1941. *Amer. J. Physiol.,* **132:** 737.
62. KETY, S. S. 1958. *In: Circulation* (*Proc. Harvey Tercentary Congress*) , p. 331. Oxford: Blackwell.
63. KETY, S. S., and SCHMIDT, C. F. 1948. *J. Clin. Invest.,* **27:** 484.
64. KLINE, R. F., and BRITTON, S. W. 1945. *Fed. Proc.,* **4:** 41.

65. LASSEN, N. A. 1959. *Physiol. Rev.,* **39:** 183.
66. LEGALLOIS, cited by HEYMANS. 1950. *Physiol. Rev.,* **30:** 381.
67. LENNOX, W. G., and GIBBS, E. L. 1932. *J. Clin. Invest.,* **11:** 1155.
68. LHERMITTE, J., and AJURIAGUERRA, DE. 1946. *Sem. Hôp. Paris,* **22:** 1945.
69. LITTEN, M. 1880. *Z. Klin. Med.,* **1:** 131.
70. LOWENBERG, K.; WAGGONER, R. W.; and ZBINDEN, T. 1936. *Ann. Surg.,* **104:** 801.
71. MABRY, C. D. 1959. *J. Pediat.,* **55:** 211.
72. MAYER, S. 1878. *Med. Centralbl.,* **16:** 579.
73. METZ, B. 1949. *Fed. Proc.,* **8:** 109.
74. MORRISON, L. R. 1946. *Arch. Neurol. Psychiat.,* **55:** 1.
75. NEIGHBORS, D., and GARRETT, C. C. 1931. *Texas J. Med.,* **27:** 513.
76. OPITZ, E., and SCHNEIDER, M. 1950. *Ergebn. Physiol.,* **46:** 126.
77. PETROFF, J. R. 1931. *Z. Ges. Exp. Med.,* **75:** 1.
78. PIKE, F. H.; GUTHRIE, C. C.; and STEWART, G. N. 1908. *J. Exp. Med.,* **10:** 490.
79. REISS, M. 1931. *Z. Ges. Exp. Med.,* **79:** 345.
80. REISS, M., and HAUROWITZ, F. 1921. *Klin. Wschr.,* **8:** 743.
81. RIGHETTI, H., cited by HEYMANS. 1950. *Physiol. Rev.,* **30:** 375.
82. ROSTORFER, H. H., and RIGDON, R. H. 1947. *Biol. Bull.,* **92:** 23.
83. SAMSON, F. E., JR., and DAHL, N. 1956. *Fed. Proc.,* **15:** 161.
84. SCHIFFER. 1869. *Centralbl. Med. Wissensch.,* Nos. 37 and 38: 579, 593.
85. SCHMIDT, C. F. 1928; 1932; 1934; 1936. *Amer. J. Physiol.,* **84:** 202; **102:** 94; **110:** 137; and **114:** 572.
86. ———. 1943. *The Cerebral Circulation in Health and Disease.* Springfield, Ill.: Thomas.
87. SCHMIDT, C. F., and PIERSON, C. J. 1934. *Amer. J. Physiol.,* **108:** 241.
88. SELLE, W. A. 1941. *Proc. Soc. Exp. Biol. Med.,* **48:** 417.
89. ———. 1944. *Amer. J. Physiol.,* **141:** 297.
90. SELLE, W. A., and WITTEN, T. A. 1941. *Proc. Soc. Exp. Biol. Med.,* **47:** 495.
91. SHAFFER. 1903. *Centralbl. Nervenk. Psychiat.* (new series), **14:** 485.
92. SPRONCK, C. H. D., cited by HEYMANS. 1950. *Physiol. Rev.,* **30:** 381.
93. STENON, N., cited by HEYMANS, *ibid.*
94. STRATTON, G. M. 1919. *Sci. Monthly,* **8:** 421.
95. SUGAR, O., and GERARD, R. W. 1938. *J. Neurophysiol.,* **1:** 558.
96. THORNER, M. W., and LEWY, F. H. 1940. *J.A.M.A.,* **115:** 1595.
97. TUREEN, L. L. 1936. *Arch. Neurol. Psychiat.,* **35:** 789.
98. VAN DER MOLEN, H. R. 1939. *Ned. T. Geneesk.,* **83:** 4921.
99. VAN HARREVELD, A., and MARMONT, G. 1939. *J. Neurophysiol.,* **2:** 101.
100. VULPIAN, A., cited by HEYMANS. 1950. *Physiol. Rev.,* **30:** 381.
101. WEINBERGER, L. M.; GIBBON, M. H.; and GIBBON, J. H., JR. 1940. *Arch. Neurol. Psychiat.,* **43:** 615, 961.

102. WELSH, J. H. 1943. *J. Neurophysiol.,* **6:** 329.
103. WERTHEMIER, E., and DUBOIS, C. 1911. *C. R. Soc. Biol. (Par.),* **70:** 304.
104. WILSON, J. L., *et al.* 1948. *Pediatrics,* **1:** 581.
105. WINDLE, W. F. 1944. *Psychosom. Med.,* **6:** 155.
106. WINDLE, W. F., and BECKER, R. F. 1942. *Proc. Soc. Exp. Biol. Med.,* **51:** 213.
107. ———. 1943. *Amer. J. Obstet. Gynec.,* **45:** 183.
108. WINDLE, W. F.; BECKER, R. F.; and WEIL, A. 1944. *J. Neuropath. Exp. Neurol.,* **3:** 224.
109. WOLFF, H. G. 1936. *Physiol. Rev.,* **16:** 545.
110. WOLFF, H. G., and LENNOX, W. G. 1930. *Arch. Neurol. Psychiat.,* **23:** 1097.
111. YANT, W. P., *et al.* 1934. *Pub. Health Bull.* (U.S. Public Health Service), No. 211.

CEREBROSPINAL FLUID

PRESSURE

In 1960 Small *et al.* (20) reported the effect on anesthetized dogs of the inspiration of 8 per cent oxygen in nitrogen mixtures. Cerebrospinal fluid, arterial blood, and central venous pressures were all measured simultaneously with modern pressure transducers. The peak increase in cerebrospinal fluid pressure, occurring at four minutes on the average, was 108 per cent over the control. Mean arterial blood pressure increased 31 per cent and venous pressure 69 per cent at the same time. Vasodilation in the brain as well as increased blood pressures, both arterial and venous, were suggested as the causes of the rise in cerebrospinal fluid pressure. Earlier experimenters have reported similar findings in both dogs and cats. Most have found an early rise in short bouts of severe hypoxia (2, 15, 17). With longer exposures the terminal increase may be lessed marked or absent (1, 7, 23, 25). Edstrom and Essex (3) found the rise occurring for thirteen to thirty-three minutes following the breathing of pure nitrogen gas until near collapse.

According to present concepts (10, 21), hypoxia can cause cerebral vasodilation and increased cerebral blood flow. Since brain and cerebrospinal fluid are incompressible, in order for the cranium to accommodate the extra volume of blood there must be a shift of fluid from the cranial cavity. In the process cerebrospinal fluid pressure is apparently elevated, and cerebrospinal fluid absorption into the venous outflow is probably increased temporarily until a new equilibrium is reached.

Not all of the points in the above explanation have been directly substantiated in experiment. However, both Edstrom and Essex (3) and Loehning *et al.* (13) have seen the brain volume of anesthetized dogs increase during or after hypoxia (0–10 per cent oxygen mixtures). White *et al.* (23) found increased cranial volume in anesthetized cats even when the brains were exsanguinated following the experimental period. The latter result suggests increased cerebral intercellular fluid, increased extracellular fluid, or both. Most workers have not found the frank edema that this would entail, nor has the reversal of intracranial changes been as difficult as this would suggest.

Changes in cerebrospinal fluid pressure similar to those in anoxic hypoxia have been observed under conditions of toxic hypoxia brought on by carbon monoxide poisoning. In anesthetized dogs and cats Forbes *et al.* (4) found abrupt rises in pressure when the concentrations of carbon monoxide in inspired air were increased. Maurer (15) also saw pressures increased 170 per cent over the control in anesthetized cats. Sjostrand (18) placed windows in the cranium of anesthetized cats for observations during exposure to carbon monoxide. He found increases in brain volume and vasodilation in the pial circulation accompanying the elevations of intracranial pressure. All of these changes were readily reversible.

Observations of human subjects exposed to atmospheres containing carbon monoxide have shown increased pressures in the cerebrospinal fluid and increased dilation of retinal vessels (4, 14, 16).

BLOOD-CEREBROSPINAL FLUID BARRIER

It has been observed by several workers (5, 6, 8, 12) that the pH of the cerebrospinal fluid in anoxic hypoxia is increased. The increase has been attributed to the parallel increase in the blood pH directly due to the hypocapnia induced by the hypoxic hyperpnea. Several workers (5, 6, 9) have reported a paradoxical rise in pH of the cerebrospinal fluid accompanying a hypoxia not entailing hyperpnea (chemoreceptor denervation or artificial respiration). Furthermore, Stone *et al.* (22) have shown that the rise in cerebral pH is attended by an increased lactic acid concentration in the cerebral tissue which may regress in recovery without a further change in the pH. Gokhan and Winterstein (6) suggested the phenomenon to be due to increased clearance of the cerebral tissues of acid metabolites occurring during the hypoxic increase in cerebral blood flow. This interesting explanation has yet to be verified by further research.

The penetration into the cerebrospinal fluid of tissue constituents not normally present there or of artificially tagged components of the blood plasma during hypoxia has been studied. Wiemers *et al.* (24) in 1950 found that radioactive thorium does not readily enter the cerebrospinal fluid either normally or as a result of extreme hypoxia in rats and kittens (10,000–11,000 meters, or 33,000–36,000 feet) . On the other hand, Slobody *et al.* (19) have found in dogs that the slope of the curve relating concentration of albumin (tagged with radioactive iodine) to time in hypoxia to be five times that during the control periods. The hypoxia was severe: breathing oxygen-nitrogen mixtures having 3–5 per cent oxygen or decompression to simulated altitude between 25,000 and 35,000 feet (7,600 and 10,700 meters) . Similar penetration has been found by Lending *et al.* (11) by glutamic oxalacetic transaminase and lactic dehydrogenase during exposure to simulated altitudes of 27,000–37,000 feet (8,200–11,300 meters) in puppies. Obviously the degree of hypoxia has been extreme in these experiments, and caution should be used in applying the results to the milder forms of hypoxia usually seen.

In carbon monoxide poisoning the increased penetration of the blood-cerebrospinal fluid barrier has been signaled mainly by increases in protein concentration in the cerebrospinal fluid (14, 16) in some instances.

REFERENCES

1. BEDFORD, T. H. B. 1943. *J. Physiol.,* **102:** 334.
2. BERGERET, P., and GIORDAN, P. 1938. *J. Physiol. Path. Gen.,* **36:** 1050.
3. EDSTROM, R. F. S., and ESSEX, H. E. 1956. *Neurology (Minneap.)* , **6:** 118.
4. FORBES, H. S.; COBBS, S.; and FREMONT-SMITH, F. 1924. *Arch. Neurol. Psychiat.,* **11:** 264.
5. GOKHAN, N., and WINTERSTEIN, H. 1953. *Hoppe Seyler Z. Physiol. Chem.,* **295:** 71.
6. ———. 1958. *Pflueger Arch. Ges. Physiol.,* **266:** 318.
7. GRANDPIERRE, R.; FRANCK, C.; and VIOLETTE, F. 1952. *C. R. Soc. Biol. (Par.)* , **146:** 1246.
8. HERTZMANN, A. B., and GESELL, R. 1928. *Amer. J. Physiol.,* **87:** 15.
9. INGRAHAM, R. C., and GELLHORN, E. 1939. *Amer. J. Physiol.,* **126:** P543.
10. LASSAN, N. A. 1959. *Physiol. Rev.,* **39:** 183.
11. LENDING, M.; SLOBODY, L. B.; and MESTERN, J. 1961. *Neurology (Minneap.)* **11:** 520.
12. LEUSEN, I.; and DEMEESTER, G. 1960. *Arch. Int. Physiol.,* **68:** 389.

13. LOEHNING, R. W.; UEYAMA, H.; and UEDA, I. 1962. *Anesth. Analg.* (*Cleve.*) , 41: 529.
14. LUPS, S., and HAAN, A. M. F. H. 1954. *The Cerebrospinal Fluid,* p. 250. New York: Elsevier Publishing Co.
15. MAURER, F. W. 1941. *Amer. J. Physiol.,* 133: 180.
16. MERRITT, H. H., and FREMONT-SMITH, F. 1937. *The Cerebrospinal Fluid,* p. 215. Philadelphia and London: W. B. Saunders Co.
17. NOELL, W., and SCHNEIDER, M. 1942. *Pflueger Arch. Ges. Physiol.,* 246: 201.
18. SJOSTRAND, T. 1948. *Acta Physiol. Scand.,* 15: 351.
19. SLOBODY, L. B., *et al.* 1957. *Amer. J. Physiol.,* 190: 365.
20. SMALL, H. L.; WEITZNER, S. W.; and NAHAS, G. G. 1960. *Amer. J. Physiol.,* 198: 704.
21. SOKOLOFF, L., and KETY, S. S. 1960. *Physiol. Rev.,* 40 (Suppl. 4) : 38.
22. STONE, W. E.; MARSHALL, C.; and NIMS, L. F. 1941. *Amer. J. Physiol.,* 132: 770.
23. WHITE, J. C., *et al.* 1942. *Arch. Surg.* (*Chic.*) , 44: 1.
24. WIEMERS, K.; MAURER, W.; and NIKLAS, A. 1950. *Z. Ges. Exp. Med.,* 115: 688.
25. WOLFF, H. G., and LENNOX, W. G. 1930. *Arch. Neurol. Psychiat.,* 23: 1097.

THE AUTONOMIC NERVOUS SYSTEM

A comparatively limited amount of work has been reported on the effect of hypoxia on the autonomic nervous system. Much more work is needed. It was held by Cannon[2] for many years that the sympathetico-adrenal system played an important role in the adaptation of an animal to hypoxia; a part of his "emergency theory" was built on this concept. Cannon felt that hypoxia was capable of producing an increase in the flow of epinephrine and explained many of the phenomena produced by hypoxia by this mechanism. He suggested (personal communication) , for example, that the retardation of gastric emptying produced by hypoxia (p. 213) could be accounted for by an increased release of epinephrine.

According to Sawyer *et al.* (11) , if normal cats are exposed to an oxygen tension of 6 per cent, they will withstand this degree of hypoxia for at least an hour without collapsing. Cats which have had the greater part of their autonomic nervous system removed, however, will collapse within 15–38 minutes. McDonough (6) found that sympathectomized dogs breathing 4 per cent oxygen suffered respiratory failure in 102 minutes, whereas control animals continued to

[2] The reader is referred to the sections which deal with the effect of hypoxia on the adrenals (p. 244) and on the blood sugar (p. 65) .

breathe up to 145 minutes. These findings support Cannon's early views.

Gellhorn and his associates have made a number of studies on the autonomic nervous system during hypoxia. Ury and Gellhorn (12), working with rabbits, reported that 6–8 per cent oxygen raised the threshold for pupillary reflex dilatation produced by weak stimulation of the sciatic nerve. They suggested the possibility that this might have been produced by inhibition of the parasympathetics and pointed out that, if this were true, both excitatory and inhibitory processes in the central nervous system would be diminished under the influence of hypoxia.

In 1940 Feldman, Cortell, and Gellhorn (4) studied the effect of hypoxia on the parasympathetic and on the sympathetic centers. Evidence was presented (from results obtained by work on the vago-insulin and sympathetico-adrenal system) that under the influence of hypoxia both parasympathetic and sympathetic centers are excited. Two years later Gellhorn, Cortell, and Carlson (2), studying the effect of hypoxia (oxygen-nitrogen mixtures between 4.5–8.1 per cent oxygen) on autonomic and somatic responses elicited by stimulation of the hypothalamus, medulla, and spinal cord in narcotized cats, found that the autonomic centers in the central nervous system are less sensitive to hypoxia than are somatic centers.

Safford and Gellhorn (10) in 1945, working with rats on age and autonomic balance, found a diminished excitability of the sympathetico-adrenal system with increased age.

In 1959 Woods and Richardson (13), studying the effects of acute hypoxia on cardiac contractility in anesthetized and vagotomized dogs, observed that breathing 100 per cent nitrogen produced a marked increase in heart force and in blood pressure. Experiments with dogs after bilateral adrenalectomy, thoracic sympathectomy, and a total preganglionic blocking indicated that the responses to acute hypoxia are mainly due to sympathetic nerves.

Studies have been made of the effect of total sympathectomy on red blood cell formation, on hemoglobin production, and on polycythemic response to hypoxia. Orahovats and Root (9) in 1953 studied the effect of total sympathectomy on red blood cell formation and on hemoglobin production in six normal and six totally sympathectomized dogs. The experimental group produced red blood cells and hemoglobin at approximately the same rates as did the control group. It was concluded that the sympathetic nervous system is not essential for regeneration of red blood cells or hemoglobin in the anemic dog.

In similar experimentation, Grant and Root (3) studied the polycythemic response of completely sympathectomized dogs to discontinuous hypoxia (twenty-seven to seventy-three days). The polycythemic response did not differ from that of the control animals. They also concluded that the peripheral sympathetic nervous system of the dog is not essential for the polycythemic response to anoxic hypoxia.

Some clinical investigations have been made of the effect of altitude on the autonomic nervous system. It is believed by Monge (8) and by Aste (1) that residents of high altitudes show a hypertonus of the autonomic nervous system. Monge, after stimulation of the oculo-cardiac reflex, observed an increased tonus of the vagus nerve. Compression of the solar plexus gave a similar response of the sympathetic nerve. Aste, by intravenous injection of atropine in twenty-five soldiers who lived in the high Andes, also demonstrated a hypertonus of the vegetative nervous system. According to McFarland (7), Dr. Crane, then chief surgeon at the Cerro de Pasco Mines in Peru, found that in order to produce an effect on the circulation equal to that seen at lower levels it is necessary to inject twice the amount of atropine.

Keys *et al.* (5) have pointed out that hypoxia disturbs the stability of the balance between the sympathetic and parasympathetic nervous systems. There is an initial tendency for the sympathetic system to dominate, but this gives way to parasympathetic dominance, which is well marked.

In summary, it may be said that hypoxia is capable of producing a wide-spread influence on the autonomic nervous system. The effects of hypoxia on the alimentary tract, on the kidneys, on the sphincter pupillae of the eye, and, perhaps, on the other tissues probably can be explained, in part at least, by its effect on the nerve supply to these various organs.

REFERENCES

1. ASTE, cited by C. M. Monge, *et al.* 1935. "Fisiologia andina—circulation," *An. Fac. Ciencias Med. Lima,* 17: 1.
2. GELLHORN, E.; CORTELL, R.; and CARLSON, B. 1941. *Amer. J. Physiol.,* 135: 641.
3. GRANT, W. C., and ROOT, W. S. 1953. *Amer. J. Physiol.,* 173: 321.
4. FELDMAN, J.; CORTELL, R.; and GELLHORN, E. 1940. *Amer. J. Physiol.,* 131: 281.

5. KEYS, A.; STAPP, J. P.; and VIOLANTE, A. 1943. *Amer. J. Physiol.,* 138: 763.
6. MCDONOUGH, F. K. 1939. *Amer. J. Physiol.,* 125: 530.
7. MCFARLAND, R. A. 1937. *J. Comp. Psychol.,* 24: 147.
8. MONGE, C. M., *et al.* 1935. "Fisiologia andina—circulation," *An. Fac. Ciencias Med. Lima,* 17: 1.
9. ORAHOVATS, P. D., and ROOT, W. S. 1953. *Amer. J. Physiol.,* 173: 324.
10. SAFFORD, H., and GELLHORN, E. 1945. *Proc. Soc. Exp. Biol. Med.,* 60: 98.
11. SAWYER, M. E. M.; SCHLOSSBERG, T.; and BRIGHT, E. M. 1933. *Amer. J. Physiol.,* 104: 184.
12. URY, B., and GELLHORN, E. 1938. *Proc. Soc. Exp. Biol. Med.,* 38: 426.
———. 1939. *J. Neurophysiol.,* 2: 136.
13. WOODS, E. F., and RICHARDSON, J. A. 1959. *Amer. J. Physiol.,* 196: 203.

MEDULLARY CENTERS

According to Gasser and Loevenhart (4), the views which have been held regarding the effect of decreased oxidation on the activity of the medullary centers may be classified as follows: (*a*) Stimulation cannot be produced by decreased oxidation. (*b*) Stimulation may be produced by decreased oxidation, but only indirectly—as by increasing the stimulating effect of carbon dioxide or by causing formation or accumulation of acid metabolic products. (*c*) Decreased oxidation itself, under proper conditions, may stimulate the medullary centers.

The third view was first advanced by Rosenthal (17) in 1882. Gasser and Loevenhart (4) felt that they had proved definitely that this view was correct. Their work was done in 1914, and since that time, of course, the function of the carotid bodies has been discovered.

It was shown by Kussmaul and Terrer (10), as early as 1857, that when the blood supply to the brain is completely suppressed, the respiratory center is first stimulated and then depressed. Grove and Loevenhart (8) in 1911 reported that the respiratory center is more sensitive to hydrocyanic acid than the vasomotor center and that the latter is apparently more sensitive than the cardioinhibitory center.

In 1914 Gasser and Loevenhart (4), reporting studies on the effect of oxygen want on medullary centers, pointed out that stimulation of these centers by hypoxia depends upon three factors: (*a*) the suddenness of the oxygen want, (*b*) the extent to which the oxygen was decreased, and (*c*) the condition of the center. Hypoxia was produced by the administration of carbon monoxide and by sodium cyanide, and the latent periods of the stimulation of the medullary centers were determined. The latent periods were found to be so short that the stimulation could not be attributed to the accumulation of acid products. They concluded that oxygen want itself is a stimulus to the medullary centers.

The hypoxia produced by carbon monoxide first stimulated the centers and then depressed them. They were stimulated and then depressed in the following order: respiratory center, vasomotor center, and cardioinhibitory center. Their work also gave support to the theory that the activity of the medullary centers depends on the condition of their oxidative processes.

Gasser and Loevenhart (4) pointed out that if cerebral anemia is produced by clamping the cerebral arteries (19), the medullary centers respond in the same manner as they do when subjected to anoxic hypoxia and, further, that the same relative irritability of the centers has been shown by investigators working on the effect of increased intracranial pressure (3, 15).

In 1919 Lutz and Schneider (11) reported that oxygen want stimulates the respiratory center in man, and in the same year Haldane *et al.* (9) also came to the conclusion that oxygen want per se can act as a stimulus to this center. These reports were made before the function of the carotid bodies was discovered. It is now thought that oxygen want stimulates the respiratory center indirectly through the chemoreceptors. It is known, then, that oxygen want, either directly or indirectly, is capable of stimulating the medullary centers. It should be emphasized, however, that the medulla oblongata as a whole is much less sensitive to lack of oxygen than are the phylogenetically younger parts of the central nervous system, such as the cerebral and cerebellar cortices.

It is in order to consider briefly the effect of hypoxia on each center:

Respiratory center.—The effect of hypoxia on this center has been discussed in some detail in the section which deals with hypoxia and respiration, and it need not be repeated here. (See chapter viii, p. 129.)

Vasomotor center.—It has been known for a long time that if an animal is subjected to hypoxia the vasomotor center is stimulated and that if the hypoxia is severe a considerable rise of blood pressure may occur. Mathison (14) in 1911 showed that not only oxygen want but also an excess of carbon dioxide in the arterial blood causes stimulation of the vasomotor center. Hypoxia presumably acts either by direct stimulation of the center or reflexly through the sinoaortic nerves (2). When these nerves are severed (and the vagi cut), hypoxia produces a fall in systemic blood pressure. The work of Loevenhart and his associates on this center has been mentioned previously.

Gellhorn and Lambert (6) have pointed out that the present concept of the mode of action of oxygen deficiency and carbon dioxide excess is the same for both respiration and circulation. Carbon dioxide causes stimulation of the "isolated" respiratory and vasomotor centers. These authors call attention to the fact that the reactions of these centers to carbon dioxide is, however, different from that of other nerve centers.

Bernthal and Woodcock (1) in 1951 reported experiments on dogs with denervated carotid and aortic bodies. They concluded that oxygen want simultaneously exerts two separate and opposite influences upon vasomotor neurons, one excitatory and the other depressant and, further, that the activity of the center during hypoxia reflects the algebraic sum of the opposing influences.

Cardioinhibitory center.—In 1910 Mathison (13) observed that irregular cardiac slowing occurred frequently during asphyxia in animals with intact vagi. He felt this was caused by stimulation of the cardioinhibitory center. Gasser and Loevenhart, as previously mentioned, also found that this center was stimulated by oxygen want.

Cardioaccelerator center.—It will be assumed for the sake of convenience in this discussion that there is an accelerator center, although its existence has not been conclusively proved. Nolf and Plumier (16), after work with dogs, believed that they had obtained some evidence of increased tonus in the accelerator cardiac nerves during asphyxia. Mathison (12), on the other hand, showed that during asphyxia the acceleration which immediately preceded the heart block was not due to stimulation of the accelerator center.

Some evidence has been presented by Sands and De Graff (18) that in progressive anoxic hypoxia the stimulating effects, up to the period of the crisis (which they found to be produced by 9 per cent oxygen), can be accounted for by the fact that hypoxia either depresses the vagi or stimulates the accelerator mechanism. In progressive hypoxia, when the vagi are cut, cardiac acceleration is often, although not always, absent; this indicates that the accelerator mechanism may be stimulated. The effect is much the same as that obtained if small doses of epinephrine are administered.

Lutz and Schneider (11), having produced hypoxia in man by use of both low pressures and low percentages of oxygen, believed they had evidence that hypoxia stimulated the accelerator center and that this took place before the cardioinhibitory center was stimulated. They admitted, however, that they could offer no real experimental proof.

It must be emphasized that it is often difficult to interpret experimental results when working on the centers regulating heart rate, since it is known that the heart may be accelerated in at least four different ways: (a) by stimulation of accelerator nerves (or center), (b) by decreasing vagal tone, (c) by secretion of epinephrine, and (d) by an increase in the temperature of the blood (5). Since cardiac acceleration may be produced by several factors, conclusions from experimental procedures must be drawn with special care.

Vomiting center.—It has been known for many years that anoxic hypoxia may produce vomiting; for example, many, although not all, individuals who ascend to high altitudes may vomit. There are many factors (some psychic) which seem to cause vomiting, and it is difficult to prove by exactly what mechanism hypoxia stimulates it.

Mechanism of medullary center effects.—The mechanism by which oxygen want affects medullary centers is as yet unknown. The extensive researches during the past few years on the functions of the aortic and carotid bodies have thrown a good deal of light on this problem, but more work is still needed. There is considerable controversy regarding the relative importance of the various factors which are known to influence the chemoreceptors.

Not only are the chemoreceptors influenced by oxygen want, but the nerve cells of the centers, too, may be affected. Gesell (7) presented evidence many years ago that the cells of the respiratory center could be directly influenced by changes in the hydrogen-ion concentration of the blood. Moreover, Gellhorn and his associates (6) have shown that carbon dioxide may influence certain centers in the medulla. It has also been demonstrated, beyond much doubt, that anoxic hypoxia causes a depression of the isolated respiratory center and perhaps other centers as well.

Finally, these vital medullary centers may be affected by oxygen want, either reflexly through the chemoreceptors or by direct action of the cells of the centers, in ways which at present are not recognized.

Since, normally, the medullary centers are under strict control of higher neural organizations—for example, the hypothalamic and pontine autonomic centers—it would be of interest to repeat, on the bulbospinal animal, much of the work reported on the effect of hypoxia on the medullary centers.

REFERENCES

1. BERNTHAL, T., and WOODCOCK, C. C., JR. 1951. *Amer. J. Physiol.,* **166**: 45.
2. BOUCKAERT, J. J., *et al.* 1941. *Arch. Int. Pharmacodyn. Ther.,* **65**: 63.
3. EYSTER, J. A. E. 1906. *J. Exp. Med.,* **8**: 565.
4. GASSER, H. S., and LOEVENHART, A. S. 1914. *J. Pharmacol. Exp. Ther.,* **5**: 239.
5. GASSER, H. S., and MEEK, W. J. 1914. *Amer. J. Physiol.,* **34**: 48.
6. GELLHORN, E., and LAMBERT, E. H. 1939. *The Vasomotor System in Anoxia and Asphyxia.* Urbana, Ill.: University of Illinois Press.
7. GESELL, R. 1925. *Physiol. Rev.,* **5**: 551.
8. GROVE, W. E., and LOEVENHART, A. S. 1911. *J. Pharmacol. Exp. Ther.,* **3**: 131.
9. HALDANE, J. S.; KELLAS, A. S.; and KENNAWAY, E. L. 1919. *J. Physiol.,* **53**: 181.
10. KUSSMAUL, A., and TERRER, A. 1857. *Untersuch. Naturl. Mensch. Tiere,* **3**: 1.
11. LUTZ, B. R., and SCHNEIDER, E. C. 1919. *Amer. J. Physiol.,* **50**: 327.
12. MATHISON, G. C. 1910. *J. Physiol.,* **41**: 416.
13. ———. 1910. *Heart,* **2**: 54.
14. ———. 1911. *J. Physiol.,* **42**: 283.
15. NAUNYN, B., and SCHREIBER, J. 1881. *Arch. Exp. Path. Pharm.,* **14**: 1.
16. NOLF, P., and PLUMIER, L. 1904. *J. Physiol. Path. Gén.,* **6**: 241.
17. ROSENTHAL, J., cited by L. HERMANN (ed.), *Handbuch der Physiologie.* **4**, Part II, 261. Leipzig: F. C. W. Vogel, 1882.
18. SANDS, J., and DE GRAFF, A. C. 1925. *Amer. J. Physiol.,* **74**: 416.
19. STEWART, G. N., *et al.* 1906. *J. Exp. Med.,* **8**: 289.

PSYCHOLOGICAL PROCESSES

The mind.—(*a*) Acute hypoxia: Under certain conditions, the grade of hypoxia may be so acute that loss of consciousness can occur without any warning. This could happen, for example, when an individual is overwhelmed by a noxious gas, such as when a miner walks into a pocket of methane or carbon monoxide gas. Unless a person is removed promptly from such an atmosphere, he will, of course, die. These circumstances are fortunately rather rare.

It is in order to discuss somewhat less severe grades of hypoxia. It has been said (6) that acute hypoxia resembles alcoholic intoxication;

the symptoms are headache, mental confusion, drowsiness, and muscular weakness and inco-ordination. A person exposed to a low-oxygen tension often passes through an initial stage of euphoria, accompanied by a feeling of self-satisfaction and a sense of power. The oxygen want stimulates the central nervous system so that the subject may become hilarious and sing or shout, and manifest other emotional disturbances.

After a certain length of time this initial stimulation is followed by depression; emotional outbursts of a different nature appear; and the personality frequently changes for the worse. Hilarity gives way to moroseness and quarrelsomeness, and the person may become pugnacious or dangerously violent. These latter symptoms are especially likely to occur in hypoxia produced by carbon monoxide poisoning. A striking example of this is given by Haldane (27), who relates that an inspector of mines who had been affected by carbon monoxide gas came out of the mine and shook hands cordially with the bystanders; but when the doctor in attendance offered him his arm, he regarded this as an insult and challenged him to a fight.

Hypoxia quickly affects the higher centers, causing a blunting of the finer sensibilities and a loss of sense of judgment and of self-criticism. The subject feels, however, that his mind is not only quite clear but unusually keen. He develops a fixity of purpose and continues to do what he was doing when hypoxia first began to affect him, in spite of the fact that it may lead to disaster. This fixity of purpose is highly dangerous, especially when such an individual is responsible for the lives or others, such as is true of an airplane pilot.

Individuals who suffer from oxygen want and manifest a fixity of purpose often make no effort to remove themselves from the zone of danger. This is well illustrated by a report of Foster and Haldane (24). Sir Clement le Neve Foster, who was chief government inspector of mines in Great Britain, inspected a mine in which a disaster had occurred and became himself a victim of carbon monoxide poisoning. He has given a dramatic account of his experience. He could have walked away from the danger zone, which he himself knew; but he lost his initiative, so that instead he sat down and wrote farewell messages, in which he repeated the word "good-bye" a number of times. It is of further interest that once or twice he was inconsistent in spelling the word.

Another example which shows, among other things, loss of interest and initiative is that of Longstaff (43). The purpose of his expedition to the Himalyas was to find the highest point by ascertaining the height of the various peaks by means of the theodolite. He lost interest in his observations and failed to check his results carefully and critically when he was at great heights, so that his figures were of no value upon his return. He missed, therefore, the main object of his expedition.

Barcroft himself experienced, and relates a third incident in his monograph (7). He had planned to incarcerate himself for a week in a low-pressure chamber. On the fifth day his wife called to see him and asked him about the barometric pressure. He stated that he had been at a simulated altitude of 18,000 feet (5,485 meters) and was now at 15,000 feet (4,570 meters) but, "after all, it made no difference." His wife realized at once that his judgment of what was important had vanished, and the experiment was ended at that point.

The experience of Haldane *et al.* (28) in a low-pressure chamber at about 22,000 feet (6,705 meters) is instructive in showing the workings of the mind under conditions of acute hypoxia. Kellas was an experienced mountaineer and was better acclimated than Haldane. At a simulated altitude of 22,000 feet, Haldane, who found that he could no longer write or make observations, handed his notebook to Kellas. Haldane insisted that the low pressure be maintained, although later he had absolutely no remembrance of it. At a barometric pressure corresponding to 20,000 feet (6,095 meters), he was handed a mirror and for some time peered at the back of it. Finally, Haldane consented that the pressure be raised, and at 14,000 feet (4,270 meters), his mind became clear and he noticed the power return to his legs. Haldane admitted himself that his insistence upon keeping the pressure so low was irrational and that he had not intended to do so at the beginning of the experiment.

Birley (12) has reported several interesting examples of altered senses of judgment of British aviators during the war of 1914–18. One pilot who had been flying at great height found later that he had taken eighteen photographs on the same plate. In another instance, a pilot at 19,000 feet (5,790 meters) cordially waved to an enemy craft and took no further action, although his observer vehemently protested.

Pugh and Ward (57) relate a more recent instance of the peculiar behavior which may be manifested at high altitudes. One individual, having returned from a climb to 28,700 feet (8,744 meters), collapsed and lay exhausted on the ground. The comment made by one of his companions was, "Poor old Tom, he's had it." No sympathy was shown him nor any help offered. Surely this callousness would not have been shown at lower levels.

These dramatic instances give an understanding of the effects of hypoxia on the mind which is clearer than any long or technical discussion could be. They particularly emphasize the fact that under conditions of oxygen want critical judgment is quite likely to be lost and that initiative, too, may entirely disappear.

b) Aftereffects of acute hypoxia: If the exposure to acute hypoxia has not been too long or too severe, the aftereffects, although often producing unpleasant symptoms, are transient in nature and of no especial consequence. The most common complaint is that of headache; this may come on during the time the subject is actually exposed to hypoxia or may develop a few hours later. It may be rather intractable and not alleviated by the ordinary analgesic drugs, but after a few hours it subsides of its own accord. Besides headache, other symptoms referable to the central nervous system—such as nausea, muscular weakness, and emotional disturbances—may manifest themselves after return to sea level.

It is generally thought that repeated exposure to oxygen want can have a cumulative effect. Armstrong (2) has stressed this and has described a condition which develops in airplane pilots only, which he has termed "aeroneurosis." He has defined this as a chronic functional disorder characterized by gastric disturbances, nervous irritability, mental fatigue, and increased motor activity. The exact etiology of this condition is unknown, and oxygen want might be only one factor in its production.

If the subject has been exposed to severe hypoxia for too long a time, the aftereffects are often of a formidable nature and may end in death. If death does not ensue, the hypoxia may cause changes in the brain resulting in permanent disability. There are instances on record which indicate that this has happened after prolonged administration of nitrous oxide anesthesia (17, 70).

Thompson and Corwin (67) in 1938 reported an interesting and heroic study on the posthypoxic period. Thompson subjected himself to acute hypoxia in a chamber for several hours; for the most part, he was kept at a simulated altitude which ranged from about 11,500 feet (3,500 meters) to 17,000 feet (5,180 meters). After his removal from the chamber, he was in a stuporous or semicomatose state and showed rather alarming posthypoxic symptoms. When his respiration failed and artificial respiration became necessary, no concern was expressed, although he was quite aware of its significance. His motor responses were slow, and activity required a great amount of effort; still greater effort was needed for initiation of effort. There were no delusional or hallucinatory experiences. He stated that it was difficult to tell when the symptoms actually disappeared, but it was several days; and, as a matter of fact, a week or more following the exposure he was still making mistakes in routine laboratory experiments. His observations agreed with those of Haldane, that mental and physical aberrations may appear after exposure to hypoxia.

c) Aftereffects of carbon monoxide poisoning: Grave aftereffects are not uncommon following exposures to carbon monoxide. Whether this is due to the fact that it produces both hemic and histotoxic hypoxia is unknown. The patient does not recover at once, as he does following short exposures to anoxic hypoxia; or, if he does recover, he may regain only partial consciousness and then lapse again into unconsciousness. Marked spastic conditions of the muscles and an occasional epileptiform seizure have been described. The patient may linger on for days in a semicomatose condition with spastic muscles and, occasionally, opisthotonus. When consciousness supervenes, loss of memory, mental incapacity, or even mania sometimes occur. If the patient survives the first few days, the symptoms will generally pass away, and he will recover, except in those instances where organic changes have taken place within the central nervous system. Following severe exposure to carbon monoxide poisoning, the patient may act as if he were practically decerebrated, as has been pointed out by Drinker (19).

d) Chronic hypoxia: While the effect of acute hypoxia on the body resembles alcoholic intoxication, that of chronic hypoxic simulates fatigue, both mental and physical (6). Since the effect of oxygen want on psychologic processes is under consideration, our discussion will be limited chiefly to the effects on the mind.

People living at high altitudes for long periods become acclimated. The matter of acclimatization has been discussed in a separate section (see p. 162). During acclimatization certain compensatory factors greatly aid the body in withstanding low partial pressures of oxygen, so that the subject can live with a greater degree of comfort and do his work more easily. These compensatory factors, however, are not equally effective in all individuals. The mental and physical health of some individuals often remains indifferent; they become irritable and do not get along with their fellow men; they may show a mild mental depression and often lack the ability to concentrate. Mental tasks are harder under conditions of oxygen want, and mistakes are more frequent. Recovery from mental fatigue, too, is slower than it is at lower altitudes. Many of these people, furthermore, are unable to obtain a refreshing sleep; their nights are often restless and disturbed by unpleasant dreams. This lack of restful sleep tends also to keep their health constantly under par. A return to lower altitudes, of course, will restore normal health to these people, and, indeed, they often find it necessary to take periodic sojourns at sea level.

Miscellaneous studies.—Within the limits of this monograph it is not feasible to discuss in detail the wealth of work which has been reported on various psychological studies made during oxygen want. Many of these have been made on aviators, but miscellaneous experimental studies not necessarily in the interests of aviation have been made on other human subjects. In the discussion which follows, the studies made on aviators will be considered first.

1. Studies made on aviators[3]: Until the year 1914, little work had been reported on the effect of hypoxia on psychologic processes, but during the war of 1914–18 numerous psychologic studies were made on aviators by a number of workers (1, 3, 4, 12, 16, 18, 21, 23, 32, 38, 47, 56, 65, 68, 71).

Dunlap (21) has summarized the findings of these early studies on pilots as follows: (*a*) The primary and important psychologic effects of oxygen want are on voluntary co-ordination and attention. (*b*) Sensitivity and perception remain efficient until hypoxia curtails the ability of the subject to attend to stimuli. (*c*) There is no reduction in speed of simple reactions. (*d*) There is no falling-off of rapidity in discrimination except that due to deficiency of motor control. (*e*) Memory and other higher mental processes are not affected until muscular inco-ordination produces distractibility or until the ability to attend to details of learning is decreased. Finally, it is suggested that the effects of hypoxia produce a change in the integrative action of the nervous system rather than any change in the irritability or efficiency of any part.

Bagby (4) in 1921 reported some of the significant results of the work done in the Medical Research Laboratory of the United States Army. The subjects used in these experiments were exposed to hypoxia by the use of the Henderson rebreathing apparatus. He summarized the findings as follows:

a) Motor performance: Progressive hypoxia caused muscular tremor, inco-ordination, and overdischarge. These became worse as rebreathing proceeded, because of a loss of integration of the central nervous system.

b) Attention phenomenon: Hypoxia increased the subject's distractibility, so that a marked reduction developed in the ability to simultaneously carry on a number of discrete tasks. When the hypoxia

[3] Reports of the early work done on aviators may be found in *Air Service Medical* (Washington, D.C.: U.S. Government Printing Office, 1919), Part II, chap. vii, "Psychology Department," pp. 293–330.

became severe, the subject was unable to concentrate on any task in a normal manner.

c) Condition of resting muscles: The observations were made on the left hand; the muscles first relaxed, then became tense, and finally became twitchy.

d) Removal of inhibitions: The subjects often manifested uncontrolled anger, but in milder forms they showed an attitude of resentment. The type of reactions varied, since some of them became silly and even went into fits of uncontrollable laughter.

e) Self observation: Many subjects stated that they could "pull themselves together" for a short time but then they "wanted to rest."

The various psychologic studies made on airplane pilots have been of both academic, and of practical, value. Some of these tests have demonstrated the importance of the factors of fatigue, staleness, and ill-health in these individuals. Certain psychologic tests, moreover, can be used as an aid in the selection of airplane personnel. It is true, of course, that nowadays these airmen are not subjected to hypoxia as they were, for example, during the war of 1914–18. Now either they are equipped with oxygen masks or the cabin of their aircraft is pressurized. However, equipment failure could, of course, cause these men to be subjected to severe grades of hypoxia.

2. Miscellaneous studies: Barcroft (8) relates that a few mental tests were given to the members of his South American party (1921–22) at Cerro de Pasco, which lies at an altitude of 14,200 feet (4,330 meters). The conclusion was that the tests were too simple to be of real value. It was observed, however, that the amount of mental effort necessary to do the tests was more pronounced than the loss of accuracy with which they were done.

Hingston (34), medical officer to the 1924 Mount Everest Expedition, gave simple mathematical tests to members of the party at 7,000 feet (2,130 meters), 14,000 feet (4,270 meters), 16,000 feet (4,875 meters), and 21,000 feet (6,400 meters). Apparently by making increased effort, the men did very well on these tests. McFarland believes that the tests probably were too simple to show subtle incapacities. It is to be remembered also that the tests were made on fairly well-acclimated subjects.

Lowson (44) in 1923 reported some studies made on the effect of oxygen want on certain psychologic processes. He concluded that until the diminution of oxygen reached 50 per cent of the normal no significant alteration in behavior occurred in the average subject; beyond this, however, the changes were rapid and great.

Tanaka (66) in 1928, working with a low-pressure chamber under

Haldane's direction at Oxford, reported work done on six subjects. He tested speed in simple and complex sorting, addition, memory, and strength of grip at different altitudes up to 21,000 feet (6,400 meters). He concluded: (a) that hypoxia caused a deficiency in both mental and physical work; (b) that there was considerable difference as to the altitude at which changes occurred; (c) that hypoxia caused a greater deficiency in mental than in physical work; (d) that hypoxia affected especially the quality of work; and (e) that the usual critical point where sudden changes occurred was 428 mm. Hg, which corresponds to an altitude of about 15,000 feet (4,570 meters).

McFarland (48) in 1932 made exhaustive studies of oxygen want on psychologic processes. In this work he used a spirometer and oxygen mixtures ranging from 11.43 (about 17,000 feet—5,180 meters) to 7.68 per cent (about 28,000 feet—8,535 meters). He came to the following conclusions: (a) Simple sensory and motor responses were not seriously impaired until the oxygen want was so severe that the subject approached collapse—about 24,000 feet (7,135 meters) or an oxygen percentage of 8.87. Vision and kinesthesis (muscle sense) were the first to be affected, and hearing, the last. (b) Choice reactions appeared to be impaired before simple reactions. (c) Neuromuscular control was impaired before the loss of capacity in more highly organized functions, such as choice reactions. (d) There was a loss of memory with oxygen percentages as low as 9.05. (e) Concerning the effect on attention, hypoxia apparently both facilitates attention by eliminating extraneous factors and handicaps it by undermining voluntary co-ordination. (f) Hypoxia impairs higher mental powers. (g) Hypoxia affects feelings or moods; depending on the length of time the individual is subjected to hypoxia and other factors, it may stimulate or depress. (h) It was concluded, also, that significant data relative to the basic patterns of personality could be obtained under severe oxygen want.

McFarland (49) in 1937 reported observations on psychological studies made during sudden ascents to 15,000 feet (4,570 meters) and 16,500 feet (5,025 meters) on trans-Andean planes and during slower ascents by train, also in the Andes, to somewhat lower altitudes. From his observations he concluded that the rate of ascent was an important variable and that there was a significant impairment of both simple and complex psychological functions at these altitudes. He found that the mental tests which involved complex reactions were most affected by high altitudes; the motor tests were affected less; and the sensory tests least of all.

3. Studies made on subjects undergoing acclimatization: In a sub-

sequent paper McFarland (50) reported sensory and motor tests on ten subjects undergoing acclimatization during a three-month period at various levels up to an altitude of 20,140 feet (9,135 meters). The following sensory and motor tests were given: (*a*) auditory thresholds—for eight frequencies, (*b*) phoria test for ocular muscle balance, (*c*) fatigue of accommodation and convergence, (*d*) measurement of after images, (*e*) color-naming test, (*f*) simple and choice reaction time, (*g*) dotting test of neuromuscular co-ordination, and (*h*) mirror test. He found a variability of response for both the individual and the group at 15,440 feet (4,700 meters) and above and a significant difference in the means for the group at 17,500 feet (5,330 meters) and above.

He also reported (51) on the following psychologic tests, using the same subjects and the same altitudes: (*a*) speed of apprehension for words, (*b*) judgments of duration, (*c*) repetition of auditory patterns, (*d*) perseveration tests, (*e*) memory tests, (*f*) code transliteration, and (*g*) Thorndike C.A.V.D. intelligence test.

At 15,440 feet differences in the means and variabilities of the mental tests were observed; these became more marked at higher altitudes. There was a close parallel between the periods of greatest discomfort in adaptation to the altitude and the psychosomatic changes or psychologic complaints.

It appears from the observations of McFarland that in fairly well-acclimated subjects psychologic processes, for practical purposes, are not affected until an altitude of approximately 15,440 feet (4,700 meters) is attained. It will be recalled in this connection that Barcroft stated that at Cerro de Pasco (14,200 feet—4,330 meters) mental tests gave indeterminate results. Any psychologic tests made, moreover, on acclimated subjects on Pike's Peak (14,100 feet—4,300 meters) probably would not show any positive results.

4. Most common alterations in psychologic behavior: It is of distinct interest to call attention to the ten most common alterations in psychologic behavior which McFarland reported. These observations were made on members of the International High Altitude Expedition to Chile. In order of frequency, they were as follows: (*a*) greater effort to carry out tasks, (*b*) more critical attitude toward other people, (*c*) mental laziness, (*d*) heightened sensory irritability, (*e*) sensitivity on certain subjects, (*f*) dislike of being told how to do things, (*g*) difficulty in concentrating, (*h*) slowness in reasoning, (*i*) frequent recurrence of ideas, and (*j*) difficulty in remembering.

These alterations in behavior reported by McFarland coincide with the early observations of Barcroft, Haldane, and others. It must be remembered, however, that McFarland's observations were made on ten rather highly selected subjects. The identical alterations in behavior in the same order of frequency might not be found in an unselected group of subjects.

McFarland reported that no significant correlations between mental tests and biochemical determinations were found. The correlation between mental tests and physiological measurements at high altitude, however, revealed a number of positive relationships.

Pugh and Ward (57) have reported observations made on mental activity during one of the more recent Mount Everest expeditions. They relate that at about 21,000 feet (6,400 meters) some members of the expedition did not experience noticeable impairment of mental activity. For example, one individual solved crossword puzzles readily, and Pugh himself relates that he did gas analysis for six hours and made few errors. All of these individuals were, of course, well acclimated to great heights.

At altitudes over 22,500 feet (6,855 meters), however, considerable impairment of mental faculties was apparent. At 26,000 feet (7,925 meters), mental and physical depression were noted. There was retardation of thought and action, and a noticeable diminution of excellence of insight and judgment.

Barach (5) in 1943 made observations on impairment of emotional control caused by hypoxia. He reported that the affective response may be depressive in nature or may take the form of exhilaration, the mood varying with the nature of the individual. In a rather small series, he found euphoria in 50 per cent of his subjects, but about the same number showed a dullness. Von Tavel (69) in the same year noted a predominantly euphoric reaction in only 10–20 per cent of his subjects. Obviously more work is needed in the field of emotional control during hypoxic states. The problem is of distinct practical interest, since depressive states are so often found in a number of clinical conditions.

Useful consciousness.—Hall (29) has defined useful consciousness during hypoxia as that state in which the individual remains attentive and is able to perform useful or purposeful acts. He has pointed out that the end point of useful consciousness can be determined with greater definiteness than can that of total loss of consciousness. Gell (25) has defined it slightly differently. He states that useful consciousness is a term expressing the length of time between the period when the subject's oxygen supply is totally deprived (at various altitudes) and the onset of physical or mental deterioration. Gell points out that it is determined primarily by altitude but is influenced somewhat by the inherent tolerance of the individual and markedly affected by the amount of physical activity.

The interval of useful consciousness at great altitudes is very short. Gell (25) states that at 40,000 feet (12,190 meters) useful consciousness lasts thirty seconds or less; at 35,000 feet (10,670 meters), from forty-five to sixty seconds; at 30,000 feet (9,145 meters), from twenty to ninety seconds; and at 25,000 feet (7,620 meters), from two to three minutes.

Under conditions of explosive decompression, such as might be produced by a meteor piercing a pressurized cabin, the interval of useful consciousness in the range of altitude between 25,000 feet and 65,000 feet (19,810 meters) is greatly diminished. According to Luft (45) at an altitude of 45,000 feet (13,715 meters), the interval would be about fifteen seconds. The reason for this is that during decompression the oxygen reverses its direction of flow; that is, it passes from the blood back into the lungs. This process continues until equilibrium is reached with the oxygen of the atmosphere.

The three workers previously mentioned, Hall, Gell and Luft, have all emphasized the practical importance to aviation of accurate appraisal of the factors which influence useful consciousness in flyers under the stress of hypoxia. Mackenzie *et al.* (46) have also stressed the significance of such studies, and Ruff and Strughold (60), too, have recognized their extreme importance.

Several workers (31, 35, 36, 46) have used writing tests to determine the end point of useful consciousness. Hemingway (31) in 1944 subjected thirty-one individuals, who wore oxygen masks, to a simulated altitude of 35,000 feet (10,670 meters). At this altitude, the oxygen supply line was disconnected, and air was breathed. The subjects started writing immediately but were unable to write longer than from fifty-five to eighty seconds (average of 72.6 seconds). The average arterial oxygen saturation was 56.6 per cent. The author felt that there was practically no danger in performing this test.

Ivy (36) in 1946 used a similar technic; that is, he cut off the oxygen supply of subjects at different altitudes and observed how long they continued to write. He stated that 26,000 feet (7,925 meters) was the critical altitude in that none of the forty-nine subjects at this altitude was able to continue writing longer than fifteen minutes. He obtained the following results: Useful consciousness was present for 3.0 minutes at 28,000 feet (8,535 meters); 2.4 minutes at 30,000 feet (9,145 meters); 1.8 minutes at 32,000 feet (9,755 meters); 1.4 minutes at 36,000 feet (19,975 meters). These periods are somewhat longer than those given by Gell. Ability to write persisted at arterial oxygen saturation greater than 66 per cent. Ivy felt that an arterial oxygen saturation of 75 per cent was the lowest safe limit for voluntary directed movement.

In the same year, Hoffman *et al.* (35) studied the interval of useful consciousness by using a simple task, namely, card-sorting. The time of useful consciousness was determined by the appearance of the first error made in the sorting. The average time of useful consciousness was 110 seconds at 28,000 feet (8,535 meters); 73 seconds at 30,000 feet (9,145 meters); 46 seconds at 35,000 feet (10,670 meters); and 35 seconds at 38,000 feet (11,580 meters). The period of useful consciousness was found to be approximately three-fourths of the total time that consciousness was retained. On the average, the arterial oxygen saturation was 64 per cent at the appearance of the first error.

Hall (29) in 1949 used the interval of useful consciousness (by the subjects' response to signals) to determine tolerance to altitude. Ten healthy young men while breathing air were subjected to the following altitudes: 30,000, 35,000, 37,000, 40,000, and 42,000 feet, corresponding to 9,100, 10,700, 11,300, 12,300, and 12,900 meters, respectively. Four subjects were bled, so that the oxygen capacities of the blood were lowered from an average of 15.3 gm. to 13.3 gm. of hemoglobin per 100 ml. of blood. In five subjects, the oxygen capacities of the blood were increased from 15.6 to 17.0 gm. of hemoglobin per 100 ml. of blood by blood transfusion. The interval of useful consciousness while breathing air at 35,000 feet (10,700 meters) was determined on each subject. It was concluded that changes induced in the oxygen capacity of the blood modified tolerance to altitude when useful consciousness was used as the index.

In 1951 Hall and his collaborator (30), working with human subjects, found that the addition of certain amounts of carbon dioxide to ambient air at low barometric pressures of 225 mm. Hg and 179 mm. Hg increased the duration of useful consciousness. It is of interest, too, that the interval of useful consciousness may be significantly improved by the ingestion of glucose. Riesin *et al.* (59) found that thirty-nine control subjects lost useful consciousness, on an average, at the end of 185.7 seconds at a simulated altitude of 27,000 feet (8,200 meters). In contrast, thirty-eight volunteers who had ingested glucose previous to the experiment retained effective consciousness, on an average, for 261 seconds.

Acclimatization and useful consciousness: In 1945 Mackenzie *et al.* (46), using a writing test, determined the interval of useful consciousness in fifty-five men, the majority of whom had been partially acclimatized. Simulated altitudes from 25,000 feet (7,600

meters) to 36,000 feet (11,000 meters) were used. The non-acclimatized group at 30,000 feet (9,100 meters) did not do as well as the
partially acclimatized group at 33,000 feet (10,000 meters). In the
former group the period of useful consciousness was 94 seconds,
whereas in the latter it was 106 seconds. It has been shown (11,33)
that a few-weeks stay at the moderate altitudes of 6,600 and 10,200
feet (2,000 and 3,100 meters, respectively) may cause a lengthening
of the time of useful consciousness in man at extreme altitudes of
25,000 feet (7,600 meters) and 26,200 feet (8,100 meters).

It should be pointed out that the interval of useful consciousness
depends in a large measure upon the type of test used. Most of the
tests employed have been of extremely simple nature, such as writing
or simple card-sorting. It seems to the authors that more challenging
tests should be used, for example, problems in mental arithmetic.

While considerable work has been done on determining the interval of useful consciousness in unacclimatized individuals, more
studies are needed on subjects who are well-acclimatized to reasonably
high altitudes.

Memory and learning ability.—During the past two decades or
so, studies have been made on memory and on learning ability of
animals which had been subjected to severe grades of hypoxia (and
asphyxia) for varying periods of time previous to tests for these
psychologic functions.

1. Studies on animals: In 1944 Becker and Windle (10) asphyxiated guinea pigs at birth, resuscitated them, and, at four to six weeks
of age, subjected them to learning tests. Twenty-three of the thirty-six
experimental animals used showed definite pathologic changes; nineteen showed inferior maze-learning ability. Jensen, Becker, and
Windle (37), four years later, subjected fifteen young adult male
guinea pigs daily (except Sundays) to a simulated altitude of 30,000
feet (9,145 meters). After 100 hours of exposure, the animals were
tested for retention of learning; no significant differences were found.
They were tested also after 150, 200, and 250 hours of exposure. The
most pronounced changes in learning occurred after 250 hours of
exposure. Four experimental animals were unable to relearn the
problem in twenty trials, although some experimental animals, after
200 hours of exposure, had relearned the problem after ten trials. It
should be remarked that a simulated altitude of 30,000 feet represents a very severe grade of hypoxia.

Bunch (14) in 1952 reported observations made on a large group
of rats of the effects of pre- and postnatal hypoxia upon memory and
learning ability at maturity. Pregnant animals were exposed to a

simulated altitude of 30,000 feet (9,145 meters) for two hours. One hundred of the offspring learned the maze (multiple-T-14 unit water maze) problem as adults and were compared with 100 control animals. The hypoxic rats were significantly inferior to their controls in the measure of learning.

Richardson (58) in 1954 produced asphyxia in rats for periods from one to twenty minutes by preventing initiation of respiration before removing full-term fetuses from the uterus. Beginning at sixty-five days of age, they were tested on the Hebb-Williams closed maze; the experimental animals made more errors than the controls. It was concluded that oxygen deprivation at the time of birth tends to reduce the rat's ability to transfer prior learning to new situations.

In 1957 Cassin and Fregly (15) subjected newborn dogs (less than twenty-four hours old) to pure nitrogen for periods varying from eleven to eighty-one minutes. The animals were revived by artificial respiration, and oxygen was given under positive pressure. They all showed some degree of central nervous system insult lasting from five to forty-eight hours, but from one to six months later, no gross motor or behavioral aberrations were observed. Nevertheless, psychologic tests, problem-solving (open-field maze) and auditory discrimination (shuttle box), showed subtle behavioral differences.

2. Studies on man: Dougal and Fiset (20) in 1950 performed psychologic tests on men who had been subjected repeatedly to a simulated altitude of 10,000 feet (3,050 meters). The authors concluded that the relative deficit of oxygen at that altitude inhibits partly the normal functioning of the higher centers, especially the learning process.

Kossmann (41) in 1947 reported a case history of a flyer who experienced severe anoxic hypoxia during a bombing mission. His nervous system apparently was physiologically damaged, for even three weeks following the episode, he showed impairment of memory and slowing of cerebration. However, eighteen and a half months later, he presumably had made a complete recovery, for his memory and intelligence tests appeared normal.

Pugh and Ward (57) have commented on possible aftereffects in human beings who have been exposed to great heights for an appreciable period. The authors called attention to eight mountain climbers who had climbed to an altitude of 28,000 feet (8,535 meters) without oxygen. They pointed out that all these individuals later enjoyed careers of distinction and occupied positions that could not have been attained by men who suffered any significant degree of mental deterioration. There was one possible exception; one individual who had spent five nights at an altitude of 25,000 feet (7,620 meters) complained of some loss of memory.

Obviously, studies of memory and learning ability made on both man and animals following exposure to hypoxia or asphyxia are of great practical importance. It is known, for example, that the human fetus, either *in utero* or during birth, may be subjected to asphyxia or hypoxia or both. It is known, also, that hypoxia produced by carbon monoxide poisoning may cause permanent brain injury and that nitrous oxide given in high concentrations during anesthesia may do likewise. It is not in the province of this monograph to pursue further these interesting and important clinical problems. Suffice it to say that more studies should be made on animals. It would be highly desirable if such experiments could be made on the higher apes.

Dreams.—Since dreams are deemed important by psychoanalysts and since they are often mentioned in the literature which deals with high altitudes, the effect of hypoxia on dreams will be considered briefly.

Most writers emphasize the disturbances of sleep experienced by unacclimatized subjects at high altitudes. It has been pointed out by Monge (53) that native Andeans accustomed to living at great heights complain of restless sleep and disturbing dreams when they suffer an attack of chronic mountain sickness (Monge's disease). Dr. Crane, who served as medical officer for the Cerro de Pasco Copper Corporation, observed that newcomers to Cerro de Pasco, at altitudes from 12,000 to 14,200 feet (3,660 to 4,330 meters), experienced restless sleep and fantastic dreams, which were often apprehensive in character.

Probably the most comprehensive observations on the effect of high altitudes on dreams are those made by McFarland (51). He has presented in some detail the dream experiences of members of the International High Altitude Expedition to Chile. He relates that, prior to the ascent to the high-plateau region, dreams of the members were generally associated with home situations and with vivid experiences close at hand; they were also concerned with sexual or anxiety situations.

When the members of the expedition first ascended high altitudes, that is, before acclimatization took place, they experienced dreams which were fantastic and illusory in nature—they presumably had the usual experience of newcomers to high altitudes. When they reached their high-altitude stations (from 17,500 feet—5,330 meters to 21,140 feet—6,440 meters), and were by this time presumably fairly well acclimated, they dreamed infrequently, and there was little consciousness of sex.

An interesting observation was that dreams which accompanied the greatest physiological disabilities were usually the most vivid and fantastic. McFarland has expressed it thus: "Variations in the general physiological state, therefore, appeared to be equally as important as inner conflicts or motives, considered by many to be the basic course of dreams." The psychoanalysts probably would find it hard to reconcile this with their concept of the significance of dreams. It is pertinent to mention that several illnesses, especially those associated with gastrointestinal disorders of any kind, may produce disturbing dreams. Sufferers from migraine often experience unpleasant dreams the night preceding an acute attack. This lends evidence to the statement made by McFarland.

Reaction time.—It is necessary to distinguish between "simple-reaction time" and "choice-reaction time." The former designates the time which elapses from the moment the stimulus is given until the response occurs. Choice-reaction time, however, requires judgment; since the subject must choose whether or not he is to respond to a given stimulus, more synapses are involved, and the time is normally longer than simple-reaction time.

A number of studies have shown (9) that anoxic hypoxia produces only slight retardation of simple-reaction time until an altitude of about 20,000 feet (6,095 meters) is reached; this is about the point of collapse in the unacclimatized subject. In 1911 Durig and Reichel (22), performing experiments on Monte Rosa (altitude of 15,000 feet—4,570 meters) on subjects who had been there eight days, and again after sixteen-days sojourn, reported a possible loss in auditory-reaction time, although they admitted their results were indeterminate. In 1893 Mosso (54) had reported somewhat similar results. In 1935 Jongbloed (40), using a low-pressure chamber, found that at a simulated altitude of about 16,404 feet (5,000 meters) choice-reaction times were significantly lengthened. Stern (64) in 1926 found that newcomers at Davos, at altitudes of 5,100 feet (1,585 meters) and 8,400 feet (2,560 meters), showed a prolonged reaction time, which was shortened by oxygen inhalation.

Tanaka (66) in 1928, using a low-pressure chamber, and McFarland (48) in 1932, using a Douglas bag, observed a significant loss in speed and accuracy in choice-reaction time above 15,000 feet (4,570 meters) and 18,000 feet (5,485 meters). However, Bonnardel and Liberson (13) in 1932 at an altitude on the Jungfraujoch of 11,333 feet (3,454 meters) found no significant changes in either visual or auditory reaction time.

McFarland (50) feels that slow reaction times which have been reported below 14,000 feet (4,270 meters) probably have been observed following a rapid ascent, so that the element of fatigue is added. In 1937 he (49) reported determinations of choice-reaction times of six subjects at Lima, Peru (about sea level), and Morococha (altitude 14,890 feet—4,540 meters). Expressed in hundredths of a second, the mean for the six subjects at Lima was 53.7 and at Morococha, 60.3.

Studies made on acclimatized subjects: In a later paper McFarland (51) reported studies made of sensory and motor responses in subjects during acclimatization in the Chilean Andes. No significant differences were observed in the simple-reaction tests until an altitude of about 20,140 feet (6,135 meters) was reached. Variability of responses was, however, reliably increased at 17,500 feet (5,330 meters). Choice-reaction time was significantly impaired at 17,500 feet.

In a subsequent paper (52), studies made of simple- and choice-reaction time on native miners in the Chilean Andes at an altitude of 17,500 feet were reported. The reaction time was prolonged, and the responses were more variable in these men than in workmen at sea level. The differences were statistically significant.

Neuromuscular control.—Hingston (34), medical officer to the 1924 Mount Everest Expedition, reported mild tremor of eyelids and fingers at 14,000 feet (4,270 meters) in one subject and at 21,000 feet (6,400 meters) in another. In 1925 Stern (63) found an increase in hand tremor at Davos, at altitudes of 5,100 feet (1,585 meters) and 8,400 feet (2,560 meters). Loewy and Wittkower (42) in 1933 described an increased reflex irritability in seven of nine subjects at similar altitudes and also noted unusually active responses to Chvostek's sign and Trousseau's phenomenon. It would seem that the findings of these latter workers should be rechecked, since the altitude was so moderate.

Jongbloed (39) found that at a barometric pressure of 150 mm. Hg (about 39,000 feet—11,880 meters) animals showed catatonic reactions similar to those produced by bulbocapnine. McFarland (48), using a Douglas bag, observed, at a simulated altitude of 17,500 feet (5,330 meters), increased muscular tremors and a loss of neuromuscular control in handwriting tests. He reported, further, that at a simulated altitude beyond 19,500 feet (5,940 meters) the loss of efficiency was sudden and great. Goralewski (26) in 1935, using a low-pressure chamber and requiring the subjects to reproduce geometrical figures and sentences, noticed an impairment in this ability in a number of subjects at oxygen percentages of 14–18 (about

10,000–3,000 feet—3,050–910 meters) ; this impairment was increased at lower oxygen pressures.

In 1946 Muido (55) studied the effect of hypoxia on eye–hand co-ordination by use of the pursuit meter (apparatus *ad modium* Abramson) . Three individuals were subjected to a simulated altitude of about 19,500 feet (6,000 meters) in a low-pressure chamber. An appreciable deterioration of co-ordination was found. Russell (61) in 1948, also using the low-pressure chamber, studied the effect of mild hypoxia for thirty-five minutes on simple psychomotor skills, namely, finger dexterity and arm–hand co-ordination. He found: (*a*) a decrease in level of performance which appeared immediately after the introduction of mild hypoxia; (*b*) a rapid adjustment following this decrement as the period under mild hypoxia increased; and (*c*) following this adjustment, an improvement with continued practice under the mild hypoxic conditions.

More recently, Shepard (62) subjected ten normal individuals to a simulated altitude of 20,000 feet (6,095 meters) for ten minutes. All subjects showed significant changes in psychomotor performance.

In summary: appreciable degrees of acute hypoxia may produce deleterious effects on neuromuscular control. These effects, in a measure at least, resemble those produced by alcohol.

Acclimatization and neuromuscular control: McFarland (50) , working with subjects during acclimatization, found that in the dotting test for neuromuscular co-ordination there was no sign of loss of efficiency until an altitude of 15,440 feet (4,700 meters) was attained.

Observations made on natives at high altitudes: McFarland (52) used the dotting test for determination of neuromuscular co-ordination on natives of the Chilean Andes residing at an altitude of about 17,000 feet (5,180 meters) . The difference between the means of men working at sea level and those of the natives at high altitudes on this test of neuromuscular co-ordination was not statistically significant. Responses of the natives of high altitudes, however, were more variable.

Effect of hypoxia on handwriting: Many investigators have studied this problem, since it is a practical and easy method of studying muscular control. In general, it may be said that the more severe the hypoxia, the greater the loss of the ability to write normally. Figure 11 shows specimens of handwriting at different oxygen percentages up to 7.68, approximate altitude of 28,000 feet (8,535 meters) . It is readily seen that as the hypoxia progresses in severity the handwriting becomes less and less legible (48) .

Type of paralysis produced by hypoxia: In severe hypoxia, an ascending type of paralysis is produced. The legs first lose their power, so that the subject is unable to stand; as the paralysis ascends, the arm muscles soon become affected; the neck muscles are the last of all to be involved. That hypoxia produces an ascending type of paralysis was dramatically illustrated by Coxwell when he made his famous balloon ascent with Glashier. Coxwell's muscles, except those of his neck, were, for the most part, paralyzed; he could still move his head and so was able to grasp the rope valves with his teeth. By so doing, he saved his life and that of his companion.

Another dramatic instance of muscular paralysis due to oxygen want is the experience of Tissandier, sole survivor of the three-man ascent in the balloon "Zenith." At great heights he realized that he needed oxygen but could not husband the strength to raise the mouthpiece of the oxygen container to his lips.

Finally, it may be mentioned that individuals suffering from carbon monoxide poisoning often become paralyzed, so that although they are conscious and wish to leave the zone of danger, they are physically unable to do so.

Résumé of effect of hypoxia on psychologic processes.—Since a brief review has been presented of many of the observations made on psychologic processes during hypoxia, little need be said by way of summary. The various psychologic tests are presumably of most practical importance for airplane pilots. One important finding is the great individual variation which may occur. This indicates, of course, the need for careful selection of pilots.

There was a time when psychologic tests for pilots were probably more important than they are now, since most planes, both military and commercial, have pressurized cabins. There are situations, however, in which hypoxia of varying degree may occur, for example, in case of failure of the mechanism which controls the pressure in the plane. Under these conditions, both pilots and passengers would be subjected to hypoxia—the degree, of course, depending upon the height at which the plane was flying. If failure occurs at extreme altitudes, the length of the period of useful consciousness becomes a very important matter. It is true that at times not much can be done to avert disaster, but often every second of consciousness will help. However, in the event of explosive decompression at high altitudes, the period of useful consciousness is perhaps only about fifteen seconds.

It has been pointed out previously, nerve tissue is the least capable of withstanding hypoxia, and the nerve cells of the cerebrum are the

the pencil numerals are just th
last two figures of th chronoscope
reading. Ink numerals are
th exact durations of sound
reactions by subtraction of pencil
record from last in order, adding
100 when necessary.

NORMAL

Curious slowing up of reflex.
Seemed to be an appreciable delay
before I could get response going. It was
like a slight "hitch" Seemed to be a
slight vertigo in upper frontal part of
head. Seemed to be slightly further away from
than hitherto.

11.61% O$_2$—16,500 FT. ALTITUDE

Unreasonable feeling of amusement
rather silly feeling. quite bucked
up after a period of lethargy.
amused out of proportion by
feeling that the higher I got
th better I got. amused at
thought of silly better +
better etc. do it a bit hysterical.

11.02% O$_2$—18,000 FT. ALTITUDE

Seem to get fatigued
rapidly during course of
test. March save myself
by brief rest between
each exertion to strike key

10.25% O$_2$—20,000 FT. ALTITUDE

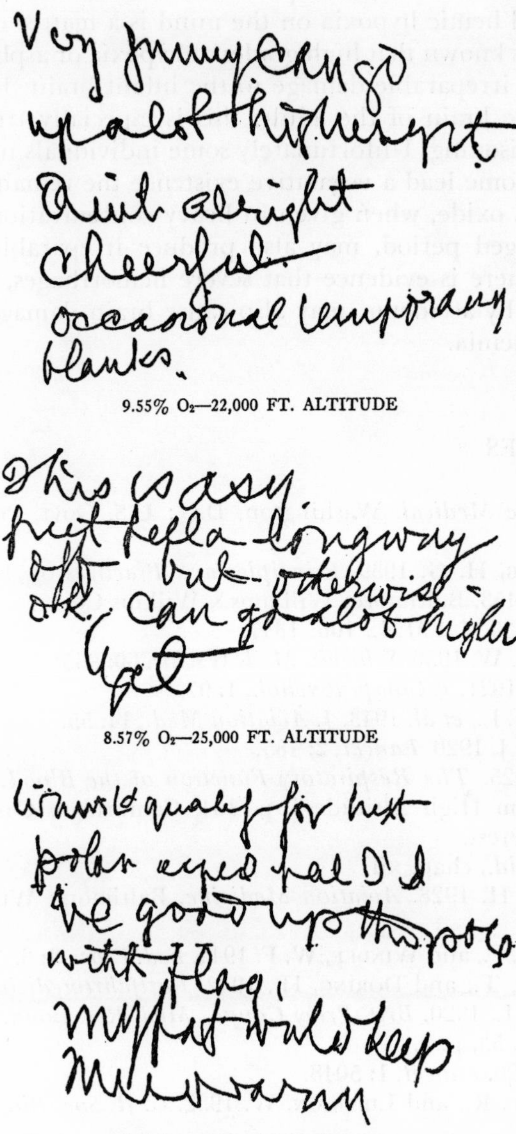

9.55% O₂—22,000 FT. ALTITUDE

8.57% O₂—25,000 FT. ALTITUDE

7.68% O₂—28,000 FT. ALTITUDE

FIG. 11.—Specimen of handwriting at the oxygen percentages and corresponding altitudes indicated. (From R. A. McFarland, "The Psychological Effects of Oxygen Deprivation on Human Behavior," *Arch. Psychol.* [N.Y.], 145 [1932], 110–11.)

first to be affected in oxygen deprivation. The effect of severe grades of anoxic and hemic hypoxia on the mind is a matter of cogent importance. It is known that high grades of hypoxia or asphyxia at birth may produce irreparable damage to the infant brain. Hypoxia, too, may affect the brain of the adult; this is especially true of carbon monoxide poisoning. Unfortunately some individuals never recover, and indeed, some lead a vegatative existence the remainder of their lives. Nitrous oxide, when given in heavy concentrations for a relatively prolonged period, may also produce irreparable damage to the brain. There is evidence that severe hemorrhages, such as may be produced by accidents, may also cause brain damage due to the prolonged anemia.

REFERENCES

1. *Air Service Medical.* Washington, D.C.: U.S. Govt. Printing Office, 1919.
2. ARMSTRONG, H. G. 1939. *Principles and Practices of Aviation Medicine,* p. 453. Baltimore: Williams & Wilkins Co.
   ———. 1936. *J.A.M.A.,* **106:** 1347.
3. BAERTSCHI, W. 1930. *Schweiz. Med. Wschr.,* **60:** 965.
4. BAGBY, E. 1921. *J. Comp. Psychol.,* **1:** 97.
5. BARACH, A. L., *et al.* 1943. *J. Aviation Med.,* **14:** 55.
6. BARCROFT, J. 1920. *Lancet,* **2:** 485.
7. ———. 1925. *The Respiratory Function of the Blood,* Part I, "Lessons from High Altitudes," p. 164. Cambridge: Cambridge University Press.
8. ———. *Ibid.,* chap. xii.
9. BAUER, L. H. 1928. *Aviation Medicine.* Baltimore: Williams & Wilkins Co.
10. BECKER, R. F., and WINDLE, W. F. 1944. *Fed. Proc.,* **3:** 3.
11. BENZINGER, T., and DORING, H., 1942. *Luftfahrtmedizin,* **7:** 141.
12. BIRLEY, J. L. 1920. *Brit. Privy Counc., Med. Res. Counc., Spec. Rept. Ser.,* No. 53, p. 5.
   ———. 1920. *Lancet,* **1:** 5048.
13. BONNARDEL, R., and LIBERSON, W. 1932. *C. R. Soc. Biol.* (*Par.*), **194:** 1265.
14. BUNCH, M. E. 1952. *Science,* **116:** 517.
15. CASSIN, S., and FREGLY, A. R. 1957. *Fed. Proc.,* **16:** 20.
16. CORBETT, C. D. W., and BAZETT, H. C. 1920. *Brit. Privy Counc., Med. Res. Counc., Spec. Rept. Ser.,* No. 53, p. 18.
17. COURVILLE, C. B. 1936. *Medicine,* **15:** 129.
   ———. 1938. *Ann. Surg.,* **107:** 371.

18. DOCKERAY, F. C., and ISAACS, J. 1921. *J. Comp. Psychol.,* 1: 115.
19. DRINKER, C. K. 1938. *Carbon Monoxide Asphyxia,* p. 133. New York: Oxford University Press.
20. DUGAL, L. P., and FISET, P. E. 1950. *J. Aviat. Med.,* 21: 362.
21. DUNLAP, K. 1918. *J.A.M.A.,* 71: 1392.
———. 1919. *Science,* 49: 94.
22. DURIG, A., and REICHEL, H. 1911. *Physiologische Ergebnisse der im Jahr 1906 durchgeführten Monte Rosa Expedition, Denkschr. der Akad. der Wissenschaften.* Vienna.
23. FLACK, M. 1920. *Brit. Privy Counc., Med. Res. Counc., Spec. Rept. Ser.,* No. 53.
24. FOSTER, C., and HALDANE, J. S. 1905. *The Investigation of Mine Air,* p. 177. London: C. Griffin & Co.
25. GELL, C. F. *In:* H. G. ARMSTRONG (ed.), *Aerospace Medicine,* p. 156. Baltimore: Williams & Wilkins Co., 1961.
26. GORALEWSKI, C. 1935, 1936. *Mitt. Arbeitsphysiol.,* 9: 94, 392.
27. HALDANE, J. S. 1922. *Respiration,* p. 127. New Haven, Conn.: Yale University Press.
28. HALDANE, J. S.; KELLAS, A. S.; and KENNAWAY, E. L. 1919. *J. Physiol.,* 53: 181.
29. HALL, F. G. 1949. *J. Appl. Physiol.,* 1: 490.
30. HALL, F. G., and HALL, K. D. 1951. *Proc. Soc. Exp. Biol. Med.,* 76: 140.
31. HEMINGWAY, A. W. 1944. *J. Aviat. Med.,* 15: 298.
32. HENMON, V. A. C. 1919. *J. Appl. Psychol.,* 3: 103.
33. HETHERINGTON, A. W.; LUFT, U.; and IVY, J. H. Dec. 1947. Symp. Milit. Physiol., Research and Develop. Board. Digest Ser. 4, G. E. 61/1.
34. HINGSTON, R. W. G. 1925. *Geog. J.,* 65: 4.
35. HOFFMAN, C. E.; CLARK, R. T.; and BROWN, E. B., JR. 1946. *Amer. J. Physiol.,* 145: 685.
36. IVY, A. C. 1946. *Fed. Proc.,* 5: 319.
37. JENSEN, A. V.; BECKER, R. F.; and WINDLE, W. F. 1948. *Arch. Neurol. Psychiat.,* 60: 221.
38. JOHNSON, H. M., and PASCHAL, F. C. 1920. *Psychobiol.,* 2: 193.
39. JONGBLOED, J. 1934. *Arch. Neerl. Physiol. L'homme Animaux,* 19: 538.
40. ———. 1935. *Klin. Wschr.,* 14: 1564.
41. KOSSMANN, C. E. 1947. *J. Aviat. Med.,* 18: 465.
42. LOEWY, A., and WITTKOWER, E. 1933. *Arch. Ges. Physiol.,* 233: 622.
43. LONGSTAFF, T. G., cited in J. BARCROFT. 1925. *The Respiratory Function of the Blood.* Part I, "Lessons from High Altitudes." Cambridge: Cambridge University Press.
44. LOWSON, J. P. 1923. *Brit. J. Med. Psychol.,* 13: 407.
45. LUFT, U. C. *In:* H. G. ARMSTRONG (ed.), *Aerospace Medicine,* p. 137. Baltimore: Williams & Wilkins Co., 1961.
46. MACKENZIE, C. G., *et al.* 1945. *J. Aviat. Med.,* 16: 156.

47. McComas, H. C. 1931. *Sci. Monthly,* **12:** 36.
48. McFarland, R. A. 1932. *Arch. Psychol.,* No. **145.**
49. ——. 1937. *J. Comp. Psychol.,* **23:** 191.
50. ——. *Ibid.,* p. 227.
51. ——. *Ibid.,* **24:** 147.
52. ——. *Ibid.,* p. 189.
53. Monge, C. 1929. *Les Erythremies de l'altitude.* Paris: Masson et Cie.
54. Mosso, A. 1893. *Life of Man on the High Alps.* London: Fisher.
55. Muido, L. 1946. *Acta Physiol. Scand.,* **12:** 99.
56. Paton, S. 1918. *J.A.M.A.,* **71:** 1399.
57. Pugh, L. G. C., and Ward, M. P. 1956. *Lancet,* **271:** 1115.
58. Richardson, J. W. 1954. *Proc. Soc. Exp. Biol. Med.,* **86:** 341.
59. Riesin, A. M.; Tahmisian, T. N.; and Mackenzie, C. G. 1946. *Proc. Soc. Exp. Biol. Med.,* **63:** 250.
60. Ruff, S., and Strughold, H. H. 1942. *Compendium of Aviation Medicine.* Translated and reproduced by U.S. Alien Property Custodian.
61. Russell, R. W. 1948. *J. Exp. Psychol.,* **38:** 178.
62. Shephard, R. J. 1956. *J. Appl. Physiol.,* **9:** 343.
63. Stern, E. 1925. *Klin. Wschr.,* **4:** 21.
64. ——. 1926. *Deutsch Med. Wschr.,* **8:** 1.
65. Stratton, G. M. 1919. *Sci. Monthly,* **8:** 421.
66. Tanaka, H. 1928. *Rept. Aero. Research. Inst.* (Tokyo Imperial University), **3:** 128.
67. Thompson, J. W., and Corwin, W. 1938. *Arch. Neurol. Psychiat.,* **40:** 1233.
68. Thorndike, E. L. June, August, 1919; January, 1920. "The Selection of Military Aviators," *U.S. Air Service,* 1 & 2: 14–17; 28–32; 29–31.
69. Von Tavel, F. 1943. *Helv. Physiol. Pharmacol. Acta,* **1:** 1.
70. Yant, W. P., *et al.* 1934. *Pub. Health Bull.* (U.S. Public Health Service), **211.**
71. Yerkes, R. M. 1919. *Psych. Rev.,* **26:** 94.

THE FUNCTIONING OF SMALL UNITS OF THE NERVOUS SYSTEM

Nerve fiber.—A number of studies have been made on the survival time of nerves during hypoxia (and asphyxia) in cats, dogs, rabbits, and frogs (36, 37, 53, 86).

In 1930 Gerard (36) reported experiments on the response of the nerve fiber to oxygen lack. He found that in the course of asphyxia action potentials led from the exposed region first rise and then fall to zero. He concluded from his experiments that asphyxia initially causes prolongation of action potentials, followed later by a depression of potential magnitude, a prolongation of refractory period, and fiber block. The time required for asphyxiation of a nerve depends on the temperature and the type of nerve; the higher the metabolism, the faster the block. When oxygen was readmitted to an asphyxiated nerve, the action potential rose rapidly within five to ten minutes to high values. The maximum response for fast stimulation may be five to six times as great as the pre-asphyxial ones, but for slow stimulation, as much as twelve times as great.

Lehmann (53) in 1937, working with excised nerves (peroneal, phrenic, and saphenous) of the cat under controlled conditions of hydrogen-ion concentration, found that when they were immersed in pure nitrogen, a typical sequence of irritability changes occurred. There was a lowering of the threshold of excitability first, followed by a progressive failure of irritability of the nerve fiber. The after-potentials disappeared before the spike—ten minutes on the average for the former, and thirty minutes for the latter. The normal functional state was restored if the hypoxia did not last too long.

Wright (86) found that the average survival times of twenty-eight rabbit nerves, ten cat nerves, and three dog nerves were 24, 33, and 33 minutes, respectively. He pointed out that the survival time of a nerve is a constant for each species. A number of workers (1, 8, 10, 27, 32, 34, 88) have experimented on various animals to determine the length of time a nerve functions after ischemia. On the whole, it was found that the time varies in different animals. It has been shown by Wright (87) and others (3) that hypoxia causes progressive depolarization and blocking of impulses in nerve tissue when a critical degree of depolarization is reached.

In 1931 Lewis, Pickering, and Rothschild (57) produced ischemic blocking of human nerves and reported that anesthesia always starts in the distal part and spreads proximally. They found, also, that the nerve is more sensitive to asphyxia in its proximal, than its distal, part and, further, that long nerves are affected earlier than short ones. A number of investigators have confirmed these findings (6, 41, 48, 73, 88), but some workers have questioned them (10, 68, 84). It was shown by Thorner and Brink (74) in 1940 that if the human ulnar nerve is deprived of its circulation for a period not exceeding thirty minutes, a succession of events occur similar to those outlined by Lehmann (53), that is, first a lowering of the threshold of excitability and then a progressive failure of irritability.

In 1948 Grandjean and his co-workers (39, 40) and Zwahlen and Grandjean (89) investigated the effect of altitude on nervous excitability. The studies showed that, in general, the threshold of sensory structures was increased; motor nerves, however, were unaffected.

Hypoxia and asphyxia and synaptic conduction.—Most of the studies reported on the effect of hypoxia on the synapses have involved stagnant hypoxia; that is, the circulation was arrested. Under this condition, there is, of course, considerable accumulation of carbon dioxide in the tissues.

As early as 1905 Tuckett (75), by producing anemia of the superior cervical ganglion, observed that the ganglion cells possessed greater resistance than those of the spinal cord. Schröder (66), however, was one of the first to study systematically the effects of anemia on sympathetic ganglia. In 1913 Cannon and Burket (22) pointed out that cells of the mesenteric plexus had a high resistance to complete anemia. Eccles (31), studying electric responses of the superior cervical ganglion, observed that a very small minute-blood supply is sufficient to maintain functional ganglionic activity.

Sugar and Gerard (71) have emphasized that synaptic conduction through the cervical sympathetic ganglion can withstand considerable hypoxia. In support of this view, they cite their own histochemical researches (70), the work of Bronk and Larrabee (19), and that of Bargeton (5). Bronk and Larrabee (19), working with the stellate ganglion, reported that it could be deprived of its circulation for about thirty minutes before it began to lose its capacity to respond. Deprivation of its circulation for approximately sixty minutes, however, caused cessation of its functioning.

In a subsequent study, Bronk *et al.* (18, 20) investigated the effect of hypoxia on conduction of impulses along axons and on transmission of impulses through synapses. Arresting the circulation of the ganglion caused transmission through it to fail in about thirty to forty minutes. Within two minutes after stopping the circulation, the oxygen tension fell to less than 5 per cent of its initial value, as shown by placing an oxygen electrode on the ganglion. However, even with a very small rate of oxygen consumption or with virtually none, transmission of the impulse was maintained for some time—in some pathways for as long as thirty minutes. This observation was in agreement with the work of Eccles. Indeed, it was shown that even after seven and a half hours of interruption of the circulation, one fourth, or more, of the synaptic pathways transmitted impulses.

Bargeton (5) in 1938, working with the superior cervical ganglion of the cat, found that in striking contrast to the cells of the central nervous system, the sympathetic ganglion cells showed a marked resistance to deprivation of blood. He showed that complete suppression of blood supply resulted in gradual disappearance of activity of the ganglion; within ten or fifteen minutes, there was total disappearance of activity, but a large degree of functional recovery returned after the ganglion had been completely deprived of blood for as long as seventy minutes.

Working with isolated, perfused heads of dogs, Heymans (42) in 1947 found that stimulation of the pre-ganglionic fibers of the superior cervical ganglion induced mydriasis during complete arrest of the circulation of the head up to forty-five minutes.

It is obvious that sympathetic ganglia show a marked resistance to oxygen deprivation.

Asphyxiation and synaptic potentials: Bonnet and Bremer (14), studying synaptic potentials in the frog's spinal cord during reflex activity, found that the potentials were depressed by asphyxiation. This work was confirmed by Brooks and Eccles (21). Van Harreveld (78), working on central synaptic conduction and asphyxia, reported that the cells in the spinal cord showed considerable resistance to asphyxia.

Tendon reflexes.—It was shown by Porter (62) in 1912 that hypoxia may abolish the flexor reflex in spinal cats. In 1932 King *et al.* (47) demonstrated that hypoxia inhibits the knee jerk. Jokl (44) in 1939 studied tendon reflexes at altitude. He reported that reflexes were normal until an altitude of 6,000 feet (1,800 meters) was reached. Beyond this height, they became diminished and remained so up to an approximate altitude of 15,000 feet (4,500 meters). It seems that this altitude represents a critical level, for above it tendon reflexes become increased, which, according to Jokl, indicates an early disturbance of nervous control. The author also stated that a second critical level exists at about 29,000 feet (8,840 meters); at this altitude, loss of consciousness, muscular cramps, paralysis, and death may occur. It is generally believed, however, that the symptoms described by Jokl frequently occur at 25,000 feet (7,620 meters) or less in unacclimatized individuals.

Van Harreveld and his colleagues have published a number of studies on the effect of asphyxiation of the spinal cord. In 1939 Van Harreveld and Marmont (82) produced asphyxiation in the spinal cords of cats by raising the dural pressure above the arterial. After fifty-five minutes of asphyxiation, the tendon reflexes returned for forty-eight hours and then disappeared.

In subsequent papers (76, 78), Van Harreveld concluded that to abolish all reflex activity in spinal cats an average of three minutes and twenty-two seconds of asphyxia is needed. In later papers (79, 80), he reported that reflex activity is increased at the beginning of asphyxia of the cord and that a flexion reflex persists longer than the knee jerk. Van Harreveld and Tyler (83) studied the metabolism of spinal cord tissue after asphyxiation and found that the metabolic changes paralleled the temporary return of reflex function.

The chronaxie.—Not many physiologists would concede that the chronaxie is a true measure of excitability of tissues. The term is becoming obsolete. The consensus now is that only the determination of the strength-duration curve gives an accurate measurement of the excitability of tissues. Be that as it may, the term "chronaxie" is still found in the literature.

A number of studies have been made on the effect of hemic hypoxia on the excitability of the different areas of the cerebral cortex.

Rizzolo (65) in 1927 ligated both carotid and both vertebral arteries in a series of dogs and determined the effect of stagnant hypoxia so produced on the chronaxie of the cortex of the brain. He subjected another group of animals to repeated hemorrhages (hemic hypoxia) and made similar studies. He concluded that in neither group was there any modification of the chronaxie. This was true even in animals which had suffered a pronounced hemorrhage (withdrawal of 200–300 cc. of blood from dogs, weighing 6–12 kg.). Occasionally (in two cases out of ten), however, he observed a definite prolongation of the chronaxie following a small hemorrhage (50–100 cc.) in a medium-sized dog. Richard (64), a few years later, using virtually the same technique, confirmed Rizzolo's work.

In 1936 the Chauchards (24) repeated the work of Rizzolo and that of Richard and reached the same conclusion, namely, that there was no change in the chronaxie of the cerebral cortex following ligation of both carotid and both vertebral vessels. These authors stressed the fact that, even after ligation of these four vessels, the cerebral hemispheres still received considerable blood; they felt that this explained absence of change in the chronaxie. They pointed out that local anemia of the cortex produced by compression of the brain caused a prolongation of the chronaxie; if the pressure was reduced, however, and it had not been acting too long, the chronaxie returned to normal. They emphasized that complete interruption of the circulation always produced a decreased excitability of the cerebral cortex. If the circulation had been interrupted for only one and a half minutes, the chronaxie quickly returned to normal; but after two and a half minutes of complete ischemia of the cortex, the alteration of the chronaxie persisted.

Apparently all workers agree that the blood supply to the cortex may be diminished considerably before there is any change in the excitability of tissues as measured by the chronaxie. One can only speculate about the relationship between the excitability of the cortex and the normal physiologic processes which occur in the cells of the cerebrum. It would be expected, however, that there is some definite relationship.

In this connection, the interesting work of Lennox and the Gibbses (54) may be mentioned. These investigators found that unconsciousness supervenes in man if the oxygen supply to the brain is suddenly reduced so that the oxygen saturation of the blood in the internal jugular vein falls to 24 per cent or less. The subject does remain conscious, however, as long as the oxygen saturation does not fall below 30 per cent.

Studies have also been made on the effect of anoxic hypoxia on the cortical chronaxie. The Chauchards (26) in 1940, using guinea pigs, observed that a simulated altitude between about 16,400 feet (5,000 meters) and 19,700 feet (6,000 meters) produced an increase of 80 per cent in the cortical chronaxie.

Beyne *et al.* (12) in 1948 studied the cortical chronaxie in man. At a simulated altitude of over 19,700 feet (6,000 meters), a shortening of the chronaxie was noted. They also made observations on guinea pigs; using simulated altitudes from about 13,000 feet (about 4,000 meters) to 16,500 feet (5,000 meters), an increase in the chronaxie was observed. Their results with the guinea pig agreed with those reported by the Chauchards.

Boeles (13) in 1954 reported observations on the chronaxie of the first motor neuron and the motor units in pentobarbitalized cats. The excitability of the sciatic nerve and the gastrocnemius muscle showed no changes until the duration of cardiac arrest had exceeded fifteen minutes, after which reanimation was no longer possible. The excitation time of the motor area of the cortex decreased one to three minutes after the onset of hypoxia, after which it increased; within fifteen to twenty seconds, the motor area became inexcitable. When respiratory arrest persisted for more than five minutes, the inexcitability was irreversible.

Several workers (25, 72, 85) have made studies on the chronaxie of the nerve fiber. The Chauchards (25), working with guinea pigs, found a diminution in the chronaxie at a simulated altitude of about 15,000 feet (4,500 meters). The chronaxie of the extensors of the hindleg decreased much less than those of the flexors.

Asphyxiation and reciprocal innervation.—It was shown in 1939 by Van Harreveld and Marmont (82), working with cats whose spinal cords had been asphyxiated for various periods of time, that after recovery the hind legs showed an exaggerated extensor tone; this usually lasted until death (about three weeks later). The conclusion was that the high extensor tone was caused by a selective damage to the inhibiting system which normally keeps the tone in check.

Van Harreveld (77, 76) studied the problem further and found that asphyxiation was capable of abolishing reciprocal innervation. He felt that this strongly supported the assumption that asphyxia damages the inhibitory neurones more severely than the excitatory ones.

As far as the authors are aware, no studies have been reported of the effect of anoxic hypoxia on reciprocal innervation.

Conditioned reflexes.—A paucity of experiments have been reported in the literature of the effect of hypoxia on conditioned reflexes.

Andreyev (2) in 1935 ligated both common carotids and both vertebral arteries in dogs and studied the changes in higher nervous activity by the method of conditioned reflexes. He observed that during the first ten to twelve days following the operation the temporary disturbances were most marked and were manifested in the complete disappearance of the conditioned reflexes. Later these were often restored. The more delicate functions of the cortex, however, as represented by the formation of long-delayed conditioned reflexes, were eliminated either permanently or for a long time.

In evaluating the effects of anemic hypoxia on conditioned reflexes, it will be remembered that, while anemia produces its effects primarily by hypoxia, it produces other changes as well.

Gantt *et al.* (33) in 1949 studied the effects of hypoxia on conditioned reflexes of two dogs, one aged eleven years and the other four years. They were exposed four hours (five or six times) to 18,000 feet (5,500 meters) and 25,000 feet (7,600 meters), by either reducing oxygen pressure or lowering the oxygen content. The responses measured were based on food or on pain. Both animals showed a marked impairment at a simulated altitude of 25,000 feet, but no change occurred at 18,000 feet in the younger dog.

The authors felt that conditional-reflex measurements can be useful in evaluating efficacy of therapy for altitude tolerance. They pointed out that conditional-reflex impairment appears when there is no other observable change.

Brain potentials.—Observations made on animals: The influence of hypoxia and asphyxia on potentials of specific brain regions has been studied in animals by a number of workers (4, 7, 9, 16, 17, 23,

30, 35, 63, 67, 71). All investigators generally agree that effective degrees of hypoxia either diminish or eliminate brain potentials. Hypoxia often produces some initial stimulation of brain potentials, but this is quickly followed by a depression.

Prawdicz-Neminski (63) in 1925 studied brain waves from the motor and visual cortices of curarized dogs and followed them after artificial respiration was suspended. No change during the dyspneic phase of asphyxia was observed, but the potentials increased through the convulsive phase and finally disappeared, although the heart was still beating. Bartley and Bishop (7) in 1933 reported that the potentials disappeared three to five minutes after ligating a superficial artery, which supplied the area of the cortex under observation. Simpson and Derbyshire (67) reported that bilateral carotid occlusion abolished potentials from the cat's motor cortex in twenty seconds. Cate and Horsten (23) in 1951, however, reported that total disappearance of the electrical activity of the brain was seen only after occlusion of all the arterial blood supply (common carotid, vertebral, and anterior spinal artery).

Sugar and Gerard (71) in 1938, studying brain potentials in cats in which an abrupt and functionally complete anemia of the brain had been produced, reported noticeable differences in the "survival time" (duration of occlusion necessary to abolish electrical activity) and the "recovery time" (interval between restoration of circulation and return of potentials) in various parts of the brain. For example, they found that following complete anemia it took fourteen to fifteen seconds for the disappearance of potentials in the cerebral cortex, whereas it took from thirty to forty seconds to make them disappear from the region of the medulla.

Van Harreveld (81) in 1947, using cats, described the EEG after ten to thirty minutes of asphyxia. After the shorter period of asphyxiation, the EEG was characterized by short (one to two seconds duration) bursts of activity with a wave frequency of 7–12 per second, repeated ten to twenty times per minute. After longer asphyxiation, the EEG was characterized by spindles of activity of longer (ten to twenty seconds) duration with a wave frequency of 12–16 per second, which were repeated with intervals varying from a few seconds to about one minute.

Gellhorn and Kessler (35) in 1942 showed that in cats and rats the effect of hypoxia on brain potentials is greatly aggravated during hypoglycemia. This action on brain potentials can be offset by the inhalation of pure oxygen.

Kessler and Gellhorn and their associate (46) a year later studied the effect of hypoxia on the EEG of unanesthetized rats during rapid ascent. When a level of 190 mm. Hg was reached, a period of temporary silence of the cortex ensued. During the period of recovery, the appearance of large spindles of a frequency of 8–10 per second occurred. If the ascent was not rapid, the period of temporary silence was not always manifested, although the spindles might be found. The authors observed that the occurrence of spindles was confined mostly to barometric pressures varying between 280 and 160 mm. Hg. When the pressure was lowered to 110–140 mm. Hg, a period of electrical silence occurred; the animals did not recover.

It is of interest that thyroid preparations lower the threshold during hypoxia. Kessler and Gellhorn (45) found no significant changes in the EEG in normal rats exposed to 7 per cent oxygen. When a thyroid preparation (thyroid powder or thyroxin) was administered, profound changes in the EEG occurred.

Lubin and Price (58) reported that the minimal amount of acid (hydrochloric) or alkali (sodium carbonate) injected intravenously necessary to produce changes in the respiratory rate in anesthetized cats had no effect on the cortical potentials. Although in most cases intravenous injection of acid causes dilatation of the pial vessels, and and intravenous injection of alkali causes constriction, these changes are not obviously related to the alterations of cortical potentials.

Observations made on human beings: It has been shown by several workers that breathing mixtures low in oxygen can abolish brain potentials in man.

In 1934 Berger (11), working with human beings, reported that the electroencephalogram became more irregular and that larger waves were seen after about seven minutes of rebreathing from a closed bag with carbon dioxide absorbed.

Gibbs and Davis (38) in 1935 obtained electroencephalograms from subjects who became unconscious after breathing pure nitrogen. It had been previously established in resting subjects that frequencies from 10 to 20 per second normally occurred and attained a maximum of 60 microvolts. Breathing pure nitrogen caused the frequency of the predominant waves to decrease to between 1 and 5 per second but caused the amplitude to increase to about 100 microvolts. These changes occurred gradually and began before the subject lost consciousness. It was also observed that overventilation of the lungs up to the point of clouding of consciousness produced similar alterations in the electroencephalogram. When the subject was allowed to breathe room air after he had breathed pure nitrogen, a decrease in all electrical activity was noted, followed by a gradual return of the normal waves.

Davis *et al.* (29) in 1938 allowed human beings to breathe gas mixtures containing 7.8–11.4 per cent oxygen while simultaneous electroencephalograms were recorded. The average voltage increased slightly; but later it decreased, and shorter trains of alpha waves occurred. Irregular delta waves appeared at the time cyanosis was first noticed; and just before consciousness was lost, large delta waves dominated the record. These delta waves disappeared with the first breath of room air, and the normal pattern was restored in about two minutes.

Hoaglund (43) in 1938 reported that a fall in oxygen tension decreased the alpha frequency. In the same year Lennox *et al.* (56) concluded from their work that hypoxia causes a significant slowing of frequency of waves of cortical activity only when the hypoxia is so extreme that unconsciousness impends. The following year Davis and Davis (28) described the effects on patients who breathed 8 per cent oxygen until consciousness was lost. With the increase of the hypoxia, the delta waves replaced the alpha waves.

Brazier (15) in 1948, studying changes in the wave frequency of the EEG in human subjects under conditions of progressive hypoxia, reported that there occurred a progressive slowing of the alpha rhythm. More recently Luft and Noell (59) studied the cerebral manifestations of hypoxia during and after exposure to a barometric pressure of 68–70 mm. Hg, approximately 54,000 feet (16,600 meters). During what they termed a period of "failing posture," the electroencephalogram deteriorated progressively until finally there occurred an absence of brain activity.

It is apparent that the electrical activity of the cerebral cortex of man is relatively resistant to the effects of hypoxia, as witnessed by the fact that most investigators have had to use severe degrees of hypoxia before significant changes in electrical activity occurred. This is also apparently true in animals.

Carbon dioxide and brain potentials.—It has been shown by Lennox *et al.* (55) that carbon dioxide accumulation increases fast waves, and it is thought that it may, in part, contribute to the augmented high-frequency potentials seen early in hypoxia. If there is sufficient excess of carbon dioxide, however, the brain potentials may be abolished, as they are during severe hypoxia. Pollock (61) in 1949, working with cats, found that high concentrations of carbon dioxide (15 per cent carbon dioxide and 85 per cent oxygen) increase the frequency, but lower the amplitude, of the cat's normal EEG. Higher concentrations (30 per cent carbon dioxide and 70 per cent oxygen) decrease the frequency and may cause reversible irregularities to appear. In evaluating the effect of carbon dioxide on brain potentials, it must be remembered that carbon dioxide at a concentration of about 15 per cent has an anesthetic action.

Spreading cortical depression (SD) of Leao.—Leao (49, 50) described a decrease in the amplitude of cortical activity as a consequence of stimulation (electrical, chemical, mechanical, or thermal). A characteristic of this depression is its slow spread at a rate of only 1 to 3 mm. per minute. It was suggested by Leao and Morison (52) that it did not require neuronal pathways for its propagation, but that it was propagated along the blood vessels. Sloan and Jasper (69), however, concluded from their work that the disturbance must spread along the neurons by contiguity.

Leao (51) reported that acute anemia (produced by arterial occlusion) is followed by SD in 2.5–5 minutes. It is believed by Marshall (60) that hypoxia, whether produced by severe blood-pressure depression or by breathing air low in oxygen content, may trigger the reaction. He believes, further, that during asphyxia, hypoxia, or rebreathing the swelling of the brain and the marked changes in thoracic pressure may bring about a spreading cortical depression by mechanical stimulation and also increase the sensitivity of the brain to initiation of SD.

REFERENCES

1. ADRIAN, E. D. 1925. *J. Physiol.,* **61:** 49.
2. ANDREYEV, L. A. 1935. *Arch. Neurol. Psychiat.,* **34:** 699.
3. ARVANITAKI, A., and CHALAZONITIS, N. 1947. *Arch. Int. Physiol.,* **54:** 406.
4. BAILEY, P., and BREMER, F. 1938. *J. Neurophysiol.,* **1:** 405.
5. BARGETON, D. 1938. *Amer. J. Physiol.,* **121:** 268.
6. BARLOW, E. D., and POCHIN, E. E. 1948. *Clin. Sci.,* **6:** 303.
7. BARTLEY, S. H., and BISHOP, G. H. 1933. *Amer. J. Physiol.,* **103:** 173.
8. BAYLESS, F. 1937. *C. R. Soc. Biol. (Par.),* **124:** 272.
9. BEECHER, H. K.; MCDONOUGH, F. K.; and FORBES, A. 1938. *J. Neurophysiol.,* **1:** 324.
10. BENTLEY, F. H., and SCHLAPP, W. J. 1943. *J. Physiol.,* **102:** 62 and 72.
11. BERGER, H. 1934. *Arch. Psychiat. Nervenkr.,* **102:** 538.
12. BEYNE, J.; CHAUCHARD, B.; and CHAUCHARD, P. 1948. *J. Physiol.,* **40:** 113.

13. BOELES, J. TH. F. 1954. *Acta Physiol. Pharmacol. Neerl., 3:* 397.
14. BONNET, V., and BREMER, F. 1948. *J. Physiol., 40:* 117 (Abstr.) .
————. 1948. *Arch. Int. Physiol., 56:* 97.
15. BRAZIER, M. A. B. 1948. *J. Neurol. Neurosurg. Psychiat., 11:* 118.
16. BREMER, F. 1935. *C. R. Soc. Biol. (Par.)* , 118: 1241.
17. BREMER, F., and THOMAS, J. 1936. *C. R. Soc. Biol. (Par.)* , 123: 1256.
18. BRONK, D. W.; BRINK, F.; and LARRABEE, M. G. 1948. *Fed. Proc., 7:* 14.
19. BRONK, D. W., and LARRABEE, M. G. 1937. *Amer. J. Physiol., 119:* 279.
20. BRONK, D. W.; LARRABEE, M. G.; and GAYLOR, J. B. 1948. *J. Cell. Comp. Physiol., 31:* 193.
21. BROOKS, M. C., and ECCLES, J. C. 1947. *J. Neurophysiol., 10:* 349.
22. CANNON, W. B., and BURKET, I. R. 1913. *Amer. J. Physiol., 32:* 347.
23. CATE, J. T., and HORSTEN, G. P. M. 1951. *Acta Physiol. Pharmacol. Neerl., 2:* 2.
24. CHAUCHARD, A., and CHAUCHARD, B. 1936. *C. R. Soc. Biol. (Par.)* , 123: 979.
25. ————. 1940. *Ibid., 134:* 331.
26. ————. *Ibid.,* p. 421.
27. CLARCK, D.; HUGHES, J.; and GASSER, H. S. 1935. *Amer. J. Physiol., 114:* 69.
28. DAVIS, H., and DAVIS, P. A. 1939. *Ass. Res. Nerv. Ment. Dis., 19:* 50.
29. DAVIS, P. A.; DAVIS, H.; and THOMPSON, J. W. 1938. *Amer. J. Physiol., 123:* 51.
30. DERBYSHIRE, A. J., *et al.* 1936. *Amer. J. Physiol., 116:* 577.
31. ECCLES, J. C. 1935. *J. Physiol., 85:* 202.
32. FRANKENHAEUSER, B. 1949. *Acta Physiol. Scand., 18:* 1 and 75.
33. GANTT, H.; THORN, G. W.; and DORRANCE, C. 1949. *Fed. Proc., 8:* 53.
34. GASSER, H. S. 1943. *Proc. Ass. Res. Nerv. Ment. Dis., 23:* 44.
35. GELLHORN, E., and KESSLER, M. 1942. *Amer. J. Physiol., 137:* 703.
36. GERARD, R. W. 1930. *Amer. J. Physiol., 92:* 498.
37. ————. 1932. *Physiol. Rev., 12:* 469.
38. GIBBS, F. A., and DAVIS, H. 1935. *Amer. J. Physiol., 113:* 49.
39. GRANDJEAN, E. 1948. *Helvet. Physiol. Pharmacol. Acta, 6:* 489.
40. GRANDJEAN, E.; POSTERNAK, J.; and WARIDEL, H. 1948. *Helvet. Physiol. Pharmacol. Acta, 6:* 484.
41. GROAT, R. A., and KOENIG, H. 1946. *J. Neurophysiol., 9:* 275 and 463.
42. HEYMANS, C. 1947. *Abstr. of Commun. of XVII Intern. Physiol. Congr.,* p. 152. New York: Oxford University Press.
43. HOAGLUND, H. 1938. *Amer. J. Physiol., 123:* 102.
44. JOKL, E. 1939. *J. Roy. Army Med. Corps, 73:* 289.
45. KESSLER, M., and GELLHORN, E. 1942. *Amer. J. Physiol., 137:* 703.
46. KESSLER, M.; HAILMAN, H.; and GELLHORN, E. 1943. *Amer. J. Physiol., 140:* 291.
47. KING, C. E.; GARREY, W. E.; and BRYAN, W. R. 1932. *Amer. J. Physiol., 102:* 305.

48. KUGELBERG, A. 1944. *Acta Physiol. Scand.,* **8** (Suppl.) : 29.
49. LEAO, A. A. P. 1944. *J. Neurophysiol.,* **7:** 359.
50. ———. 1947. *Ibid.,* **10:** 409.
51. ———. 1951. *Electroenceph. Clin. Neurophysiol.,* **3:** 315.
52. LEAO, A. A. P., and MORISON, R. S. 1945. *J. Neurophysiol.,* **8:** 33.
53. LEHMANN, J. E. 1937. *Amer. J. Physiol.,* **119:** 111.
54. LENNOX, W. G.; GIBBS, F. A.; and GIBBS, E. L. 1935. *Arch. Neurol. Psychiat.,* **34:** 1101.
55. ———. 1936. *Ibid.,* **36:** 1236.
56. ———. 1938. *Ass. Res. Nerv. Ment. Dis.,* **18:** 277.
57. LEWIS, T.; PICKERING, G. W.; and ROTHSCHILD, P. 1931. *Heart,* **16:** 1.
58. LUBIN, A. J., and PRICE, J. E. 1942. *J. Neurophysiol.,* **5:** 261.
59. LUFT, U. C., and NOELL, W. K. 1956. *J. Appl. Physiol.,* **8:** 444.
60. MARSHALL, W. J. 1959. *Physiol. Rev.,* **39:** 239.
61. POLLOCK, G. H. 1949. *J. Neurophysiol.,* **12:** 315.
62. PORTER, E. L. 1912. *Amer. J. Physiol.,* **31:** 223.
63. PRAWDICZ-NEMINSKI, W. W. 1925. *Pflueger Arch. Ges. Physiol.,* **209:** 362.
64. RICHARD, A. 1936. *C. R. Soc. Biol. (Par.)* , **123:** 787.
65. RIZZOLO, A. 1927. *C. R. Soc. Biol. (Par.)* , **96:** 1209.
66. SCHRÖDER, R. 1907. *Pflueger Arch. Ges. Physiol.,* **116:** 600.
67. SIMPSON, H. N., and DERBYSHIRE, A. J. 1934. *Amer. J. Physiol.,* **109:** 99.
68. SINCLAIR, D. C. 1948. *J. Neurophysiol.,* **11:** 75.
69. SLOAN, N. and JASPER, J. 1950. *Electroenceph. Clin. Neurophysiol.,* **2:** 317.
70. SUGAR, O., and GERARD, R. W. 1938. *Amer. J. Physiol.,* **123:** 198.
71. ———. 1938. *J. Neurophysiol.,* **1:** 558.
72. TANAKA, H., and TOYOSHIMA, Y. 1935. *Bull. Nav. Med. Ass.,* Japan, **24:** 365.
73. THOMPSON, I. M., and KIMBALL, H. S. 1936. *Proc. Soc. Exp. Biol. Med.* **34:** 601.
74. THORNER, M. W., and BRINK, J., cited by M. W. THORNER and L. H. LEVY. 1940. *J.A.M.A.,* **115:** 1595.
75. TUCKETT. 1905. *J. Physiol.,* **33:** 77.
76. VAN HARREVELD, A. 1939. *Amer. J. Physiol.,* **128:** 13.
77. ———. 1939. *Proc. Soc. Exp. Biol. Med.,* **40:** 561.
78. ———. 1941. *Amer. J. Physiol.,* **133:** 572.
79. ———. 1944. *Ibid.,* **141:** 97.
80. ———. *Ibid.,* **142:** 32.
81. ———. 1947. *J. Neurophysiol.,* **10:** 361.
82. VAN HARREVELD, A., and MARMONT, G. 1939. *J. Neurophysiol.,* **2:** 101.
83. VAN HARREVELD, A., and TYLER, D. B. 1942. *Fed. Proc.,* **1:** 87.
84. WEDDELL, G., and SINCLAIR, D. C. 1947. *J. Neurol. Psychiat.,* **10:** 26.
85. WOROBJEW, A. M. 1934. *Fiziol. Zh. S.S.S.R.,* **17:** 972.
86. WRIGHT, E. B. 1946. *Amer. J. Physiol.,* **147:** 78.

87. WRIGHT, E. B. 1947. *Ibid.*, **148**: 174.
88. ZOTTERMAN, Y. 1933. *Acta Med. Scand.*, **80**: 185.
89. ZWAHLEN, P., and GRANDJEAN, E. 1948. *Helvet. Physiol. Pharmacol. Acta*, **6**: 471.

EFFECT OF HYPOXIA ON SENSE ORGANS

THE EYE

McFarland, Evans, and Halperin (48) in 1941; Weaver (74) in 1943; and Gellhorn and Hailman (24) also in 1943 have reviewed the literature concerning the effect of hypoxia on vision. Of the three reviews, that of McFarland *et al.* is the most extensive.

McFarland *et al.* (48) have pointed out that the retina is closely related to the brain, embryologically, morphologically, and physiologically. Furthermore, Krause (37) has shown that because the retina is anatomically a part of the brain, it has a similar metabolism. Since nervous tissue, as previously mentioned, is particularly sensitive to oxygen want, it would follow that certain functions involving the retina would be similarly affected.

Balloonists first called attention to the fact that accomodation was affected at high altitudes and further reported that they experienced difficulty in reading the mercury column, although distant vision was unaltered.

Wilmer and Berens (76), making quantitative studies of vision as early as 1918, found that judgment of distance, range of visual fields, accomodation, convergence, and retinal sensitivity were impaired at an oxygen pressure corresponding to an altitude of 20,000 feet (6,095 meters). Slight differences at 15,000 feet (4,570 meters) were noted, but none at 10,000 feet (3,050 meters). Goldman and Schubert (29) and Sauer (59) obtained similar results. Barcroft (4) relates that several members of his South American party experienced visual disturbances at Cerro de Pasco, altitude of 14,200 feet (4,325 meters).

Discrimination of light intensity.—Many observers have noticed an increase in the threshold for brightness produced by hypoxia. Bert (6) called attention to this many years ago, and reports of balloonists also emphasized it.

It has been shown by a number of workers (9, 18, 46, 47, 73) that during hypoxia the threshold for light is raised both for light-adapted and dark-adapted eyes. It was demonstrated by McFarland and Evans (47) that there is a diminution in sensitivity to light at a simulated altitude of only 7,400 feet (2,255 meters). By determining the absolute light threshold during hypoxia, these workers found that at a simulated altitude of 15,000 feet (4,570 meters) a light intensity 2.5 times greater than normal was required in order for it to be seen.

It has also been shown that the threshold for discrimination of light intensities increases during hypoxia (23, 62, 63). Gellhorn and Spiesman (26) in 1935, using oxygen mixtures from 11 to 9 per cent, corresponding to altitudes from 17,000 feet (5,182 meters) to 22,000 feet (6,705 meters), observed a decrease in visual intensity and discrimination. Schubert (62, 63) in the same year also reported a considerable increase in the threshold for brightness in experiments performed in a low-pressure chamber at simulated altitudes above 21,000 feet (6,400 meters).

Visual acuity is also lessened by hypoxia (5). McFarland and Halperin (50) have emphasized the importance of light intensity when studying visual acuity. At low-light intensities, visual acuity is greatly decreased during hypoxia; whereas, at high intensities, the effect is slight.

In what Monge (53) termed "subacute mountain sickness," he found a diminution of visual acuity and a cloudiness of vision.

Peripheral field of vision.—Wilmer and Berens (76) in 1918 found a contraction of the peripheral field of vision at about 15,000 feet (4,500 meters); more severe degrees of hypoxia intensified the contraction. Goldman and Schubert (29) in 1933 made similar investigations, using both a low-pressure chamber and low-oxygen mixtures. They also found a shrinkage of peripheral vision noticeable at about 14,000 feet (4,200 meters). Four years later, Furuya (22), working with a low-pressure chamber, obtained somewhat similar results. He noted that changes began at about 16,400 feet (5,000 meters). Kyrieleis (38), on the other hand, could not find any contraction in the peripheral field of vision at simulated altitudes as high as 26,000 feet (7,925 meters). He felt that the results obtained by some of the other workers could be explained as due to weakness of attention of their subjects, and he also criticized their methods.

Halstead (30) in 1945, subjected twenty males to a simulated altitude of 10,000 feet (3,050 meters) for five or six hours daily, six days a week for a period of from four to six weeks. About the fourth week of exposure, thirteen of the twenty subjects developed a marked and progressive impairment of peripheral vision; in some subjects, central vision was also affected. In several instances, days or weeks elapsed before return to previous levels of visual efficiency.

Four additional subjects were exposed to altitudes ranging from 15,500 feet (4,720 meters) to 18,000 feet (5,485 meters). The impairment of peripheral vision appeared earlier and was more marked.

In summary, it may be said that although there is still some controversy concerning the effect of hypoxia on the peripheral field of vision, there is fairly substantial evidence that hypoxia constricts the peripheral field.

Central field of vision.—In 1938 Evans and McFarland (17) reported that central visual acuity remained unaffected even at the peak of oxygen deprivation and that except for a region from 6 to 8 degrees about the macula, the angioscotoma widened with progressive oxygen want until it obliterated the visual field. It is of interest in this connection that Cusick *et al.* (13) in 1940 showed that at an altitude of 18,000 feet (5,485 meters) to 21,000 feet (6,400 meters) the retinal vessels dilate. (See p. 338.)

Since ephedrine sulphate is often given in conditions associated with angioscotoma brought about by venous stasis, Evans and McFarland suggested that similar medication might be of benefit to individuals who suffer from visual disturbances produced by hypoxia. It is believed, however, that the changes in the size of the vessels are not alone responsible for the angioscotoma but that hypoxia also affects the functions of the ganglia of the retina.

It has also been observed that hypoxia produces a widening of the blind spot (29).

Afterimages.—Gellhorn and Spiesman (27) in 1935, using a Douglas bag, found a lengthening of the latent period of negative afterimages following inhalation of oxygen mixtures from 11 to 9 per cent, corresponding to altitudes of about 17,000 feet (5,180 meters) to 22,000 feet (6,705 meters). It was found that the effect lasted as long as twelve minutes after readmission of air.

Two years later McFarland (42), in airplane ascents, found a lengthening of the appearance and disappearance of afterimages of 43 and 46 per cent, respectively after one flight. Using a low-pressure chamber, McFarland and his co-workers (48) found a lengthening of the latent time of the afterimage; in general, a more severe degree of hypoxia produced a greater lengthening. Simulated altitudes of 11,500 feet (3,405 meters), 14,000 feet (4,270 meters), and 17,000 feet (5,180 meters) were used.

In 1943 McFarland and his collaborators (51), using a low-pressure chamber, measured the latency of the "tertiary" visual afterimage and found that hypoxia prolonged it. They noted that this effect was consistent with the apparent dimming of the visual field at altitude.

It was noted, furthermore, that inhalation of oxygen produced only a slow recovery of this function.

Experiments on acclimatized subjects.—Working with acclimatized subjects during the International High Altitude Expedition to the Chilean Andes, McFarland (43) reported a lengthening of the latent period of the afterimage, which was statistically significant at 20,100 feet (6,100 meters). He also observed a tendency for the afterimages to persist longer.

Site of action of hypoxia on visual system.—Gellhorn and Hailman (24) point out that the retina is composed of a complex set of ganglion cells whose metabolism is probably similar to that of other parts of the central nervous system. The fact that hypoglycemia and hypoxia act synergistically on the visual threshold of the dark-adapted eye (49) bears this out.

The above authors have suggested that hypoxia could act on the visual system in one or more of three ways by affecting: (*a*) photochemical processes in the retina; (*b*) retinal synapses; and (*c*) the geniculate-striate system. They point out that the rapid recovery of light sensitivity of the dark-adapted eye following readmission of air indicates that the effect of oxygen deprivation on visual function is extraphotochemical (10, 47). Further proof that hypoxia acts on the retinal neurons and not on the photochemical system has been demonstrated by Craik (12). He rendered the eye temporarily blind by local pressure, but when the pressure was removed, afterimages were formed. Seitz and his co-worker (65, 66) have shown that if strychnine is applied locally to one eye during hypoxia, the treated eye regains a normal critical fusion frequency (CFF) and a normal angioscotoma. This shows that the retinal synapses may be more sensitive to hypoxia than are those located in the geniculate-striate system.

Although the retinal synapses are presumably more sensitive to hypoxia, it must be remembered that the final sensation and perception is greatly influenced by the reactivity of cortical neurons. Gellhorn and Hailman state that hypoxia impairs visual processes through interference with the transmission of nervous impulses from the retina to the brain, but hypoxia also causes alteration in cortical functions.

Size of retinal vessels.—Cusick *et al.* (13), in 1940 reported studies of the effect of hypoxia on the size of retinal vessels. They found that at simulated altitudes from 16,000 to 19,000 feet (about 5,500 to 6,400 meters) the diameter of retinal vessels increased 10–20 per cent, the veins dilating more than the arteries. In 1947 Duquet *et al.* (16) subjected fourteen men between the ages of eighteen and thirty-eight to hypoxia, using a decompression chamber. They found enlargement of the retinal vessels at altitudes as low as 13,100 feet (4,000 meters); the dilatation reached its maximum at 19,700 feet (6,000 meters). Their results were in agreement with those of Cusick and his co-workers.

Hickman and Frayser (33) in 1959 reported that when the arterial blood oxygen is reduced by breathing low-oxygen mixtures (10 per cent in nitrogen for approximately five minutes), the retinal venous blood oxygen falls, but less than the arterial oxygen, so that there was a decrease in the retinal arteriovenous oxygen difference. This was presumably associated with an increased retinal blood flow, since (by photographic means) the vessels were seen to dilate.

It is of interest that Dammert (14) observed that subjects suffering from high-altitude disease showed a considerable dilatation of the capillaries of the retina.

Intraocular tension.—As early as 1918, Wilmer and Berens (76) stated that there was no correlation between the intraocular tension and various cardiovascular changes produced by high altitudes. Furuya (20) in 1936, however, reported that intraocular tension always increases at high altitudes above about 13,000 to 16,000 feet (4,000 to 4,900 meters). He made his measurements on six subjects in a low-pressure chamber. Similar findings were reported two years later by Buscalossi (11), who also used a low-pressure chamber. He measured ocular tension with Schiötz's tonometer. On the other hand, Pinson (54) in 1940 reported that anesthetized rabbits subjected to a simulated altitude of 40,000 feet (12,200 meters) showed no appreciable alterations in intraocular pressure. The question arises whether the anesthetic agent influenced his results.

If hypoxia actually causes a rise in intraocular tension, it is of considerable clinical significance, since it might be hazardous for individuals suffering from glaucoma to subject themselves to high altitudes.

Color vision.—Wilmer and Berens (76) in 1918 could not find any changes in color sensitivity at simulated altitudes of 20,000 feet feet (6,095 meters) or more. On the other hand, Vishnevskiy and Tsyrlin (72) in 1935 found that retinal sensitivity to red, green, and blue light was somewhat decreased at altitude. They concluded that cone vision was affected to a greater extent than rod vision. McDonald and Adler (41), however, in 1939 found that rod vision and cone vision are equally affected by oxygen deprivation.

Velhagen (71) in 1935, using the anomaloscope, reported that many people who have normal color vision at sea level suffer a disturbance in this function at altitude. He stated, also, that slight anomalies in color vision became accentuated under conditions of oxygen deprivation and, further, that one form of congenital anomaly may be converted into another. These changes he reported took place at about 10,000 feet (3,000 meters).

Schmidt (60) a year later, also using the anomaloscope, came to a somewhat different conclusion. He felt that if there were no color blindness at sea level, there would be none at altitude. He also believed that there was no conversion of color blindness from one form to another at altitude. He felt, however, as did Velhagen, that if color blindness were present at sea level, it would be increased by oxygen want and that this probably occurred at about 10,000 feet.

Mechanism of pupillary dilatation during hypoxia.—In 1945 Gellhorn and Levin (25) studied the size of the pupils of normal and adrenalectomized cats which had been subjected to hypoxia; later, asphyxia was also produced by clamping the trachea. Pupillary size was determined on normal, sympathectomized, and completely denervated pupils. They reported that no evidence was found that adrenalin or sympathetic excitation plays a part in the dilatation of the pupil seen either in hypoxia or asphyxia. It was suggested that the dilatation had both a neural and a non-neural component. The former is probably associated with a diminution of the tone of the third nerve center; the latter, with the formation of acid metabolites.

Hodes (35), on the other hand, felt that pupillary dilatation occurred only when the animal was moribund and the dilatation was caused by direct effects of hypoxia on the iris and not by neural factors. Hoorens (36) in 1948 emphasized that hemic hypoxia, anoxic hypoxia, and asphyxia all produced a marked mydriasis. He felt their action was due in part to a central neurogenic mechanism and in part to a purely peripheral one.

Flicker fusion frequency (FFF).—The frequency at which an interrupted or flickering light is perceived as a steady light is known as the fusion frequency of flickering light (FFF). It may be determined by measuring the number of light and dark intervals, or cycles, per second at which fusion occurs. A number of workers have studied the effect of hypoxia on this phenomenon.

Seitz (64) in 1940 reported that hypoxia produced by breathing gas mixtures low in oxygen caused a considerable decrease in FFF. Lilienthal and Fugitt (39) studied the effects of small amounts of COHb (hemic hypoxia) on men already under conditions of anoxic hypoxia. Increments in COHb of the order of 5–10 per cent resulted in appreciable deterioration of FFF at altitudes of 5,000 feet (1,525 meters) and 6,000 feet (1,830 meters), which alone do not affect this phenomenon. These authors stated that FFF is usually impaired at altitudes of from 9,000 feet (2,745 meters) to 12,000 feet (3,660 meters).

Simonson and Winchell (67) found that when men breathed 14 per cent oxygen, corresponding to an approximate altitude of 10,000 feet (3,050 meters), a significant decrease of FFF developed within twelve minutes in thirteen subjects. In 1954 Rokseth and Lorentzen (57) carried out experiments on twenty-five healthy human subjects ranging in age from twenty to twenty-five years. They were subjected to a simulated altitude of 10,000 feet (3,050 meters) but were also given alcohol (doses of 0.5–0.7 g/kg body weight). In most subjects the combination of alcohol and hypoxia caused a greater decrease in FFF than did hypoxia alone. The effect appeared to be a simple additive one.

Adler and Ivy and their associates (1) in 1950 found a gradual deterioration of FFF following repeated exposure to altitude. The subjects reported an increasing "feeling of tiredness." It was felt that FFF might be used as a criterion of central nervous fatigue.

Fatigue of accommodation and of convergence.—Several workers have shown that hypoxia may cause fatigue of accommodation and of convergence. Wilmer and Berens (76), working with rebreather tests, called attention to this phenomenon in 1918; they found increased fatigability at 15,000 feet (4,500 meters). McFarland (43) in 1937 also found a significant increase in fatigue at about the same altitude in the Chilean Andes as reported by Wilmer and Berens. In the same year, Furuya (21) reported a decrease in range of accommodation which began about 16,400 feet (5,000 meters). Giardini (28) in 1949, working with eight subjects, found that a simulated altitude of about 13,000 feet (3,900 meters) produced a significant fatigue of accommodation.

Extraocular muscles.—Considerable work has been reported on the effect of hypoxia on the phorias. The literature in this field has been reviewed by McFarland *et al.* (48). In this monograph only the effect of hypoxia on orthophoric subjects will be considered.

McFarland *et al.* (43) found that the test for 40 cm. vision revealed an increase of the average deviation from orthophoria at 20,000 feet (6,000 meters), which was usually in the direction of an insufficiency of convergence. This actually was measurable at 9,200 feet (2,800 meters). He observed similar changes in a low-oxygen chamber (45).

Wilmer and Berens (76) reported a decrease in adduction, abduction, and sursumvergence (upward movement) at 20,000 feet (6,000 meters). They measured the field of binocular fixation in a group of men with normal muscle balance and discovered that 7 per cent of these men suffered deterioration during hypoxia. After testing the eyes with a stereoscope, they reported that there was a change in fusion ability in two of six persons.

Co-ordinated ocular movements.—In 1937 McFarland, Knehr, and Berens (52) reported the effect of oxygen deprivation on ocular movements during reading and during fixation. Photographic technics were used in this study. They found that in reading the eyes did not co-ordinate as well at 18,000 feet (5,485 meters) and that it took longer to read a given line. There was also a general tendency toward diminished precision of ocular fixation. Interestingly enough, they observed certain latent defects during periods of hypoxia in a number of subjects, who apparently had normal ocular muscle balance.

Effect of recompression on visual functions.—It is of interest that visual functions may be increased temporarily above the normal level after recompression. For example, Schubert (61) has found that recompression from about 23,000 feet (7,000 meters) to about 16,400 feet (5,000 meters) produced an increased sensitivity to visual discrimination. This probably may be regarded as a supernormal phase, a physiologic phenomenon not infrequently observed in nerve functions.

HEARING

In progressive anoxic hypoxia, the sense of hearing is the last to disappear. Henderson (32) in 1918 and Bagby (3) in 1921, using both the rebreather method for inducing hypoxia and the low-pressure chamber, could detect no change in hearing caused by oxygen want until either all the other, higher cerebral centers were impaired or just before collapse took place. In 1904 Aggazzotti (2), working with a low-pressure chamber, reported, however, a decrease in auditory sensitivity both in human beings and in guinea pigs at a barometric pressure of 420 mm. Hg, corresponding to an approximate altitude of 15,500 feet (4,720 meters).

Barcroft (4) reported that some of the members of his expedition suffered from auditory disturbances at Cerro de Pasco, situated at an altitude of 14,200 feet (4,300 meters); and Richter (56), during a Himalayan expedition, also noticed alteration in hearing. Raffo (55) in 1934, too, observed a decrease in auditory sensitivity in residents of the Andes at an altitude of 13,600 feet (4,150 meters).

Using a Douglas bag for inducing hypoxia, Gellhorn and Spiesman (26) in 1935 reported that, if 10 per cent oxygen or less were inhaled for ten to thirty minutes, there was an increase in the hearing threshold, which often lasted for several hours, depending upon the severity of the hypoxia, the duration of the experiment, and the sensitivity of the subject.

McFarland (42) in 1937 reported that the auditory threshold for eight different frequencies was about twice as high at Morococha, Peru, altitude of 14,900 feet (4,540 meters), as at Lima (approximately at sea level). In a subsequent paper (43) in which he reported studies made during acclimatization, he found that at 17,500 feet (5,300 meters) the threshold for the four highest frequencies was significantly increased.

Studies made on the auditory threshold on native residents in the Chilean Andes (altitudes from 15,000 to 17,000 feet—4570 meters to 5,180 meters) by McFarland (44) showed that the threshold was six to eight decibels higher than for workmen at sea level; the results were statistically significant. The variability of response was also greater in the high–altitude group.

Cochlear potentials.—Weaver *et al.* (75) in 1949 studied the effects of oxygen deprivation upon cochlear potentials in cats. They reported that only severe grades of hypoxia (4 per cent oxygen or less), corresponding to altitudes over 40,000 feet (12,200 meters), caused deleterious effects. As the hypoxia developed, the cochlear potentials underwent a rapid initial loss and then leveled off; with extreme hypoxia, the losses amounted to forty decibels or more.

Bornschein and Krejci (7) in the same year, also using cats, found that hypoxia caused a decrease of cochlear potentials and that in severe grades of hypoxia the changes produced were not always reversible. They concluded that the effect on cochlear potentials was a primary sequel of the hypoxia and not a secondary one following a disturbed circulation.

In 1953 Wing *et al.* (77), working on cochlear microphonics, observed that they were reversibly reduced when arterial oxygen content was decreased to values roughly between the limits of 6–9 volumes per cent. Davis *et al.* (15) in 1955 reported studies on cochlear potentials in guinea pigs following intracochlear injections of certain substances (sodium cyanide and sodium azide) during hypoxia. They concluded that the summating potential was affected by hypoxia and by ionic change. In the same year, Tonndorf and his coworkers (70) studied the combined effect of sound and oxygen deprivation (10–8 per cent oxygen) upon microphonics in guinea pigs. Various combinations of sounds were produced (1,000 c.p.s., 130 db.,

1 min). There was some decrease in the cochlear microphonics, the effect depending upon the degree of oxygen deprivation and on the magnitude of the simultaneous sound. It appears, then, that a rather severe grade of hypoxia must exist before there is a significant change in cochlear potentials.

Vestibular sensations.—Little work has been reported on this phenomenon. Raffo (55) in 1934 found a heightened sensitivity to artificial stimulation of the vestibular apparatus. On the other hand, Ruff and Strughold (58) in 1942 reported that hypoxia caused a decrease in vestibular sensitivity. Gellhorn and Spiesman (26) showed that vestibular reflexes in man, measured by the number of nystagmic movements following caloric stimulation, are altered to a lesser degree than certain other sensory functions, such as hearing and vision. They reported that inhalation of 10 per cent oxygen from seven to fifty minutes caused a decrease in nystagmic responses only in some of their subjects. It would seem that more work is needed on the effect of hypoxia on vestibular sensations.

TACTUAL SENSITIVITY

The effect of altitude on tactual sensitivity was studied by Loewy and Wittkower (40) following an ascent, without physical strain, from an altitude of that of Davos—5,100 feet (1,550 meters) —to one of 8,700 feet (2,650 meters). An increased effect of the dermographic and chemical stimuli was noted. The sensitivity to pressure on the skin was slightly impaired, as was the two-point threshold. The explanation they gave for their findings was that the oxygen want stimulated the vasomotor center, causing a peripheral vasoconstriction. It seems, however, that this work needs confirmation, since it is questionable whether the vasomotor center would be stimulated at 8,700 feet.

Hartmann (31), in acclimatized subjects in the Himalayas, found that below an altitude of 23,000 feet (7,000 meters) skin sensitivity was not impaired. He felt, on the basis of experimental evidence obtained from work done in a low-pressure chamber, that in non-acclimatized subjects the critical changes in skin sensitivity occur at altitudes approximately 5,000 feet (1,525 meters) lower than they would in acclimatized subjects. According to his work, then, changes would not occur in the average person until a height of about 18,000 feet (5,485 meters) was attained. This, indeed seems more likely than the findings reported by Loewy and Wittkower (above). Furthermore, Strughold (69) in 1936 found an increased threshold of sensitivity at a simulated altitude of about 18,000 feet (5,485 meters) in non-acclimatized subjects; this also confirms the findings of Hartmann.

On the other hand, Fleisch and Grandjean (19) in 1944 observed some changes in skin sensitivity at lower levels. Working with eighteen subjects at an altitude on the Jungfraujoch of 11,500 feet (3,450 meters) , they found a lowering of the threshold for pressure. This returned to normal in about a week.

TASTE AND SMELL

Little experimental work has been reported on the effect of hypoxia on taste and smell. Quantitative data are difficult to obtain. These two special senses are so closely associated that unless especial precautions are observed when experiments involving either one is performed any results reported must be accepted with hesitation.

Hingston (34) , medical officer for the 1924 Mount Everest Expedition, reported that at an altitude of 19,000 feet (5,800 meters) two members of the expedition noticed an impairment of the sense of taste. When they descended to 16,500 feet (5,100 meters) , taste was restored. Richter (56) , during a Himalayan expedition in 1932, reported alterations in taste at an altitude of 16,500 feet. His findings, therefore, corresponded with those of Hingston.

Fleisch and Grandjean (19) in 1944, working with eighteen subjects on the Jungfraujoch, about 11,500 feet (3,450 meters) , found a lowering of the threshold to tastes (bitter, sour, sweet, and salty) . At higher altitudes—over 17,000 feet (about 5,000 meters) —the threshold was raised.

No reports in the literature could be found dealing with the effect of hypoxia on the sense of smell. It may be that during the observations of the effect of high altitudes on taste just quoted, smell was also affected by the hypoxia. More, well-controlled work is needed on the effect of hypoxia on both taste and smell.

While such studies might appear to be of academic interest only, it is worthwhile recalling that occasionally patients who have suffered a skull injury lose their sense of smell. This distressing condition may be transient in nature but is sometimes permanent. It is possible that in these latter cases the skull injury may have damaged irreparably the blood vessels supplying the olfactory center, so that the loss of smell is due to a local anemic hypoxia.

PAIN

There is little data on the effect of hypoxia on pain. Stokes *et al.* (68) in 1948 studied the effect of anoxic hypoxia and of hypercapnia on perception of thermal cutaneous pain in man; fourteen males whose ages ranged from twenty to forty-five years were used. It was observed that breathing 10 per cent oxygen did not affect the pain threshold significantly.

Five per cent carbon dioxide and 7.5 per cent carbon dioxide elevated the threshold of pain; the former, by 13 per cent and the latter, by 28 per cent. It was felt that these effects were due to central action and not to any peripheral effects on the pain end-organs.

In 1961 Bullard and Snyder (8) determined the threshold of pain on two mammalian species, the rat (non-hibernating animal) and the ground squirrel (hibernating animal). The response to thermal pain in the rat was decreased by breathing 7.5 per cent oxygen and abolished by 5 per cent oxygen. The ground squirrel showed no alteration of response until the oxygen percentage was lowered to 2.5 per cent. It is known, of course, that mammalian species which hibernate withstand more severe hypoxia than do non-hibernating animals.

More work is obviously needed on the effect of hypoxia on pain.

RÉSUMÉ OF THE EFFECT OF HYPOXIA ON THE SPECIAL SENSES

From the practical point of view of the effect of hypoxia on the special senses, the effect on the eye is doubtless the most important. There is evidence that losses of accommodation and visual acuity occur at relatively low altitudes and, further, aftereffects may follow exposure to severe degrees of hypoxia. Since pilots now use oxygen masks or pressurized cabins when flying above 8,000 feet (2,440 meters), the effect of hypoxia on the eye is no longer as important as it once was.

Nearly all observers agree that the ear is the most resistant of all to hypoxia, and, for practical purposes, it probably functions until psychomotor collapse occurs. Little work has been reported on vestibular sensations. There is some evidence that hypoxia may cause a slight decrease in sensitivity.

The sense of touch is probably somewhat affected at altitudes beyond 18,000 feet (5,500 meters), but this is of no great practical importance.

There is little data on the effect of hypoxia on pain. One study on man has shown that the perception of thermal cutaneous pain is not significantly altered by breathing 10 per cent oxygen.

Nothing authoritatively can be said about taste and smell. While the effect of hypoxia on these two senses is not especially important for practical purposes, nevertheless, as previously mentioned, a careful study of the effects of hypoxia on them might provide a better understanding in certain disorders of both these senses.

REFERENCES

1. ADLER, H. F., *et al.* 1950. *J. Aviat. Med.*, 21: 221.
2. AGGAZZOTTI, A. 1904. *Arch. Ital. Biol.* (Turin), 41: 69.
3. BAGBY, E. 1921. *J. Comp. Psychol.*, 1: 97.
4. BARCROFT, J. 1925. *The Respiratory Function of the Blood,* Part I, "Lessons from High Altitudes," p. 19. Cambridge: Cambridge University Press.
5. BERGER, C., and BOJE, O. 1937. *Skand. Arch. Physiol.*, 77: 129.
6. BERT, PAUL. 1878. *La Pression barometrique.* Paris: Masson.
7. BORNSCHEIN, H., and KREJCI, F. 1949. *Mschr. Hals Nas. Ohr.*, 83: 386.
8. BULLARD, R. W., and SNYDER, J. L. 1961. *Proc. Soc. Exp. Biol. Med.*, 106: 341.
9. BUNGE, E. 1935. *Arch. Augenh.*, 109: 452.
10. ———. 1936. *Ibid.*, 110: 189.
11. BUSCALOSSI, A. 1938. *Ann. Ottal.*, 66: 292.
12. CRAIK, K. J. W. 1940. *Nature*, 145: 512.
13. CUSICK, P. L.; BENSON, O. O.; and BOOTHBY, W. M. 1940. *Proc. Mayo Clin.*, 15: 500.
14. DAMMERT, cited by C. MONGE. 1929. *Les Erythremies de l'altitude*, pp. xi–134. Paris: Masson et Cie.
15. DAVIS, H., *et al.* 1955. *Fed. Proc.*, 14: 35.
16. DUQUET, J.; DUMONT, P.; and BAILLIART, J. P. 1947. *J. Aviation Med.*, 18: 516.
17. EVANS, J. N., and McFARLAND, R. A. 1938. *Amer. J. Ophthal.*, 21: 968.
18. FISHER, F. P., and JONGBLOED, J. 1935. *Arch. Augenh.*, 109: 452.
19. FLEISCH, A., and GRANDJEAN, E. 1944. *Helvet. Physiol. Pharmacol. Acta* 12 (Suppl. III) : 35.
20. FURUYA, G. 1936. *Acta Soc. Ophthal. Jap.*, 40: 2432.
21. ———. 1937. *Acta Soc. Ophthal. Jap.*, 41: 142.
22. ———. *Ibid.* P. 415, cited in *Ber. Ges. Physiol.* (1937), 103: 465.
23. GELLHORN, E. 1936. *Amer. J. Physiol.*, 115: 679.
24. GELLHORN, E., and HAILMAN, H. 1943. *Fed. Proc.*, 2: 122.
25. GELLHORN, E., and LEVIN, J. 1945. *Amer. J. Physiol.*, 143: 282.
26. GELLHORN, E., and SPIESMAN, I. G. 1935. *Amer. J. Physiol.*, 112: 519.
27. ———. *Ibid.*, p. 620.
28. GIARDINI, A. 1949. *Riv. Med. Aero.*, 12: 511.
29. GOLDMAN, H., and SCHUBERT, G. 1933. *Arch. Augenh.*, 107: 216.
30. HALSTEAD, W. C. 1945. *Science*, 101: 615.
    ———. *Ibid.*, 102: 159.
31. HARTMANN, A. H. 1935. *Verh. Deutsch. Ges. Inn. Med.*, 47: 48.

32. HENDERSON, Y., *et al.* 1918. *J.A.M.A.,* **71**: 1382.
33. HICKMAN, J. B., and FRAYSER, R. Feb., 1959. *Sch. Aviat. Med.* (Randolph AFB, Texas) , 58–155.
34. HINGSTON, R. W. G. 1925. *Geog. J.,* **65**: 4.
35. HODES, R. 1940. *Amer. J. Physiol.,* **131**: 144.
36. HOORENS, A. 1948. *Arch. Int. Pharm. Ther.,* **77**: 464.
37. KRAUSE, A. C. 1934. *The Biochemistry of the Eye,* p. 88. Baltimore: Johns Hopkins Press.
38. KYRIELEIS, W.; KYRIELEIS, A.; and SIEGERT, P. 1935. *Arch. Augenh.,* **109**: 178.
39. LILIENTHAL, J. J., JR., and FUGITT, C. H. 1946. *Amer. J. Physiol.,* **145**: 359.
40. LOEWY, A., and WITTKOWER, E. 1933. *Arch. Ges. Physiol.,* **233**: 622.
41. McDONALD, R., and ADLER, F. H. 1939. *Arch. Ophthal.,* **22**: 980.
42. McFARLAND, R. A. 1937. *J. Comp. Psychol.,* **23**: 191.
43. ———. *Ibid.,* p. 227.
44. ———. *Ibid.,* **24**: 189.
45. ———. May, 1938. *The Effects of Oxygen Deprivation (High Altitude) on the Human Organism.* Report 13, U.S. Department of Commerce, Bureau of Air Commerce.
46. McFARLAND, R. A., and EDWARDS, H. T. 1937. *J. Aviat. Med.,* **8**: 3.
47. McFARLAND, R. A., and EVANS, J. N. 1939. *Amer. J. Physiol.,* **127**: 37.
48. McFARLAND, R. A.; EVANS, J. N.; and HALPERIN, M. 1941. *Arch. Ophthal.,* **26**: 886.
49. McFARLAND, R. A., and FORBES, W. 1940. *J. Gen. Physiol.,* **24**: 69.
50. McFARLAND, R. A., and HALPERIN, M. H. 1940. *J. Gen. Physiol.,* **23**: 613.
51. McFARLAND, R. A.; HURVICH, L. M.; and HALPERIN, M. H. 1943. *Amer. J. Physiol.,* **140**: 354.
52. McFARLAND, R. A.; KNEHR, C. A.; and BERENS, C. 1937. *J. Exp. Psychol.,* **21**: 1.
53. MONGE, C. 1929. *Les Erythremies de l'altitude.* Paris: Masson et Cie.
54. PINSON, E. A. 1940. *J. Aviat. Med.,* **11**: 108.
55. RAFFO, E. 1934. *Rev. Sud. Am. Med. Chir.,* **5**: 91.
56. RICHTER, cited by A. LOEWY. 1932. *Physiologie des Höhenklimas.* Berlin: Julius Springer.
57. ROKSETH, R., and LORENTZEN, F. V. 1954. *J. Appl. Physiol.,* **6**: 559.
58. RUFF, S., and STRUGHOLD, H. 1942. *Compendium of Aviation Med.*
59. SAUER, W. W. 1924. *Ohio Med. J.,* **20**: 629.
60. SCHMIDT, I. 1937. *Luftfahrtmedizin.,* **2**: 55.
61. SCHUBERT, G. 1932. *Pflueger Arch. Ges. Physiol.,* **231**: 1.
62. SCHUBERT, G. 1935. *Physiologie des Menschen im Flugzeug.* Berlin: Julius Springer.
63. ———. 1937. *Pflueger Arch. Physiol.,* **77**: 129.
64. SEITZ, C. P. 1940. *Arch. Psychol.,* **257**.
65. ———. *Ibid.,* **287**.

66. Seitz, C. P., and Rosenthal, C. M. 1940. *Psychol. Bull.*, **37**: 462.
67. Simonson, E., and Winchell, P. 1951. *J. Appl. Physiol.*, **3**: 637.
68. Stokes, J., III; Chapman, W. P.; and Smith, L. H. 1948. *J. Clin. Invest.*, **27**: 299.
69. Strughold, H. 1936. *Luftfahrtmedizin*, **1**: 192.
70. Tonndorf, J.; Hyde, R. W.; and Brogan, F. A. September, 1955. *USAF Sch. Aviat. Med.*, Report No. 55–32.
71. Velhagen, K., Jr. 1935. *Arch. Augenh.*, **109**: 40.
72. Vishnevskiy, N. A., and Tsyrlin, B. A. 1935. *Fiziol. Zh.*, **18**: 237.
———. 1936. Abstract in *J. Aviat. Med.*, **7**: 215.
73. Wald, G., et al. 1942. *J. Gen. Physiol.*, **25**: 891.
74. Weaver, E. M. F. 1943. *J. Aviat. Med.*, **14**: 289.
75. Weaver, E. G., et al. 1949. *Amer. J. Physiol.*, **159**: 199.
76. Wilmer, W. H., and Berens, C. 1918. *J.A.M.A.*, **71**: 1394.
77. Wing, K. G., et al. 1953. *J. Comp. Physiol. Psychol.*, **46**: 352.

CHAPTER XIX

RESISTANCE TO HYPOXIA

A great amount of research has been done in an attempt to find some procedure or therapeutic agent which would increase tolerance to hypoxia and so improve physical and mental performance at altitude. It would be highly desirable, of course, to increase resistance to hypoxia not only at altitude but also in certain clinical conditions.

Space does not permit a detailed review of all the pertinent literature. Suffice it to say that many different animals and methods have been used. Some of the work has been done on man. Only brief mention can be made of some of the typical procedures employed.

ENDOCRINE GLANDS

Adrenal glands.—It was shown by Britton and Kline (15) in 1945 that adrenalectomy decreased resistance to hypoxia in rats. Several investigators (73, 125) have demonstrated that Kendall's extract (which is a crude substance) markedly increased resistance to hypoxia. It has been shown too that adrenocorticotrophin (ACTH) enables an animal to withstand oxygen want better (79).

Sobel and Sideman (120) in 1960 found that guinea pigs treated with cortisone had increased resistance to hypoxia. In the same year DeBias and Paschkis (34) reported that resistance to hypoxia was not increased when cortisone was administered to adrenalectomized guinea pigs; however, if the thyroid was also removed, resistance to hypoxia was increased.

Gellhorn and Packer (46), working with rabbits, reported that, because adrenalin produces a hyperglycemia, tolerance to hypoxia is increased. However, indeterminate results of the effect of adrenalin on resistance to hypoxia have been reported by several workers (17, 23, 124).

It was shown by Binet and Strumza (13) that ephedrine (a synthetic compound related in chemical constitution and in physiologic

350

action to epinephrin) and related compounds delayed respiratory failure during sudden and severe hypoxia.

Thyroid.—In general, it may be stated that substances which depress cellular oxidation aid the animal organism in withstanding hypoxia. It would be expected, then, that thyroidectomy (7, 77, 121), a state of hypothyroidism (132), or substances which depress thyroid activity, such as thiourea (49, 77) and thiouracil (49, 50, 51, 64), would aid the animal in resisting the effects of hypoxia. On the other hand, elevation of metabolic rate decreases tolerance to hypoxia; examples are: hyperthyroid states (132), the thyroid stimulating hormone [TSH] (107), thyroxine, and dinitrophenol (77).

Estrogens.—Davis and Jones (32), working with rats, found that estrogens (diethylstilbestrol) increased resistance to hypoxia. However, Goldsmith *et al.* (49), also working with rats, found no effect.

Progesterone and testosterone.—Neither one of these compounds, according to Davis and Jones (32), had any effect on hypoxic tolerance.

Insulin.—It was reported by Selle (115) in 1944 that insulin decreases resistance to hypoxia. This finding would be expected, since it is known that hypoglycemia decreases tolerance to hypoxia.

Hypophysis.—It was shown by Vacca and Boeri (127) in 1953 that hypophysectomy decreased tolerance to hypoxia in rats.

CENTRAL NERVOUS SYSTEM STIMULANTS AND DEPRESSANTS

Amphetamine (alpha-methyl-phenethylamine).—In 1940 Dill *et al.* (35) worked with human subjects at simulated altitudes from 10,000 feet (3,050 meters) to 24,000 feet (7,315 meters). Just prior to the experiment, 20 mg. of amphetamine was administered subcutaneously. Their conclusion was that under some conditions of stress, if the duration was not too long, amphetamine proved useful to aviators. There was, however, no evidence of its usefulness in combating ill effects of acute hypoxia on the respiratory system. Russell (110) in 1947, also working with man, reported that amphetamine did not increase resistance to hypoxia. Kessler *et al.* (68) in 1943 observed that amphetamine increased resistance to hypoxia as shown by a study of the electroencephalogram of rats.

Cocaine.—Loehning *et al.* (80) in 1953, working with rats at simulated altitudes of 14,000 feet (4,270 meters) to 22,000 feet (6,705 meters), observed that large doses of cocaine (100 mg. to 200 mg/kg) produced a decrease in tolerance to hypoxia. Small doses (50 mgm/kg) had no effect. In a later study (81), the authors used young rats; the administration of cocaine produced indeterminate results. These reports are of interest since the Andean natives use the coca leaf extensively.

Caffeine.—Emerson and Van Liere (41), working with mice, reported that caffeine did not increase hypoxic resistance.

Chlorpromazine 10 (3 dimethylaminopropyl) -2-chlorphenothiazine hydrochloride.—This is a central nervous depressant. The effect of this drug has been studied in its relation to tolerance to hypoxia by several workers. Dawson and Hiestand (33) in 1955 used mice which were subjected to complete hypoxia. They reported that there was some increased hypoxic resistance. In 1956 Tabusse and his co-worker (122) subjected guinea pigs to a simulated altitude of 42,640 feet (13,000 meters) and found that resistance to hypoxia was decreased. They were working, of course, with an extremely low-oxygen tension. DeBias and Paschkis (34) in 1960, working with adrenalectomized animals at 27,000 feet (8,230 meters), found that chlorpromazine had no effect. These workers, too, used a fairly severe degree of hypoxia.

Diphenylhydantoin (*dilantin sodium*).—There seems to be a general agreement that this preparation increases resistance to hypoxia (40, 50, 61).

Alcohol.—It has been observed that full narcotic doses of ethyl alcohol in mice significantly increase hypoxic resistance (41).

CHANGES IN HYDROGEN-ION CONCENTRATION

Carbon dioxide.—Carbon dioxide aids in increasing resistance to hypoxia. It may benefit the organism by: (*a*) increasing minute-volume of respiration and blood pressure, (*b*) producing dilatation of the cerebral vessels, and (*c*) causing a slight shift to the right in the dissociation curve of oxyhemoglobin.

Childs and Henderson and their collaborator (27) wrote that the results obtained on Pike's Peak suggested that carbon dioxide might be beneficial at altitude. Since that time a number of workers (67, 69, 71, 104, 109) have shown that carbon dioxide, in correct proportions, increases tolerance to hypoxia in both man and animals. It has been reported (90), however, that at the extreme altitude of 40,000 feet (12,190 meters) the addition of 10 per cent carbon dioxide to inspired oxygen was without favorable physiologic effect.

Ammonium chloride.—It is now generally accepted that anoxic hypoxia is accompanied by alkalosis. It has been postulated that if a mild state of acidosis would be produced at altitude, the subject would be more comfortable and that both mental and physical performance would be improved. It is known that ammonium chloride in effective doses produces an acidotic condition of the body.

Considerable evidence has been accumulated during the past thirty years that ammonium chloride has a beneficial effect on the animal organism at altitude, either by increasing tolerance to altitude, by hastening the process of acclimatization, or by improving work capacity. This has been shown by a number of workers (1, 5, 6, 28, 37, 52, 56, 84, 109) ; all of these used man as a subject. It has been shown also that following administration of ammonium chloride, dogs more rapidly adapt to low-oxygen tensions (48).

Not all workers have reported beneficial effects from the use of ammonium chloride, as far as prevention of mountain sickness is concerned. Barron *et al.* (8) administered ammonium chloride (15 gm.) to six of twelve men who ascended by automobile to an elevation of 15,600 feet (4,755 meters) within a period of eight hours. They concluded that the ingestion of this salt was more of a handicap than an advantage, since three of the six men who took it had severe mountain sickness, while only two of the six men who served as controls were similarly affected.

As would be expected, sodium bicarbonate decreases tolerance to hypoxia (84).

In summary, although ammonium chloride is of benefit at altitude, so far as the authors are aware, this salt is used neither by the mountain climber nor by airplane crew and passengers.

Fasting.—The fasting state is usually associated with acidosis. It has been shown by several workers that fasting affects resistance to hypoxia. Langier and his collaborators (74, 78) in 1943 found that rats fasted for from twelve to twenty-four hours showed a decreased ability to withstand hypoxia. If fasted longer than that period, however, they showed an increased resistance. The authors attributed the latter finding to a lower basal metabolic rate.

Several experimenters have worked with cats. Smith *et al.* (118) found that if these animals lost from 15 to 20 per cent of their body weight, their ability to withstand hypoxia was increased up to 50 per cent. Smith and Oster (117) somewhat later, also working with cats, found that what they termed complete starvation increased their resistance to hypoxia. This probably could be explained by a decreased metabolic rate.

In 1945 King *et al.* (70), working with human beings, found that omitting lunch before a flight decreased tolerance to oxygen want.

PHYSICAL FACTORS

Hypothermia.—During the last two decades or so, it has been rather conclusively shown that during hypothermia resistance to hypoxia may be significantly increased. A good many investigators have studied this problem; work had been done on: rats (29, 31, 65, 106), mice (3, 59, 72, 83), guinea pigs (86, 88), ground squirrels (19), puppies (87), and dogs (72). The increased resistance to hypoxia doubtless is due to the lowering of oxygen consumption.

Hyperthermia.—It has been shown that hyperthermia significantly decreases resistance to hypoxia. The work was done on rats (65) and on guinea pigs (86). Since an elevation of temperature increases oxygen consumption, it would be expected that tolerance to hypoxia would be decreased.

Humidity.—There is considerable evidence, at least in mice and rats, that moist air offers an increased resistance to hypoxia (97, 98, 103). Phillips *et al.* (98) observed that mice placed in a moist saturated atmosphere at ambient temperatures between 22°–20° C. withstood hypoxia longer than control animals. The authors pointed out that a reduced temperature and an increased humidity lower energy requirements and rate of heat loss by vaporization. Some physiologists might question the explanation given for the beneficial effect of increased humidity. The same workers (97) noted that for mice in an ambient temperature of −10° C. and breathing air entirely free of moisture the maximal survival altitude was 410 mm. Hg; but, if the air was 100 per cent saturated, they survived to an altitude of 180 mm. Hg.

More work is needed on the effect of humidity on hypoxic tolerance. The problem is of clinical significance because the control of humidity is important in the management of premature infants who suffer from hypoxia.

CARBOHYDRATES

It has been shown by numerous workers (14, 16, 22, 23, 24, 30, 38, 53, 58, 59, 60, 70, 76, 85, 89, 93, 94, 95, 100, 105) that ingestion of carbohydrates increases tolerance to anoxic hypoxia. Although some investigators (12, 39, 54, 62, 114) have reported indeterminate results, there is a preponderance of evidence that carbohydrates increase hypoxic resistance. Since on a carbohydrate diet more carbon dioxide is produced, the respiratory center is stimulated, and pulmonary ventilation is increased. Carbohydrates also furnish a good source of anaerobic energy.

Campbell (22) in 1938 reported that rats fed on a pure carrot diet showed a significant protection against acute oxygen want. His work has been confirmed by other workers (30, 59, 89) but not by all (130). Campbell published several other papers (23, 24) on the effect of a carbohydrate diet on tolerance to hypoxia. He felt that his observations would have a definite clinical value, since it might be possible to work out a diet which would be beneficial for patients suffering from oxygen deprivation. In fact, he actually suggested several such diets.

Several European investigators (47, 57, 116), working with man, have reported that glucose has favorable effects in preventing mountain sickness and is also of help during mountain climbing. Pugh and Ward (102) called attention to the beneficial effects of glucose on the members of the various Mount Everest expeditions of the early nineteen-fifties.

King *et al.* (70) in 1945 reported that a significant gain in altitude tolerance was afforded by pre-flight and in-flight meals high in carbohydrate content. They felt that the adoption of diets rich in carbohydrates would be a practical procedure.

McFarland (85) reviewed the matter of possible beneficial effects of a high-carbohydrate diet at altitude and concluded that such a diet would not be of significant aid. He pointed out that pressurized cabins are now used in most planes and an increase in ceiling of 1,000–2,000 feet (305–610 meters) would have no practical importance.

Lawton (76) has pointed out the relative danger of hypoglycemia following a meal high in carbohydrates. He emphasizes that meals rich in carbohydrates are characterized by fast absorption and quick utilization. If a significant amount of hypoglycemia does occur, it might have a deleterious effect. Lawton suggests a pre-flight meal of high-protein content. Some of the protein is, of course, converted to carbohydrates, so that the subject would still receive some benefit from the carbohydrates.

MISCELLANEOUS FACTORS

Enzymes.—The effect of cytochrome C on resistance to hypoxia has been studied in rats (10, 29, 113) and mice (111). The results reported were negative. Two studies made on man (101, 108), however, appear to show some increase in resistance to hypoxia.

Studies have also been made on adenosine-tri-phosphate (ATP) and on an enzyme inhibitor, di-isopropyl-fluoro-phosphate (DFP). The latter compound had no effect on acute hypoxia (45). On the other hand, it was observed that survival time in hypoxia is closely related to the cerebral ATP concentration (112).

Vitamins.—Some studies have been made on the effect of vitamins on resistance to hypoxia. It has been reported that nicotinic acid increases tolerance to hypoxia in rats (20). Rats which are deficient in vitamin B_1 show a greater ability to withstand hypoxia than do animals on a normal diet (25, 26, 55). Although vitamin-B complex increases tolerance to altitude, vitamin B_2 or B_{12} added to the normal diet has no beneficial effect. It was observed that rats which were deficient in tocopherol (vitamin E) were less resistant to hypoxia, whereas animals treated with tocopherol showed a marked increase to hypoxia (63, 123).

Methylene blue.—Peterson (96) reported over twenty years ago that methylene blue increased the tolerance of rats to hypoxia. Beneficial effects have been reported by other workers on man (18) and on the dog (75). One worker, however, reported that this agent did not benefit man (109). It is well to recall that in large doses methylene blue is distinctly toxic.

Although methylene blue is not as effective in cyanide poisoning (histotoxic hypoxia) as are the nitrites, nevertheless it is of distinct aid. The methemoglobin formed binds the cyanide.

Adrenergic and cholinergic drugs.—In general, it may be said that cholinergic drugs increase resistance to hypoxia and adrenergic drugs have the opposite effect (41).

A number of investigators have studied the effect of the chemical mediator, acetylcholine (ACh), on resistance to hypoxia. The work was done on guinea pigs (43, 44, 122). On the whole, the results were indeterminate, since two groups of workers (43, 44) found that ACh increased resistance to hypoxia slightly, but one group (122) could find no effect.

Neostigmine, a parasympathetic-mimetic compound, has been shown to have prophylactic effects against hypoxia (40).

PRODUCTION OF POLYCYTHEMIA OTHER THAN BY ANOXIC HYPOXIA

a) Transfusion of red blood cells.—It has been demonstrated in both man (91, 92) and in animals (4, 21) that transfusion of red blood cells causes a significant increased resistance to hypoxia. At extreme altitudes, 31,000 feet [9,450 meters] (119) and 40,000 feet [12,190 meters] (130), however, transfusion of red blood cells was of no significant aid.

b) Carbon monoxide.—It was shown by Fenn (42) that if polycythemia had been produced previously by administration of small amounts of carbon monoxide, tolerance to hypoxia is increased. On the other hand, an appreciable amount of carbon monoxide in the blood may decrease resistance to hypoxia (7). This latter finding would be expected, since carbon monoxide produces an effect on the body similar to that of hemic hypoxia. Pitts and Pace (99) in 1947, working on the effect of carboxyhemoglobin on man, reported that a 1 per cent increase in the amount of carboxyhemoglobin in the blood was equivalent to an altitude increase of 335 feet.

c) Administration of cobalt chloride.—It has been known for more than three decades that the administration of cobalt chloride produces a polycythemia in animals. More recent work has confirmed the earlier findings (36). It is known also that cobalt chloride causes an increase in red blood cells in man; this preparation has been used for treating anemias in human beings (131). Polycythemia produced by cobalt enables an animal to withstand a more severe degree of hypoxia (36, 128).

It would be expected that an increase in the amount of hemoglobin would enable the animal organism to withstand hypoxia better. This would certainly be true during marginal conditions of hypoxia. It is obvious, however, that giving transfusions of red blood cells offers many technical difficulties and can hardly be considered as a practical procedure. Carbon monoxide is not a desirable agent since it has toxic qualities. Cobalt chloride is convenient to administer, but it may cause distressing gastrointestinal symptoms in many individuals. In fact, none of the three methods of producing polycythemia just mentioned is without fault.

ACCLIMATIZATION TO ANOXIC HYPOXIA

It has been known, of course, for many years that people who are acclimatized to altitude live more comfortably and are more efficient, both mentally and physically, than is the newcomer to altitude. There is much well-documented evidence that both acclimatized man and animals have a longer survival rate when exposed to acute hypoxia than the unacclimatized. Only a few studies will be cited.

It was shown by Thorn *et al.* (126) in 1946 that rats which have been acclimatized by discontinuous hypoxia to simulated altitudes of 18,000 feet (5,485 meters) and 26,000 feet (7,925 meters) had an increased survival rate compared to control rats when both were exposed to a simulated altitude of 34,000 feet (10,363 meters) for two hours.

Benzinger and Doring (11) in 1942 found that a stay for a few weeks at a height of 6,560 feet (2,000 meters) considerably increased the resistance when the individuals were subjected to a writing test at a simulated altitude of 26,240 feet (8,000 meters). In fact, they were able to write satisfactorily for ten minutes. An unacclimatized person could not live at that altitude for more than a few minutes.

Velasquez (129) in 1959 reported that natives living at 14,900 feet (4,542 meters), when subjected to simulated altitudes of 30,000 feet (9,144 meters) and 40,000 feet (12,192 meters), had much greater tolerance when subjected to certain tests than did men residing at sea level. To determine the end point of the test, in general, handwriting and ability to obey simple orders were used. This finding could, of course, be expected.

It has been pointed out by Luft (82) that even acclimatization at altitudes of 8,000 feet (2,440 meters) to 10,000 feet (3,050 meters) for ten to fourteen days is sufficient to raise the physiologic ceiling from 23,000 feet (7,010 meters) to 28,000 feet (8,535 meters). The beneficial effect lasts for over two weeks or so. This is a most interesting observation.

SUMMARY

On the whole, most of the researches concerning increasing resistance to hypoxia have proved to be largely of academic interest. Some of the agents or methods used, as has been seen, were of significant aid, especially transfusion of red blood cells, administration of cobalt chloride, a carbohydrate diet, and the ingestion of ammonium chloride. They probably would be of use during marginal conditions of hypoxia, but actually they have little practical value. None of them is without fault, as has been mentioned previously.

The authors are in agreement with Dr. Luft (82), who emphasized that the most impressive results in connection with increasing resistance to hypoxia were obtained by a relatively short stay at rather modest altitudes.

Luft points out that a sojourn from ten to fourteen days at an altitude from 8,000 to 10,000 feet will aid materially in increasing hypoxic tolerance. The beneficial effects so gained will last only about three weeks; however, if the subject exposes himself to the above-mentioned altitudes at least an hour or so a day, acclimatization will persist.

It is recognized that it would not always be convenient to acclimatize subjects initially in the manner described, but in these days of rapid travel it would not be difficult to transport individuals to high-plateau regions. Another method, of course, is to incarcerate subjects in a low-pressure chamber; obviously this method of producing acclimatization routinely leaves a great deal to be desired.

REFERENCES

1. ADLERSBERG, D., and PORGES, O. 1923; 1925. *Z. Ges. Exp. Med.,* **38:** 214; **45:** 167.
2. ADOLPH, E. F. 1948. *Amer. J. Physiol.,* **155:** 366.
3. ADOLPH, E. F., and GOLDSTEIN, J. 1959. *J. Appl. Physiol.,* **14:** 599.
4. BANCROFT, R. W. 1949. *Amer. J. Physiol.,* **156:** 158.
5. BARACH, A. L., *et al.* 1946. *J. Aviat. Med.,* **17:** 123.
6. ———. 1947. *Ibid.,* **18:** 139.
7. BARACH, A. L.; ECKMAN, M.; and MOLOMUT, N. 1941. *Amer. J. Med. Sci.,* **202:** 336.
8. BARRON, E. S., *et al.* 1937. *J. Clin. Invest.,* **16:** 541.
9. BARTLETT, R. G., JR., and ALTLAND, P. D. 1959. *J. Appl. Physiol.,* **14:** 785.
10. BENJAMIN, B.; STEINER, M.; and MILMAN, D. H. 1948. *Science,* **107:** 142.
11. BENZINGER, T., and DORING, H. 1942. *Luftfahrtmedizin,* **7:** 141.
    ———. 1943. Abstract from *Bull. War Med.,* **4:** 171.
12. BILLON, J. 1942. *Thèse Medicine.* Lyon.
13. BINET, L., and STRUMZA, M. 1938. *M. C. R. Acad. Sci.,* **207:** 543.
14. BLASIUS, W., and BAUREISEN, E. 1942. *Luftfahrtmedizin.,* **6:** 67.

15. Britton, S. W., and Kline, R. F. 1945. *Amer. J. Physiol.,* **145** (2) : 190.

16. ———. 1945. *Fed. Proc.,* **4:** 9.

17. Bronshtein, Y. E. 1944. *Amer. Rev. Soviet. Med.,* **1:** 314.

18. Brooks, M. M. 1948. *J. Aviat. Med.,* **19:** 298.
    ———. 1945. *Ibid.,* **16:** 250.

19. Bullard, R. W., and Funkhouser, G. E. 1960. *The Physiologist,* **3:** 33.

20. Calder, R. M. 1948. *Proc. Soc. Exp. Biol. Med.,* **68:** 642.

21. Campbell, J. A., Jr., 1928. *J. Physiol.,* **65:** 255.

22. ———. 1938. *Ibid.,* **93:** 31P.

23. ———. 1938. *Quart. J. Exp. Physiol.,* **28:** 231.

24. ———. 1939. *J. Physiol.,* **96:** 33P.

25. Charipper, H. A.; Goldsmith, E. D.; and Gordon, A. S. 1944. *Anat. Rec.,* **89** (4) : 44.

26. ———. 1945. *Amer. J. Physiol.,* **145:** 130.

27. Childs, S. B.; Hamlin, H.; and Henderson, Y. 1935. *Nature,* **135:** 457.

28. Christensen, E. H., and Smith, H. 1936. *Skand. Arch. Physiol.,* **73:** 155.

29. Christensen, W. R., and Clinton, M., Jr. 1947. *Proc. Soc. Exp. Biol. Med.,* **66:** 360.

30. Craven, C. W. 1951. *Amer. J. Physiol.,* **167:** 617.

31. Davidovic, J., and Wesley, I. 1959. *Amer. J. Physiol.,* **197:** 1357.

32. Davis, B. D., and Jones, B. F. 1943. *Endocrinology,* **33:** 23.

33. Dawson, J. F., Jr., and Hiestand, W. A. 1955. *Fed. Proc.,* **14:** 36.

34. DeBias, D. A., and Paschkis, K. E. 1960. *Fed. Proc.,* **19:** 154.

35. Dill, D. B., *et al.* 1940. *J. Aviat. Med.,* **11:** 181.

36. Dorrence, S. S., *et al.* 1943. *Amer. J. Physiol.,* **139:** 399.

37. Douglas, C. G.; Greene, C. R.; and Keigin, F. G. 1933. *J. Physiol.,* **78:** 404.

38. Eckman, M., *et al.* 1945. *J. Aviat. Med.,* **16:** 328.

39. Elias, H.; Kaunitz, H.; and Laub, R. 1933. *Exp. Med.,* **92:** 436.

40. Emerson, G. A. 1943. *Proc. Soc. Exp. Biol. Med.,* **54:** 252.

41. Emerson, G. A., and Van Liere, E. J. 1943. *J. Lab. Clin. Med.,* **28:** 700.

42. Fenn, W. D. 1948. *Proc. Amer. Phil. Soc.,* **92:** 144.

43. Franck, E., *et al.* 1948. *C. R. Soc. Biol.* (*Par.*) , **142:** 79.

44. Franck, E.; Grandpierre, R.; and Didon, P. 1948. *Toulouse Med.,* **49:** 10.

45. Freedman, A. M., and Himwich, H. E. 1948. *Science,* **108:** 41.

46. Gellhorn, E., and Packer, A. C. 1939. *Proc. Soc. Exp. Biol. Med.,* **41:** 345.

47. Gilbert, G. 1931. *Deutsch. Med. Wschr.,* **57:** 500.

48. Goebel, F., and Marczewski, S. 1938. *Acta Biol. Exp.* (Warsaw) , **12:** 87.

49. GOLDSMITH, E. D.; GORDON, A. S.; and CHARIPPER, H. A. 1945. *Endocrinology,* **36:** 364.

50. GORDON, A. S.; GOLDSMITH, E. D.; and CHARIPPER, H. A. 1944. *Proc. Soc. Exp. Biol. Med.,* **56:** 202.

51. ———. 1945. *Endocrinology,* **37:** 223.

52. GREENE, C. R., cited by G. S. SMYTHE. 1923. *Kamet Conquered.* London.

53. GREEN, D. M.; BUTTS, J. S.; and MULHOLLAND, H. F. 1945. *J. Aviat. Med.,* **16:** 311.

54. GREGOIRE, F.; LEBLOND, C. P.; and ROBILLARD, E. 1944. *J. Aviat. Med.,* **15:** 158.

55. HAILMAN, H. F. 1944. *Amer. J. Physiol.,* **141:** 176.

56. HARTMANN, H., and MURALT, A. VON. 1934. *Biochem. Z.,* **271:** 74.

57. HEPP, G. 1937. *Munch. Med. Wschr.,* **84:** 765.

58. HERSHGOLD, E. J., and RILEY, M. B. 1959. *Proc. Soc. Exp. Biol. Med.,* **100:** 831.

59. HIESTAND, W. A., and MILLER, H. R. 1944. *Amer. J. Physiol.,* **142:** 310.

60. HIMWICH, H. C., *et al.* 1942. *Amer. J. Physiol.,* **135:** 387.

61. HOFF, E. C., and YAHN, C. 1944. *Amer. J. Physiol.,* **141:** 7.

62. HOMBURGER, E., and HIMWICH, H. E. 1943. *Fed. Proc.,* **2:** 23.

63. HOVE, E. L.; HICKMAN, K.; and HARRIS, P. L. 1945. *Arch. Biochem.,* **8:** 395.

64. HUGHES, A. M. 1944. *Fed. Proc.,* **3:** 21.

65. ILK, S. G., *et al.* 1961. *Fed. Proc.,* **20:** 211.

66. ISIKAWA, T. 1939. *Tohoku J. Exp. Med.,* **36:** 375.

67. IVY, A. C., *et al.* Sept. 1, 1943. OMEcmr—241, Final Bimonthly Report to Com. Med. Res., O.S.R.D., p. 5.

68. KESSLER, M.; HAILMAN, H.; and GELLHORN, E. 1943. *Amer. J. Physiol.,* **140:** 291.

69. KEYS, A. STAPP, J. P.; and VIOLANTE, A. 1943. *Amer. J. Physiol.,* **138:** 763.

70. KING, C. G., *et al.* 1945. *J. Aviat. Med.,* **16:** 69.

71. KLINE, R. F. 1947. *Amer. J. Physiol.,* **151:** 538.

———. 1947. *Fed. Proc.,* **6:** 143.

72. KOTTKE, F. J., *et al.* 1948. *Amer. J. Physiol.,* **153:** 10.

73. KOTTKE, F. J., *et al. Ibid.,* p. 16.

74. LANGIER, H., and LEBLOND, C. P. 1943. *Rev. Canad. Biol.,* **2:** 474.

75. LAWSON, F. L. 1942. *Amer. J. Physiol.,* **136:** 494.

76. LAWTON, W. H. 1957. *U.S. Armed Forces M. J.,* **8:** 937.

77. LEBLOND, C. P. 1944. *Proc. Soc. Exp. Biol. Med.,* **55:** 114.

78. LEBLOND, C. P.; GROSS, J.: and LANGIER, H. 1943. *J. Aviat. Med.,* **14:** 262.

79. LI, CHOH HAO, and HERRING, U. V. 1945. *Amer. J. Physiol.,* **143:** 548.

80. LOEHNING, R. W., *et al.* 1952. *J. Pharm. Exp. Ther.,* **106:** 404.

81. ———. 1953. *Ibid.,* **108:** 80.

82. LUFT, U. C. *In:* H. G. Armstrong (ed.), *Aerospace Medicine,* p. 138. Baltimore: Williams & Wilkins Co., 1961.
83. MADDEN, R. F.; STEMLER, F. W.; and HIESTAND, W. A. 1955. *Amer. J. Physiol.,* **108:** 121.
84. MARGARIA, R., and FARAGLIA, L. 1940. *Boll. Soc. Ital. Biol. Sper.,* **15:** 1096.
85. McFARLAND, R. A. 1953. *Human Factors in Air Transportation, Occupational Health and Safety.* New York: McGraw-Hill Book Co.
86. MILLER, J. A. 1949. *Science,* **110:** 113.
87. MILLER, J. A., JR., and MILLER, F. S. 1961. *Fed. Proc.,* **20:** 214.
88. MILLER, J. A., JR.; MILLER, F. S.; and FARRAR, C. B. 1951. *Fed. Proc.,* **10:** 92.
89. NELSON, D., *et al.* 1943. *Proc. Soc. Exp. Biol. Med.,* **52:** 1.
90. OTIS, A. B., and RAHN, H. 1949. *Proc. Soc. Exp. Biol. Med.,* **70:** 487.
91. PACE, N.; CONZOLAZIO, W. V.; and LOZNER, E. L. 1945. *Science,* **102:** 589.
92. PACE, N. *et al.* 1947. *Amer. J. Physiol.,* **148:** 152.
93. PACKARD, W. H. 1905–06. *Amer. J. Physiol.,* **15:** 30.
94. ———. 1907. *Ibid.,* **18:** 164.
95. ———. 1908. *Ibid.,* **21:** 310.
96. PETERSON, J. M. 1941. *Nature,* **148:** 84.
97. PHILLIPS, N. E.; SAXON, P. A.; and QUIMBY, F. H. 1947. *Science,* **106:** 67.
98. ———. 1950. *Amer. J. Physiol.,* **161:** 307.
99. PITTS, G. C., and PACE, N. 1947. *Amer. J. Physiol.,* **148:** 139.
100. POLONOVOSKI, M. 1940. *Bull. Acad. Med.,* **123:** 688.
101. PROGER, S., and DEKANEAS, D. 1946. *J. Ped.,* **29:** 279.
102. PUGH, L. G. C., and WARD, M. P. 1956. *Lancet,* **271:** 1115.
103. QUIMBY, F. H., *et al.* 1948. *Amer. J. Physiol.,* **155:** 462.
104. RAHN, H., and OTIS, A. B. 1947. *Amer. J. Physiol.,* **150:** 202.
105. RIESIN, A. H.; TAHMISIAN, T. N.; and MACKENZIE, C. G. 1946. *Proc. Soc. Exp. Biol. Med.,* **63:** 250.
106. ROBILLARD, E., and GAGNON, M. 1953. *Rev. Canad. Biol.,* **12:** 411.
107. ROTTER, W. 1941. *Archiv. Kreislaufforsch.* (Dresden), **9:** 226.
108. RUFF, S.; FEDTKE, H.; and AMMON, R. 1950. *Z. Kreislaufforsch.,* **39:** 146.
109. RUHL, A. 1943. *Deutsch. Med. Wschr.,* **69:** 25.
110. RUSSELL, D. D. 1947. *Brit. Med. Bull.,* **5:** 43.
111. SALZBERG, H. S., and JACOBI, H. P. 1950. *Proc. Soc. Exp. Biol. Med.,* **73:** 589.
112. SAMSON, F. E., JR.; BALFOUR, W. M.: and DAHL, N. 1958. *Fed. Proc.,* **17:** 140.
113. SCHEINBERG, I. H., and MICHEL, H. O. 1947. *Science,* **105:** 365.
114. SCHUTZE, U. 1941. *Luftfahrtmedizin,* **5:** 97.
115. SELLE, W. A. 1944. *Amer. J. Physiol.,* **141:** 297.

116. SIROTINNE, N. 1938. *J. Med. Acad. Sci. Ukraine,* **8:** fasc. 2.
————. 1938–39. *d'apres Bruxelles Med.,* **19:** 499.
117. SMITH, D. C., and OSTER, R. H. 1946. *Amer. J. Physiol.,* **146:** 26.
118. SMITH, D. C.; OSTER, R. H.; and TOMAN, J. E. P. 1944. *Amer. J. Physiol.,* **140:** 603.
119. SMITH, E. L. 1944. *Fed. Proc.,* **3** (1) : 42.
120. SOBEL, H.; SIDEMAN, M.; and ARCE, R. 1960. *Proc. Soc. Exp. Biol. Med.,* **104** (1) : 31.
121. STREULI, H., and ASHER, L. 1918. *Biochem. Z.,* **87:** 359.
122. TABUSSE, L., and MADAME DE MONTRICHARD. 1956. *Med. Aero.* **11:** 306.
123. TELEFORD, I. R.; WISWELL, O. B.; and SMITH, E. L. 1954. *Proc. Soc. Exp. Biol. Med.,* **87:** 162.
124. THOMPSON, J. W., *et al.* April 25, 1944. Proc. 16th Meeting of the Associate Com. Med. Research, Nat'l Research Council, Canada, C-2064.
125. THORN, G. W., *et al.* 1945. *Endocrinology,* **36:** 381.
126. THORN, G. W., *et al.* 1946. *Bull. Johns Hopkins Hosp.,* **79:** 59.
127. VACCA, C., and BOERI, E. 1953. *Rev. Med. Aero.,* **16:** 139.
128. VAN LIERE, E. J.; FANG, H. S.; and NORTHUP, D. W. 1954. *Amer. J. Physiol.,* **179:** 503.
129. VELASQUEZ, T. 1959. *J. Appl. Physiol.,* **14:** 357.
130. WETZIG, P., and D'AMOUR, F. E. 1943. *Amer. J. Physiol.,* **140:** 304.
131. WOLF, J., and LEVY, I. J. 1954. *Arch. Intern. Med.,* **93:** 387.
132. ZARROW, M. X., *et al.* 1951. *Amer. J. Physiol.,* **167:** 171

INDEX

Date Due

PRINTED IN U. S. A.   CAT. NO. 23231